D0090554

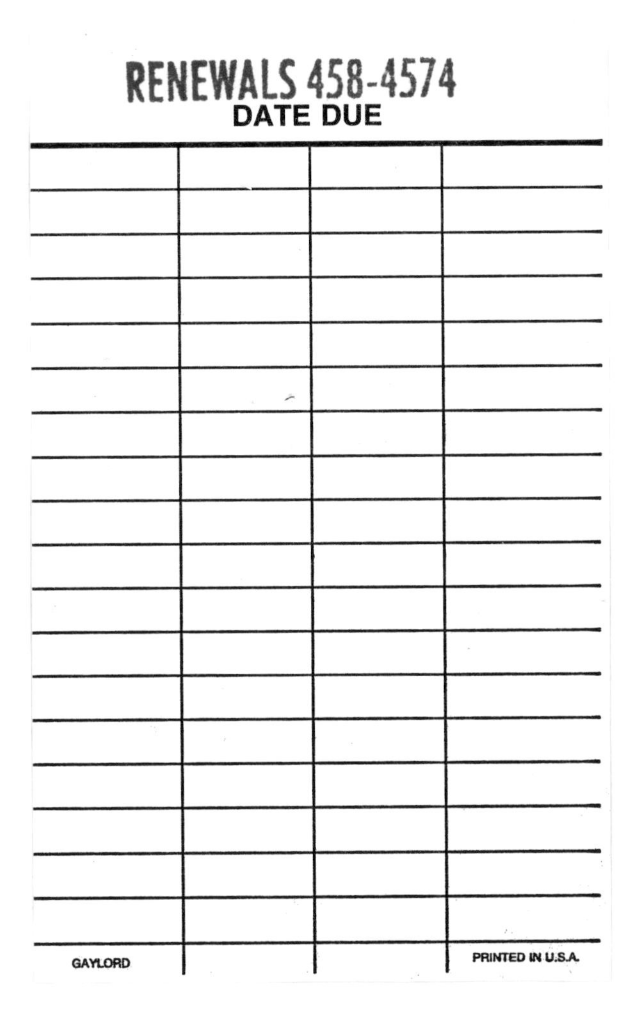
RENEWALS 458-4574
DATE DUE
GAYLORD
PRINTED IN U.S.A.

Health Informatics

(formerly Computers in Health Care)

Kathryn J. Hannah   Marion J. Ball
Series Editors

Deborah Lewis Gunther Eysenbach
Rita Kukafka P. Zoë Stavri
Holly B. Jimison
Editors

Consumer Health Informatics

Informing Consumers and Improving Health Care

With 28 Illustrations

With a Foreword by Warner V. Slack

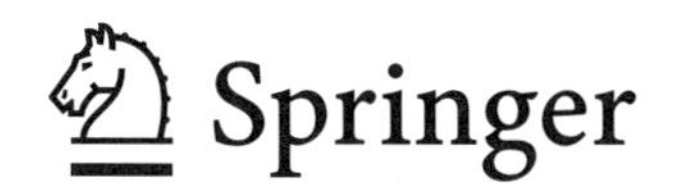

Deborah Lewis, EdD, RN, MPH
Associate Professor and Coordinator
Nursing Informatics
University of Pittsburgh School of Nursing
Pittsburgh, PA 15261
USA

Gunther Eysenbach, MD, MPH
Senior Scientist, Centre for Global eHealth Innovation
Division of Medical Decision Making and Health Care Research
Toronto General Research Institute of the UHN
and
Associate Professor
Department of Health Policy
Management and Evaluation
University of Toronto
Toronto, ON M5G 2C4
Canada

Rita Kukafka, DrPH, MA, CHES
Assistant Professor
Mailman School of Public Health
Division of Sociomedical Sciences
Department of Medical Informatics
Columbia University
New York, NY 10032
USA

P. Zoë Stavri, MLS, PhD
Assistant Professor
Oregon Health & Science University
and
Visiting Assistant Professor, part-time
Health Sciences Informatics, SOM, JHU
Chambersburg, PA 17201
USA

Holly B. Jimison, PhD
Medical Informatics Investigator
KP Center for Health Research
and
Assistant Professor
Public Health and Preventive Medicine
Oregon Health & Science University
Portland, OR 97227-1110
USA

Series Editors:
Kathryn J. Hannah, PhD, RN
Adjunct Professor, Department of Community Health Science
Faculty of Medicine
The University of Calgary
Calgary, Alberta T2N 4N1
Canada

Marion J. Ball, EdD
Vice President, Clinical Informatics Strategies
Health Sciences Informatics, SOM, JNU
Chambersburg, PA 17201
Healthlink, Inc.
Baltimore, MD 21210
and
Adjunct Professor
The Johns Hopkins University
School of Nursing
Baltimore, MD 21205
USA

ISBN 0-387-23991-X Printed on acid-free paper.

Printed in the United States of America. (BS/MVY)

9 8 7 6 5 4 3 2 1 SPIN 10942871

springeronline.com

To Emme and MeiMei

Foreword

In *Consumer Health Informatics*, Deborah Lewis and her fellow editors have assembled a group of clinicians and scientists eminently qualified to enlighten all those interested in clinical computing. I have long believed that patients represent the largest yet least well-utilized healthcare resource, and that the interactive computer can help clinicians to better understand their patients even as it empowers patients to take greater control of their own medical destinies [1,2]. It is my honor and pleasure, therefore, to add a few words of foreword to this welcome book.

I had the good fortune to spend the 1960s at the University of Wisconsin. In this wonderful atmosphere of progressive ideology and strong social conscience, two lines of reasoning evolved in my mind [1,3]. The first led to a set of controversial ideas I called "patient power," arguing that patients should be encouraged to participate as partners with their clinicians in medical decisions [4,5]. Further, I proposed that patients and clinicians alike would benefit if medical records were declassified, shared, and developed jointly by patient and clinician, and that words, such as "order" and "comply," would be better dropped from the medical lexicon and replaced with words that communicated a more collaborative process [4–6]. For centuries, the medical profession had perpetrated paternalism as an essential component of patient care, thereby detracting from what patients could contribute to the quality of their medical care and depriving them of the self-esteem that comes from mutual respect and self-reliance. The assumption was that "doctor knows best." Patient power questioned this. As Shaw once wrote, "Do not do unto others as you would that they should do unto you. Their tastes may not be the same" [7].

My second line of reasoning was that the computer could be used wisely and well in the practice of medicine. As with patient power, the idea was controversial, and those of us who were entering this new field were confronted by concerns about the computer in medicine under any circumstances. Would modern times destroy the art of medicine? Would these machines result in the disempowerment that had been associated with the industrial revolution? Yet, contrary to prevailing concerns, the computer in our laboratory instead offered the opportunity to empower the patient [1].

My colleagues and I had the idea that we could program a computer to interact directly with the patient, to engage in meaningful dialogue, to explore medical problems in detail, and to do so in a personalized, dignified, and considerate manner. There was a theoretical reason for pursuing this. Could the computer model the clinician as interviewer? But there were practical reasons as well. We hoped the interactive computer would help clinicians in the care of their patients; that using the computer would be interesting, perhaps even enjoyable for the patient; and in the back of our minds was the idea that the computer might actually help patients to help themselves with their medical problems.

We began with a computer-based history of allergies [8]. Our first patient, selected by a tired intern who had been up all night and to some extent liked the idea of being replaced by a computer, was also the most informative. He sat down at the LINC computer, borrowed from Neurophysiology [9]; the tapes churned and "HAVE YOU EVER HAD HIVES?" appeared on the screen. The characters flickered—the LINC was very slow by today's standards—lights on the console flashed on and off, and the speaker emitted an eerie, high-pitched sound. On the other side of a Sheetrock partition, people were walking in and out, and a cat was meowing. It was reminiscent of Kafka's *Castle* [10] or Koestler's *Darkness at Noon* [11]—clearly, not optimal circumstances for any medical interview, let alone one conducted by a computer [1].

Yet our patient quickly became engaged, and soon it was clear that rapport had been established between man and machine. He laughed out loud at some of the comments; and he talked to the computer, sometimes in praise and sometimes in criticism. For the first time as a patient, he was in control. Later, when the Teletype began to print his summary, in a legible but otherwise traditional format, he turned and asked, "May I read that?" and there, in a break with tradition, I encouraged him to read his record; and as he read, he discovered errors that needed correction. The computer as an interviewer had been, and would continue to be in our experience, an acceptable means to share the medical record at a time when the shared record was controversial and resisted in the traditional setting [1,6]. Here was patient power at work.

With subsequent computer-based medical histories, and later with programs designed to help patients to help themselves, we did our best to yield further control to the patient—to request permission to proceed, to respect the patient's priorities, to respect the right to decide and not to decide, to help with uncertainty, and to respect reluctance to respond—and patients were consistent in their praise of this approach [12]. Concern about the computer as a negative, depersonalizing influence proved to be unfounded; most patients found their experience to be interesting, enjoyable, and informative; and in our experience, corroborated by others, patients often found it easier to communicate with the computer about potentially embarrassing matters than to communicate the same information to their doctor [13-15]. Furthermore, when we designed the computer-printed summaries with the patient as well as the clinician in mind, patients, who were eager to read their summaries, helped us, not only to correct errors of commission and omission, but also to remove offensive wording.

Over the years, numerous studies have demonstrated that dialogue between patient and computer—well received by patient and clinician—has the potential to yield comprehensive interviews on a wide variety of medical and psychological problems [16]. Still, as a practical matter it has been hard for clinicians' offices to provide the computers, protected space, and administrative overhead required for these interviews. Computing for the patient, for interviews, for health-related information, and for a wide variety of other purposes, needed a new technology. This came with the advent of the Internet and the increasing availability of PCs with access to the Internet. And now, *Consumer Informatics*, as presented so ably in this book, is a burgeoning field. Patients and prospective patients can now participate in their health care over the Internet from the privacy of their homes; and they are availing themselves of this electronic communication in great numbers. According to a recent survey, well over 100 million people in the United States turn to the Internet for health related information [17]. For the most part, this information is presented in a didactic, non-interactive manner, but I am confident that more and more interactive programs will be available to address the individual needs of patients who use them. Increasingly, patients communicate with each other as well as with their clinicians by electronic mail [1,6]; and although currently limited to a few clinical practices, secure Web sites are now available that give patients a means to view their medications; request prescriptions, appointments, and referrals; view upcoming appointments; and view the results of their diagnostic studies [18–23]. Further, it should now be possible to deliver to people in their homes, interactive interviews that obtain their medical histories and incorporate the results of these interviews into their electronic medical records, readily available both to patient and clinician [6].

I am confident that the "digital divide" will continue to narrow, that the Internet will continue to become democratized as well as democratizing, available to more and more people from all walks of life, and that consumer informatics will improve the quality of medical care. This excellent collection of thoughtful, informative, and thought-provoking chapters shows that this process is already well underway.

Warner V. Slack, MD
Professor of Medicine, Harvard Medical School
Co-Director, Division of Clinical Computing, Department of Medicine
Beth Israel Deaconess Medical Center
November 23, 2004

References

1. Slack WV. Cybermedicine: how computing empowers doctors and patients for better health care (revised and updated edition). San Francisco: Jossey-Bass, 2001.
2. Slack WV, Safran CS, Kowaloff HB, Pearce J, Delbanco TL. A computer-administered health screening interview for hospital personnel. MD Comput 1995;12:25–30.
3. Slack WV. Patient-computer dialogue and the patient's right to decide. In: Brennan PF, Schneider SJ, Tornquist E, eds. Computers in health care: information networks for community health. New York: Springer-Verlag, 1997;55–69.
4. Slack WV. Patient power: a patient-oriented value system. In: Jacques JA, ed. Computer diagnosis and diagnostic methods. Proceedings of the Second Conference on the Diagnostic Process held at the University of Michigan. Springfield, IL: Charles C. Thomas, 1972;3–7.
5. Slack WV. The patient's right to decide. Lancet 1977;2:240.
6. Slack WV. A 67-year-old man who e-mails his physician. JAMA 2004;292:2253–61.
7. Shaw GB. *Man and Superman: A Comedy and Philosophy*. Baltimore: Penguin; 1952. (Originally published 1903)
8. Slack WV, Hicks GP, Reed CE, Van Cura LJ. A computer-based medical history system. N Engl J Med 1966;274:194–8.
9. Clark WA, Molnar CE. The LINC: a description of the laboratory instrument computer. Ann NY Acad Sci 1964;115:653–68.
10. Kafka F. *The Castle*. A new translation based on the restored text (M. Harman, trans). New York: Schocken Books, 1998.
11. Koestler A. *Darkness at Noon* (D. Hardy, trans). New York: Macmillan, 1987.
12. Slack WV. Patient-computer dialogue: a review. In: van Bemmel JH, McCray AT, eds. Yearbook of medical informatics 2000: patient-centered systems. Stuttgart, Germany: Schattauer, 2000;71-8.
13. Slack WV, Van Cura LJ. Patient reaction to computer-based medical interviewing. Comput Biomed Res 1968;1:527–31.
14. Lucas RW, Mullin PJ, Luna CB, McInroy DC. Psychiatrists and a computer as interrogators of patients with alcohol-related illnesses: a comparison. Br J Psychiatry 1977;131:160–7.

15. Locke S, Kowaloff HB, Hoff RG, et al. Computer-based interview for screening blood donors for risk of HIV transmission. JAMA 1992;268:1301–5.
16. Bachman JW. The patient-computer interview: a neglected tool that can aid the clinician. Mayo Clin Proc 2003;78:67–78.
17. HarrisInteractive. No significant change in the number of "Cyberchondriacs"—those who go online for health care information. Health Care News 2004. Available at *http://www.harrisinteractive.com/news/newsletters/healthnews/HI_HealthCareNews2004Vol4_Iss07.pdf.* Accessed November 24, 2004.
18. Sands DZ, Halamka JD. PatientSite: patient centered communication, services, and access to information. In: Nelson R, Ball MJ, eds. Consumer informatics: applications and strategies in cyber health care. New York: Springer-Verlag, 2004.
19. Gray JE, Safran C, Davis RB, et al. Baby CareLink: using the internet and telemedicine to improve care for high risk infants. Pediatrics 2000;106:1318–24.
20. Wald JS, Pedraza LA, Reilly CA, et al. Requirements for the development of a patient computing system. Proc AMIA Symp 2001;731–5.
21. Tang PC, Black W, Buchanan J, et al. Proc AMIA Symp 2003;649-53.
22. Department of Veterans Affairs. My HealtheVet. Available at *http://www.myhealthevet.va.gov/ShowDoc/MHV/help/faq.htm#q1*. Accessed March 22, 2004.
23. Earnest MA, Ross SE, Wittevrongel L, et al. Use of a patient-accessible electronic medical record in a practice for congestive heart failure: patient and physician experiences. J Am Med Inform Assoc 2004;11:410–17.

Series Preface

This series is directed to healthcare professionals who are leading the transformation of health care by using information and knowledge to advance the quality of patient care. Launched in 1988 as Computers in Health Care, the series offers a broad range of titles: some are addressed to specific professions such as nursing, medicine, and health administration; others to special areas of practice such as trauma and radiology. Still other books in the series focus on interdisciplinary issues, such as the computer-based patient record, electronic health records, and networked healthcare systems.

Renamed Health Informatics in 1998 to reflect the rapid evolution in the discipline now known as health informatics, the series continues to add titles that contribute to the evolution of the field. In the series, eminent experts, serving as editors or authors, offer their accounts of innovation in health informatics. Increasingly, these accounts go beyond hardware and software to address the role of information in influencing the transformation of healthcare delivery systems around the world. The series also increasingly focuses on "peopleware" and the organizational, behavioral, and societal changes that accompany the diffusion of information technology in health services environments.

These changes will shape health services in the new millennium. By making full and creative use of the technology to tame data and to transform information, health informatics will foster the development of the knowledge age in health care. As coeditors, we pledge to support our professional colleagues and the series readers as they share the advances in the emerging and exciting field of health informatics.

Kathryn J. Hannah
Marion J. Ball

Preface

As a parent, I recently became personally aware of the importance of consumer health informatics. After a frightening trip to the hospital with an unconscious child, I was told that her EEG was "very abnormal" and that she had a seizure disorder. Other words followed but they didn't get processed. I only heard *abnormal EEG* and *seizure disorder*. Before I could think of any questions to ask, the neurology team was gone.

Within minutes, the parade of "what ifs" began in my mind. I asked to speak to the doctors who had examined my daughter, but they had moved on to another hospital unit. A nurse paged the fellow, who said she would return to talk to me. I waited several hours and found myself entertaining more questions, and especially wishing I could remember the name of the drug they were going to be giving my daughter.

I decided to walk across the street to my office to check the Internet. I thought a quick search would give me some of the answers I needed. Knowing to look only at a "trusted site," I went directly to a national organization for persons with epilepsy. I clicked on the link for answers to questions and then on the link entitled "Children". My eyes were drawn to the bulleted points on the right side of the page:

- "300,000 children have seizures"
- "there are different types of seizure disorders"
- "many children feel loss of self-esteem and social isolation"

Further exploration of the same Web site led me to a page that discussed driving restrictions for persons with epilepsy. I couldn't help but think about how my bright five-year old daughter's life was going to be impacted by this diagnosis.

I did not quickly see a link to medication information so I left this Web site and searched using the keywords *epilepsy*, *medication*, and *children*. There were many hits. One of the first was for an attorney who assists parents whose children have been injured by seizure medications. I ultimately returned to the hospital an even more anxious parent.

With the passing of time, fear started to overtake my usual rational pattern of thought. I talked to a staff nurse and asked her how my daughter's life would be changed by epilepsy? Would my five-year old be injured by the medication? Would she become dysfunctional? Would she still be permitted to attend school?

The considerate answers she gave me based on her experience, really helped reassure me. A pediatric resident soon joined us, and I asked him the same questions. He provided the same calm reassurance. That night, the resident and the unit nurse helped me process the small amount of information I had and helped me move forward to more rational thinking. I still had many questions but now they were practical and based on my daughter's unique situation.

As my information needs changed, I was better able to focus my Internet search. I found wonderful support and answers in *BrainTalk Communities*, which is part of the Massachusetts General Hospital, Department of Neurology Web resources (http://adams.mgh.harvard.edu/NISRDG/#ptweb).

As I consider my experience of that day, I am aware that people seek information from a variety of resources and use many different approaches to process information. I am also aware that when faced with a crisis it is difficult to separate intellectual questions from situational emotions. My own experience has taught me to think differently about the role of the care provider and how important high-quality, accessible information resources are for healthcare consumers in times of crisis. The Internet is a powerful resource when it provides access to accurate and personally meaningful information. There are situations when a conversation with a healthcare provider is the best resource, but that is not always possible in today's healthcare environment.

As a developer of consumer health information resources, I am convinced that we must create new consumer-provider communication paradigms that capitalize on the strengths of information technologies to meet the needs of individual healthcare consumers. The designers of healthcare Web sites need to work with knowledgeable consumers and healthcare providers to ensure that high-quality information is thoughtfully presented. I also believe that clear, direct, and hopeful messages should be brought forward to prominent placement on Web sites for healthcare consumers who are seeking information in times of crisis. We have a wonderful opportunity to build resources to meaningfully help people process information when they need it most.

These chapters present information that represents the current science of consumer health informatics and provide examples of model programs that seek to build new information sharing strategies. As professional organizations and consumer health working groups make important contributions to consumer health informatics, the growing library of literature will help shape the field. A number of healthcare informatics' educational programs have integrated consumer health informatics content, and governmental agencies have set agendas that promote research and development in this field.

Through the chapters that follow the reader will gain insights into the definitions for consumer health and health informatics through theory-based approaches. "Best-practice" strategies for development and evaluation, and model initiatives in consumer health informatics are presented. The text includes authors and editors from interdisciplinary backgrounds who have presented, as fully as possible, the depth and breadth of consumer health informatics expertise. We are fortunate to have the knowledge and expertise that they provide in the pages that follow.

I have shared my own experience to illustrate the importance of access to high-quality, individualized information that is available in an environment of consumer-provider information-sharing, as well as the importance of including the consumer in the design and development process. We have much to gain by the efforts of so many who are researching, teaching, and living the experience of access to consumer health information. It is my hope that the wonderful contributions made in this book will lead to greater insights and produce more research to strengthen and guide the science of consumer health informatics.

Deborah Lewis, EdD, RN, MPH

Acknowledgments

We thank our family and friends who contribute their time and enduring patience for our careers.

We thank our colleagues who have contributed to this text and to the field of Consumer Health Informatics.

We thank Michelle Schmitt, Marion Ball, and Springer for making this work a reality.

We acknowledge the healthcare consumer, and the patients, and family members, who use Consumer Health Informatics resources daily to seek answers.

We remember Rob Kling for his invaluable contribution to the field of Social Informatics.

Deborah Lewis, EdD, RN, MPH
Gunther Eysenbach, MD, MPH
Rita Kukafka, DrPH, MA, CHES
P. Zoë Stavri, MLS, PhD
Holly B. Jimison, PhD

Contents

Contributors

Richard Appleyard, PhD
Associate Professor, Department of Medical Informatics and Clinical Epidemiology, Web Services Manager, Information Technology Group, Oregon Health & Science University, Portland, OR, USA

Joyce E.B. Backus
Lead, Web Management Team, Public Services Division, National Library of Medicine, Bethesda, MD, USA

Haile Berhe
Lead Programmer, CHESS Project, Center for Health Systems Research and Analysis, University of Wisconsin-Madison, Madison, WI, USA

Eric W. Boberg
CHESS Project, University of Wisconsin-Madison, Madison, WI, USA

Patricia Flatley Brennan, RN, PhD
Lillian Moehlman-Bascom Professor of Nursing, Professor, Industrial Engineering, University of Wisconsin, Madison, WI, USA. E-mail: pbrennan@engr.wisc.edu

Betty L. Chang, DNSc, FNP, FAAN
Professor Emerita, UCLA School of Nursing, University of California, Los Angeles, CA, USA

James J. Cimino, MD
Professor of Biomedical Informatics and Medicine, Columbia College of Physicians and Surgeons, New York, NY, USA

Gunther Eysenbach, MD, MPH
Senior Scientist, Centre for Global eHealth Innovation, Division of Medical Decision Making and Health Care Research, Toronto General Research Institute of the UHN; Associate Professor, Department of Health Policy, Management and Evaluation, University of Toronto, Toronto, ON, Canada

Charles P. Friedman, MS, PhD
Professor of Medicine, Director of the Center for Biomedical Informatics, Director of the Pittsburgh Biomedical Informatics Training Program, University of Pittsburgh, Pittsburgh, PA, USA

Denise Goldsmith, RN, MS, MPH
Program Manager, Nursing Informatics, Patient Care Services/Information Systems, Beth Israel Deaconess Medical Center, Boston, MA, USA

David H. Gustafson, MS, PhD
Research Professor, Industrial Engineering, CHESS Project Director, University of Wisconsin-Madison, Madison, WI, USA

James H. Harrison, Jr., MD, PhD
Associate Professor, Department of Pathology, Faculty in Residence, Center for Biomedical Informatics, University of Pittsburgh, Pittsburgh, PA, USA

Robert P. Hawkins
Maier-Bascom Professor, School of Journalism and Mass Communication, University of Wisconsin-Madison, Madison, WI, USA

Holly B. Jimison, PhD
Medical Informatics Investigator, KP Center for Health Research; Assistant Professor, Public Health and Preventive Medicine, Oregon Health & Science University, Portland, OR, USA

Bonnie Kaplan, PhD
Lecturer, Yale Center for Medical Informatics, President, Kaplan Associates, Hamden, CT, USA

Rita Kukafka, DrPH, MA, CHES
Assistant Professor, Mailman School of Public Health, Division of Sociomedical Sciences, Department of Medical Informatics, Columbia University, New York, NY, USA

Eve-Marie Lacroix, MS
Chief, Public Services Division, National Library of Medicine, Bethesda, MD, USA

Deborah Lewis, EdD, RN, MPH
Associate Professor and Coordinator, Nursing Informatics, University of Pittsburgh School of Nursing, Pittsburgh, PA, USA

Yves A. Lussier, MD
Director, Biomedical Informatics Core, Northeast Research Center in Biodefense and Emerging Infectious Diseases; Assistant Professor, Department of Biomedical Informatics and Department of Medicine, Columbia University College of Physicians and Surgeons, Columbia University, New York, NY 10032, USA

Fiona McTavish, MS
Deputy Director, CHESS Project, University of Wisconsin-Madison, Madison, WI, USA

Betta Owens, MS
Director, CHESS Research Consortium, University of Wisconsin-Madison, Madison, WI, USA

Suzanne Pingree
CHESS Project, University of Wisconsin-Madison, Madison, WI, USA

Cornelia M. Ruland, RN, PhD
Director, Center for Shared Decision Making and Nursing Research, Rikshospitalet National Hospital, Oslo, Norway

Charles Safran, MD
President, American Medical Informatics Association, Associate Clinical Professor of Medicine, Harvard Medical School, Chairman and CEO, Clinician Support Technology, Newton, MA, USA

Daniel Z. Sands, MD, MPH, FACMI
Assistant Clinical Professor of Medicine, Harvard Medical School, Chief Medical Officer and VP of Clinical Strategies, Zix Corporation, Center for Clinical Computing, Beth Israel Deaconess Medical Center, Boston, MA, USA

Steve Sawyer, BS, MS, MD, DBA
Associate Professor, School of Information Sciences and Technology, Pennsylvania State University, University Park, PA, USA

Roy Schoenberg, MD, MPH
President, CareKey Incorporated, Boston, MA, USA

Catherine Arnott Smith, PhD
Assistant Professor, School of Information Studies, Center for Science and Technology, Syracuse University, Syracuse, NY, USA

P. Zoë Stavri, MLS, PhD
Assistant Professor, Oregon Health & Science University; Visiting Assistant Professor, part-time, Health Sciences Informatics, SOM, JHU, Chambersburg, PA, USA

Meg Wise, PhD
Center for Health Systems Research and Analysis, University of Wisconsin, Madison, WI, USA

1 Consumer Health Informatics

Deborah Lewis, Betty L. Chang, and Charles P. Friedman

Over the last few decades, consumer involvement in health care has been dramatically transformed. Not the least of these transformations has been consumers' active participation in decision making about their own health and the health of their family members. The advent and growing popularity of the Internet and its searchable World Wide Web have revolutionized consumers' access to information. The sheer volume of Internet-based information on virtually any subject has been a source of both satisfaction and frustration for healthcare consumers.

In the not-so-distant past, health information for patients was delivered from the perspective of the medical world. This model was understandable, as patients traditionally looked to their healthcare providers as the primary, and possibly only, source of information on health and disease. Although this approach may have been valuable in reducing access to misinformation, it also limited the range of information available to patients or consumers and placed the patient in a less engaged role. During the past decade, involving consumers in the process of health care has been increasingly emphasized, with an appreciation for the positive impact on outcomes that follows. This paradigm shift from physician-centered to patient-centric care and the impact of Internet access to health information has formed the basis for the development of consumer health informatics. This chapter presents several definitions that have been advanced for consumer health informatics and provides an overview of the process of consumer health information delivery.

Toward a Definition of Consumer Health Informatics

To begin, it is helpful to define what is meant by "health consumers." The American Medical Informatics Association, Consumer Health Informatics Working Group, and the International Medical Informatics Association, Nursing Informatics Interest Group [1,2] have defined a health information consumer as a person who seeks information about health promotion, disease prevention, treatment of specific conditions, and management of various health conditions and chronic illnesses. Consumers of health information have consisted not only of persons with specific health conditions and their friends and family, but also of the public concerned about promoting optimal health.

As noted earlier, several definitions exist for consumer health informatics. According to the U.S. General Accounting Office, consumer health informatics is "the use of modern computers and telecommunications to support consumers in obtaining information, analyzing their unique health care needs and helping them make decisions about their own health" [2].

Consumer health informatics has been defined by Gunther Eysenbach as "the branch of medical informatics that analyses consumers' needs for information; studies and implements methods of making information accessible to consumers; and models and integrates consumers' preferences into medical information systems" [3, p. 3].

Tom Ferguson defines consumer health informatics as "the study, development, and implementation of computer and telecommunications applications and interfaces designed to be used by health consumers" [4, p. 2].

Although this is likely not a complete collection of all definitions of consumer health informatics, these key definitions acknowledge the importance of the use of computer and information technology to support the process of health information delivery in an integrated manner to healthcare consumers. They also consistently focus on the importance of meeting the consumer's personal information needs.

Consumer health informatics is differentiated from the existing field of medical informatics by Houston et al. "First, because of its frequent patient-centered approach, consumer health informatics may have an even stronger overlap with public health. In addition, the design of consumer health informatics applications require more frequent input from patients and consumers" [5, p. 1, sub 4,6].

Tom Ferguson describes the importance of addressing the personal information needs of modern healthcare consumers: "When they have a serious medical concern, they (healthcare consumers) don't just accept whatever treatment their local doctor offers. They'll spend hours and hours on the Internet learning about their condition, communicating with other patients and clinicians who share their interests, and tracking down every lead they can find on the best new treatments" [6]. Dr. Ferguson has delineated 10 levels in which consumers participate in the access and use of health care information [7, pp. 1–2], as follows:

Level 1. e-Patients search for health information.

Seventy-three million American adults currently use the Internet to look for information regarding their health concerns. Four out of five of their online sessions begin with a search engine. Patients give themselves online crash courses on their newly diagnosed diseases and disorders. They prepare for doctors' appointments and look up information on the drugs and other treatments that their doctors recommend. They look for new ways to control their weight. But above all, they search for information that might help others. According to a recent Pew Internet & American Life survey, more e-patients search for medical information for friends and family members (81%) than for themselves (58%) [7, pp. 1–2].

Level 2. e-Patients exchange e-mail with family members and friends.

Online patients reach out via e-mail to those they know and love, reporting on their health problems and concerns, and seeking information, advice, and support from their personal network of friends and family members. Their loved ones typically respond with sympathy, understanding, and support. They recommend specific resources: doctors, treatment centers, Web sites, books, and support groups. They refer e-patients to "second-level" contacts, for example, another friend who knows about the topics of concern to them. They also use e-mail to coordinate face-to-face visits and assistance [7, pp. 1–2].

Level 3. e-Patients seek guidance from online patient-helpers.

When faced with a new diagnosis of a serious medical problem, e-patients may seek out and communicate with an experienced online self-helper with the same condition, for example, the Webmaster of a site devoted to their concern. There are thousands of these condition-specific online patient helpers on the Internet, and they are not difficult to find. Patient-helpers can usually recommend the best online resources for a particular condition. In addition, they typically provide a type of uniquely practical and reassuring "been-there-done-that" advice that may be difficult or impossible to obtain elsewhere [7, pp. 1–2].

Level 4. e-Patients participate in online support groups.

Many e-patients facing serious medical challenges participate in Internet support communities devoted to a single medical condition (e.g., breast cancer or depression). These groups usually communicate via postings on Web-based forums or electronic mailing lists. Participants share their thoughts, feelings, personal stories, and experiences and ask and reply to questions. They also exchange information on medical studies and clinical trials, discuss current treatment options, and recommend treatment centers and professionals with special expertise in the shared condition [7, pp. 1–2].

Level 5. e-Patients join with other online self-helpers to research their shared concerns.

The members of some Internet support communities organize themselves into online work groups, reviewing the medical literature on their disorder and providing lists of frequently asked questions (FAQs) for the newly diagnosed. Some online support groups conduct informal research on their shared concerns. A few have even developed and carried out their own formal research studies or have partnered with professional researchers to conduct medical research, with group members serving as research subjects [7, pp. 1–2].

Level 6. e-Patients use online medical guidance systems.

At some sites, e-patients can type in the names of all the drugs they are currently taking and receive a report of all possible drug interactions. At others, they can read reviews of a drug their doctor has proposed, written by dozens of patients who have actually used it. There are sites where patients can answer a series of questions about their symptoms and receive a listing of possible diagnoses, along with a list of the medical tests and observations that could help them decide which might be most likely. Further, a number of online physician directories are available where e-patients can find detailed information about individual doctors and hospitals, for example, patient evaluations, surgical success rates, and reports of malpractice settlements. I have come to think of such sites as early prototypes of what my colleague Richard Rockefeller has called medical guidance systems—information technology (IT) systems that use computing power to help e-patients make good medical decisions. In the future, such systems could make it possible for e-patients to play an even more knowledgeable and responsible role in contributing to their own medical care.

Within these first six levels, e-patients operate primarily in the world of lay medicine and self-managed care, with little or no involvement with health professionals. The four levels that follow involve interactions between e-patients and health professionals [7, pp. 1–2].

Level 7. e-Patients interact with volunteer online health professionals.

Online patients sometimes send their e-mailed questions to health professionals they have found on the Internet. Or they may visit Web sites (e.g., *drgreene.com* or *drweil.com*) at which physicians or other health professionals offer to answer visitors' medical questions. Hundreds of health professionals currently provide such services. Many sites (e.g., *http://www.goaskalice.columbia.edu*) list hundreds of previously asked questions and answers in a searchable or browsable format [7, pp. 1–2].

Level 8. e-Patients use the paid services of online medical advisors and consultants. Some e-patients take advantage of the online-only services now offered by a growing number of professionals: They may pay a physician or a nurse to answer their e-mailed questions. They may seek an online second opinion from a physician specializing in their condition. They may sign up for a series of e-mailed counseling sessions with an e-therapist. They may employ the services of an online medical researcher. Or they seek the advice of an online personal trainer, nutritionist, or weight loss coach. Because level 8 medical professionals do not require face-to-face contact, they can offer their services to anyone with an Internet connection [7, pp. 1–2].

Level 9. e-Patients engage in electronic conversations with their local clinicians. Growing numbers of e-patients exchange e-mail with their local brick-and-mortar physicians. The content of these communications frequently resembles that of a provider–patient phone call. Patients ask questions to help them prepare for, or follow up on, a clinical visit. But because e-mail is more convenient and less time pressured, e-patients need not worry about interrupting their busy doctors. Patients who communicate with their doctors via e-mail may find it easier to pose thoughtful questions, introduce new topics, and report on the results of their online searches. Some providers now offer more sophisticated online patient services, for example, threaded patient–physician messaging, online advice nurses, online support communities, shared access to the patient's electronic medical records, online appointment scheduling, and online prescription refills [7, pp. 1–2].

Level 10. e-Patients receive one-way electronic messages from their clinicians. Some health professionals use the Net to send their patients unrequested messages that are not interactive, for example, targeted suggestions for behavioral change or patient education materials of the doctor's choosing. In most cases, the effectiveness of these offerings can be increased by presenting them in an "opt-in" manner, by adding a "talk back" option, or both, moving the interaction to level 9. Although such one-way communications may be acceptable to older or less sophisticated patients, some experienced e-patients think of unsolicited one-way messages as spam and may find them offensive [7, pp. 1–2].

Toward a Model for Consumer Health Informatics

Drs. Lewis and Friedman [8] have proposed a model for consumer health informatics (Fig. 1.1) that places the consumer at the center of the process of information transformation. This model illustrates how relevant and valid information—integrated appropriately into an environment of shared decision making—can improve both the satisfaction with the process of care delivery and measurable outcomes reflected in consumers' health status. Information technology, as a mode of message/information transfer, serves to assemble and process the information and act as a catalyst for feedback. Healthcare consumers work with their healthcare providers to assemble and understand the retrieved information in the context of their personal health concerns. The ideal system output is an informed healthcare consumer who is making health choices based on personal health goals that lead to improved health outcomes. The model is graphically represented in Fig. 1.1.

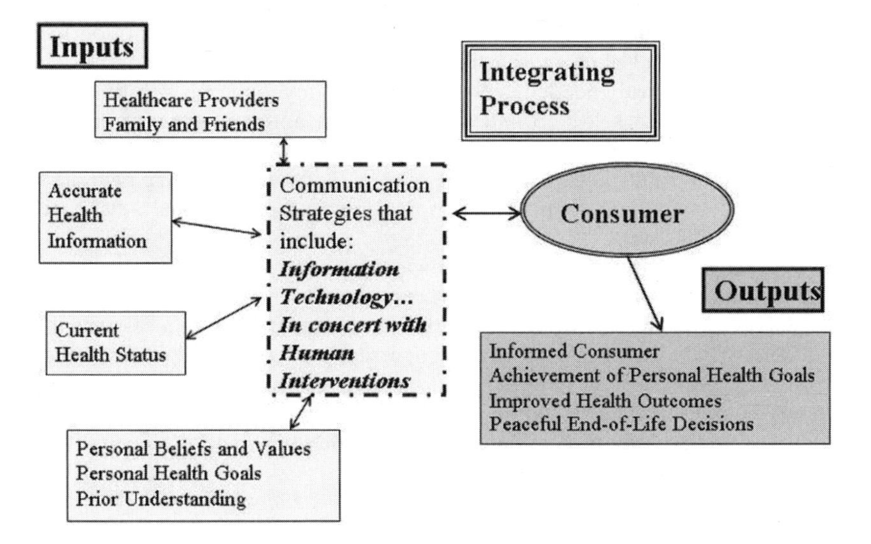

FIGURE 1.1. A model for consumer health informatics. (The consumer in this figure is meant to represent persons of all genders, races, and ethnicities.)

One Consumer's Experiences and Perceptions: Jason G. Cooper, MS

Consumer health informatics is best illustrated through the actual experiences of a healthcare consumer. We recognize Jason Cooper for his willingness to share his story and for the understanding that it brings to our study of consumer health informatics.

Case Study

I was diagnosed with Crohn's in 1993—a life-altering event for anyone with this chronic disorder. Instead of entering the military as an officer, I was medically discharged and decided to attend graduate school. Although I didn't know it then, this is where my education with community health informatics would begin.

Wanting to learn more about this disease, I searched for health resources. Beginning with my mother's books (she's a nurse), I read for hours on end. Most of these books dealt with people who were extremely sick from inflammatory bowel disease (IBD), which served to do nothing more than frighten me. Sadly, nothing informatively satisfying was given to me when diagnosed. I was prescribed Azulfidine, given a one-page brochure, and sent on my way.

At the time, the Internet was just beginning to blossom into the public and private sectors. After a couple of years of unsuccessfully "dealing" with my condition alone, I decided to seek help from my peers. Online discussion groups, varying Web sites, and the Crohn's and Colitis Foundation of America's (CCFA's) "Ask the Physician" forum are where I spent many hours. By far, these were the most enlightening experiences—learning that others had similar food interaction problems; learning that I was not alone; and, asking volunteer gastroenterologists specifics about prescription medications, diet, and a myriad of other questions.

I had found what I truly needed years before when my diagnosis was first made: an information resource, a self-help and support group, and a healthcare professional willing to lend personal advice. For those suffering with many chronic ailments, these are three very important issues: educating oneself, knowing there are peers that are experiencing the same and supporting one another, and professional advice without the need for an office visit.

In retrospect, an information kiosk at the gastrointestinal (GI) doctor's office where I was diagnosed, to address all of these concerns, would have helped considerably. The Internet has come a long way since 1993 and advances in informatics research will open more doors for patients to self-inform. I am currently pursuing a Ph.D. at Duke University and I am focused on IBD diet and wellness research. I believe the future of community health informatics will be to assist individuals in learning, finding applicable resources, and seeking professional advice outside the standard office visit.

As a fellow informatician, I perceive the principal challenges to be:

- Electronic Health Record (EHR) standardization, which without we cannot confidently deliver complete and accurate health information.
- Standardizing the delivery of patient health information outside the current care paradigm (i.e., Web delivery of tests, findings, and billing; Web and e-mail reminders for normal visits, special visits, bills, and insurance; and personalized health-related news and information).
- Enriching patient education and compliance.

I believe that we can address these challenges and change the way information is delivered by:

- Widely standardizing the EHR (IEEE, ISO, other standards organizations, and e-health leaders).
- Implementing e-capable (Internet, mobile devices, etc.) health information distribution.
- Educating patients on diverse levels such as hard-copy brochures (perpetual method), information kiosks in specialty clinics and community/family medicine clinics, e-health delivery, and e-health education (oneself, loved ones, or academia).

On a closing note, my heartfelt understanding is shared with those indomitable sufferers of IBD—Crohn's disease or ulcerative colitis, as well as those with irritable bowel syndrome (IBS). I've been through 11 years, lots of Crohn's medications, countless procedures, and a bowel resection . . . yet I continue to dream of a cure of these troubling disorders. I plan to dedicate time and effort for research toward quality-of-life issues and patient education. I also applaud the tireless work and contributions of researchers, educators, philanthropists, and the innumerable healthcare professionals.

Summary and Issues

Healthcare consumers are actively involved it seeking health information and in using the information they are finding to make decisions about their health. People seek healthcare information from a variety of sources, which include print and electronic resources, healthcare providers, other consumers, and their families and friends. The information may be delivered in a variety of print and media-based formats, through electronic access, that is, Internet-based delivery, telephone delivery, e-mail and chat, access to electronic databases, and other formats too numerous and constantly evolving to mention. It is important that access to health information is consumer centered and accessible for the person involved and for his or her provider, and that the process of consumer health information delivery focuses on the personal information needs of the healthcare consumer. To meet the unique information needs of healthcare consumers and support the process of optimal health outcomes consumer health informatics applications need to support the synergy between patient and provider.

The example provided by Jason Cooper illustrates the need for integrated systems that support healthcare consumers' access to the information combined with access to healthcare providers working and interested to discuss, validate, and assist consumers in understanding the information in the context of their own health concerns. In the course of creating consumer health informatics tools, consumers, providers, and informaticians must pay attention to ethical and social issues so that together they shape the future as they would like it to be, in terms of both how technology is used and what kinds of regulations are put in place. Certification and self-regulation, instead of only government regulation, are needed to ensure information accuracy and to help users evaluate the credibility of information providers and information sources [9, p. 312].

In this text we are presenting the science of consumer health informatics. Each chapter makes a unique contribution to this effort. We are ever aware that any discussion of consumer health informatics should represent the science of healthcare informatics within the context of the healthcare consumer we seek to serve. The text is organized to move the reader from a discussion of definitions for consumer health and health informatics through theory-based approaches for design to a presentation of "best-practice" strategies for development and evaluation. The text ends with discussion of model initiatives in consumer health informatics. Critical issues are examined that challenge providers, consumers, and informaticians who seek to create and use consumer health informatics applications.

References

1. International Medical Informatics Association, N.I.I.G., International Medical Informatics Association, Nursing Informatics Interest Group, 2004. *http://www.imia.org/ni/archive.htm*
2. The American Medical Informatics Association, C.H.I.W.G. AMIA, 2004. *http://www.amia.org/working/chi/main.html*
3. Eysenbach G. Recent advances: consumer health informatics. Br J Med 2000;320:1713.
4. Ferguson T. What is consumer health informatics? In: Tom Ferguson, MD, ed. The Ferguson Report. Austin, 2001.
5. Houston TK, Chang BL, Brown S, et al. Consumer health informatics: a consensus description and commentary from American Medical Informatics Association members. Proc AMIA Symp 2001;269–73.
6. Ferguson T. Online patient-helpers and physicians working together: a new partnership for high quality health care. [see comment]. Br Med J 2000;321:1129–32.
7. Ferguson T. What e-patients do online: a tentative taxonomy. In: Tom Ferguson, MD, ed. The Ferguson Report. Austin, 2002.
8. Lewis D, Friedman CP. Consumer health informatics. In: Ball MA, Hannah KJ, Newbold SK, Douglas JV, eds. Nursing Informatics: Where Caring and Technology Meet. New York: Springer-Verlag, 2000.
9. Kaplan B, Brennan PF. Consumer informatics supporting patients as co-producers of quality. J Am Med Inform Assoc 2001;8:309–16.

2
Empowered Consumers

PATRICIA FLATLEY BRENNAN and CHARLES SAFRAN

People play a critical role in achieving health for themselves, the people they care about, and the communities within which they live. Consumers of health services create and maintain healthy lifestyles, develop healthy communities, and, in collaboration with healthcare professionals, manage disease and its recovery. Similar to their professional counterparts, lay people engaged in health care also benefit from informatics solutions that permit them ready access and judicious application of health information, clinical recommendations, and interpersonal support. The purpose of this chapter is to characterize lay people as patients and consumers of health services, examine their recognized and implicit roles in health and health care, and explore how consumer health informatics (CHI) innovations support an empowered, engaged consumer.

An ideology of empowerment—granting of power to a dependent group or enhancing an individual's ability for self-determination—pervades contemporary American culture. CHI proceeds from this ideology and, in turn, facilitates its realization in health care. CHI innovations provide information about their health concerns, assist consumers in finding others who share their concerns, and afford them platforms to promulgate characterizations of health problems that are more person-centered rather than industry-centered. CHI innovations also help consumers navigate the complex healthcare system and access the professional recommendations and evidenced-based practice guidelines that aid in disease management. CHI innovations have the potential to support knowing participation in healthcare practices. In this chapter, we explore ideas central to collaboration in health care, examine the roles of lay persons, and evaluate the rich, ever growing set of informatics innovations for the extent to which they empower consumers to take charge of their health and actively participate in decisions about healthcare delivery.

Collaboration in Health Promotion and Disease Management

Accomplishing personal and population health objectives and the goals of healthcare delivery requires the active participation of many individuals, including clinicians, research scientists, healthcare administrators, policy makers, and financiers. Lay persons play a central role in the health and healthcare process, not only as the identified recipients of professional health services but also as initiators of positive personal health behaviors, who organize and manage home-based care for themselves and others, and as citizens engaged in the collaborative practices such as proper sanitation and clean air promotion that ensure the health of their communities. Philosophies of partnership and consumerism aptly characterize the active, engaged roles assumed by lay people as they join with health professionals to set and accomplish healthcare goals.

Philosophies of partnership and consumerism reflect the ideological shift among health professionals and policy makers, and lay persons themselves, in the ways lay persons are perceived to participate in health and health care. Partnership expands the roles of patient from the once widely accepted connotation of dependence, passivity, and compliance to one of active engagement. Considering lay persons as *partners* with healthcare providers shifts the balance of power for decision making and choice from one clearly situated within the purview of skilled professionals with specialized knowledge to one arising from a clinical alliance characterized by shared expectations, mutual problem solving, and joint decision making. Experiences within the mental health sector demonstrated that active engagement of patients in planning and carrying out treatment resulted in outcomes far superior to those arising under more traditional, clinician-directed care [1] and led to a reconceptualization of patients from passive recipients into actively engaged clients. This change in perception spread throughout the entire healthcare sector, resulting in a shifting of the concept of patient from one who receives care to one who actively participates in care options.

Consumerism emerged in the 1960s as a social movement characterized by the right to act based on informed choice, active participation, and full engagement in critical processes. Rights may be granted by one group holding power in a situation or marketplace to another, or may be wrested from those holding power by those desiring participation. Both pathways are evident in the history of health care. Consumerism results in a redefinition of what constitutes participation and who has rights to information, as well as what information is considered central and relevant.

We restrict the term "patient" to the roles assumed by lay people engaged in a care partnership with a specific health professional. This relationship is characterized by mutual respect, commitment to shared goal setting and treatment planning, and an accountability of both parties for the treatment plan and its implementation. "Consumers of health care" are, broadly, all persons, sick or well, who seek information and take action in accord with personal preferences, life situations, and individual health goals, and may, but do not always, include a specific relationship with an identified healthcare provider.

The shift in naming lay persons from patients to consumers reflects not only a perceptual change but also the real changes in the distribution of work in health care that shifted from a professional model of service delivery to a collaborative model of care engagement. Care migrated from the hospital and clinic to the home and community, spurred on as much by financing incentives such as prospective payment as by the evidence that community-based care augmented and could even be superior to institution-based treatment. This changing of the care site vested more responsibility in lay people to take on some of the work once viewed as solely a professional pursuit, such as monitoring health status and delivering clinical therapeutics. Thus, achievement of health and accomplishment of healthcare goals rests not only on the ministrations of health professionals but essentially also on the active participation of patients and informal caregivers.

Expansion in the connotation of patients and recognition of their essential contribution to ensuring the accomplishment of healthcare goals occurred concurrently with rapid growth in society's and sciences' understandings of health, disease, and therapeutics. Recognition of the role played by heredity and a lifetime of health behaviors led to the realization that accomplishing health goals rested not only on the judgments and actions that occurred during an encounter with a professional but was also found within the everyday choices and behaviors in the life of each individual. Therefore, information needed by consumers to create and maintain health, and recover from disease, needed to address not only those dimensions relevant in the health service encounter but also those practices and choices that, made in the course of everyday living, were most likely to lead to long-term well-being.

One more change in the healthcare milieu contributed to the expanded role of lay people, and consequently to expansion of their information needs. Despite growth in understanding of the biological basis of illnesses, personal preferences assumed increasing importance as guides for the selection of treatment choices. Increased sophistication in therapeutics now can present patients and clinicians with several equally appealing treatment approaches that differ in factors related more to individual preferences and values than to physiological considerations. For example, in selecting cancer treatment approaches, consideration of the patient's willingness to tolerate certain side effects may shift the intervention choice toward one approach over an equally effective but potentially more noxious alternative. Only through exploration of patients' values and preferences can these considerations be understood and meaningfully applied to the clinical decision. Thus, in addition to factual information about disease etiology and treatment options, people need strategies that help them reflect on the meaning of illness and the consequences of its management in their lives. CHI innovations provide great assistance in this arena. Careful understanding of the nature and context of consumers is essential in the design and deployment of CHI innovations.

Who Are the Consumers?

A perspective on health and health care that encompasses health-promoting lifestyles, healthy communities, active participation in health care, and clarification of personal values necessitates consideration that all persons, sick or well, hold vested interests in health, health care, and health information and therefore are constituents of CHI. Critical characteristics of these constituents, such as their ages, genders, ethnic and cultural identities, and socioeconomic situations, influence their health states, their access to health care, and the ways they are likely to use CHI innovations [2–4].

"Consumer" is not a uniform characteristic of all people; rather, consumers are distinguished by their very diversity. Clearly, some consumers act in self-interest, making choices and engaging in health-enhancing behaviors. Some constituent consumers, such as parents, informal caregivers, and friends, act as *agent*s for others, advocating for their needs, ministering personal care services, and seeking and interpreting information for them. Thus, the phrase "consumers" refers to a rich and diverse collection of individuals with a self-defined need for health information and role in ensuring the accomplishment of their own health goals or those of others.

For most people, health concerns and the need for health information occur at home, away from the resources and supports of healthcare institutions. Fear and questions may arise unpredictably at times when health professionals are unavailable. Concerns arise regarding managing illnesses and the accouterments of care in the context of family living environments. Home-dwelling consumers thus integrate their health practices and healthcare experiences subject to the influences of the structure of their environments, the social rules of living in their community, and diurnal variation of their lives [5]. CHI innovations are used in these contexts, capitalizing on and competing with the resources and tenor of environments much different from the typical healthcare situation.

Contemporary consumers are "wired" consumers. Approximately 125 million Americans have access to the Internet, and about 80% of these have sought health information at least once [6]. People of all ages, including children and elders, access health information on the Internet. Women are more likely than men to seek health information on the Internet, and the promise of privacy makes this medium particularly useful for those who prefer to explore health concerns in private. Although many consumers need information about specific medical conditions or health concerns, others look for information about health insurance, health promotion, and the quality assessment of their local hospitals and clinicians [7]. Thirty to forty percent of consumers have Internet access from their homes; the remainder use public computers connected to the Internet from schools, libraries, and workplaces. Unlike electronic mail or online telephone directories which are accessed almost daily, consumers look for health information on an as-needed basis.

Achieving personal and community health goals, and ensuring full value of modern therapeutics, relies on the active engagement of consumers. The Internet has promise to reach all citizens where they live and work, and, importantly, where they encounter health concerns and must cope with health problems. Yet, although the Internet and a host of contemporary technologies provide content, skills training, and linkages with others who share similar concerns, technologies in and of themselves are not empowering—empowerment emerges from the ways the technologies are used by the people they are designed for and the healthcare professionals who serve them.

Empowerment: Using Technology to Enhance Consumer Participation in Health and Health Care

Empowerment is a characteristic of groups and individuals that energizes them with the knowledge and confidence to act in their own behalf in a manner that best meets identified goals. Closely aligned conceptually with consumerism and assertiveness, empowerment is distinguished by its contextual nature—that is, empowerment emerges not in a vacuum, but as a realignment of a power structure in which power, once vested in one group or person, becomes claimed, and even shared, by others. Empowerment results in a redefinition of concerns, infusing once dominant paradigms of thought with the values and perspectives of new groups or individuals. Empowerment is visible through the actions and rhetoric of those involved. These actions and visibility occur on the level of both public health (the health of communities and groups) and personal health.

Public health empowerment can best be seen through the actions of self-help groups and collectives who claim the right to define health concerns in terms of those most affected by them (such as mentally ill persons or the elderly) rather than those who seek to care for them. Communities and collectives participate as equal partners with governments and the healthcare industry in setting health priorities and investing in community-level health enterprises. Melville [8], citing a political science view of empowerment, identifies five key dimensions of empowerment: information, access, choice, representation, and redress of grievances. Thus, *social groups* who are empowered have information about health concerns, access to and choice among resources, representation in decisions about the structure and deployment of those resources, and redress for their concerns regarding how resources are used. CHI innovations that provide comprehensive information about health concerns, support access and choice, and strategies for engaging in the dialogs needed for representation in decision making and redress of concerns facilitate public health empowerment.

The ideology of empowerment of *individuals* also provides a useful starting point for examining how CHI enables consumers to actively manage their own health concerns and participate in their own health care. On an individual level, empowerment is ". . . a social process of *recognizing*, *promoting*, and *enhancing* peoples' abilities to meet their own needs, solve their own problems and mobilize the necessary resources in order to feel in control of their lives" [9]. In this sense, then, empowerment characterizes the manner in which patients and clinicians approach care, with mutual expectations, rights, and responsibilities. Empowerment represents a change in philosophy for both care providers and patients alike, requiring the former to abandon the authoritative control once held and the latter to assume a greater level of deliberate self-involvement in the care process.

Empowerment does work; there is good evidence that coaching patients using empowerment strategies leads to broadened, less pejorative definitions of illness as well as improved self-management by lay persons. However, without concomitant responses from care delivery systems, and clinical providers themselves, the benefits of empowerment are unlikely to emerge [10].

For consumers to be fair and equal participants in empowered partnerships with clinicians requires that they have adequate knowledge; set realistic goals; access systematic problem solving, coping, and stress management tools; obtain social support; and maintain self-motivation. In turn, clinicians and care delivery systems must bring to the situation a commitment to collaboration, content, and communication strategies; attention to the comprehensive needs of the individual; confidentiality; and continuity along the care concerns of the individual [10]. Although some dimensions of empowerment emerge only in the interpersonal context of care, information technology, specifically CHI innovations, can ensure the ubiquitous availability to society and lay persons of the tools and communication channels necessary to support empowerment.

CHI, the deliberate application of medical informatics technologies to serve the needs of lay persons, proceeded from many philosophical origins [11,12]; regardless of the implicit or explicit motivation of the initiators, CHI innovations have the capacity to support empowerment of lay persons in managing their own health concerns and acquiring the necessary healthcare resources to achieve health goals. The information technology requirements to support empowerment include four key functions: access to comprehensible, reliable, and relevant health information; communication with peers and professionals; access to personal care management tools including self-monitoring and decision support systems; and ubiquitous access to clinical records. The past 20 years has witnessed a plethora of experimental and prototype Internet-based resources that attempt to fulfill these requirements.

Consumer Health Informatics as a Means Toward Empowerment

Almost since the Internet began, lay people and their family caregivers have looked to exploit its capacities to achieve health and healthcare goals. The Electronic Grandparent project of the mid-1970s used simple terminal connections to link elders in a senior center and children in a daycare center, promoting intergenerational communication [13]. In 1982, the Cleveland Free-Net opened as an experimental use of early electronic bulletin board technology designed for rapid consultation between family medicine trainees and their off-site faculty mentors. Unexpectedly, lay people learned that they, too, could post questions and have them answered by the family medicine experts. By 1985, in San Francisco, there were more than 25 public bulletin board services for people with AIDS, allowing those coping with this complex, emerging disease easy access to peers who could offer self-management advice and the few professionals who had some knowledge about how to treat an unusual health problem. The 1990s witnessed rapid growth in the deliberate use of Internet-based systems designed to promote self-management and educate consumers about health, wellness, healthcare options, and disease management strategies [14,15]. The widespread availability of the World Wide Web led to the creation of health-related Internet resources (health-related Web sites), ensuring direct access by consumers to professional and research biomedical literature and to commercial health information management providers, such as WebMD®. Recent developments in Web-enabled access to clinical records systems provided an opportunity for healthcare systems to provide patients with access to their clinical records, thus expanding the portfolio of CHI tools.

Key Types of Consumer Health Informatics Innovations

CHI encompasses a variety of applications of Internet-based computer technology employed to meet the information, self-care, and health service participation of patients, family members, and well persons. CHI tools are used to deliver advice and instruct professional support and include health-related Web sites and mobile/wireless computing tools. These also allow patients to record and sometimes analyze relevant clinical concerns. Some CHI applications assist patients in making complex decisions [16] while others provide coaching and advice on clinical management of patient problems [17,18].

Interactive health communication technologies (IHC) is the term employed by the Science Panel on Interactive Communications Technologies (SciPICT) to encompass the variety of Internet-based CHI innovations [19]. IHCs include health-related Internet resources, specialized Internet-accessible clinical care services, and Internet-supported communication and information management with care providers. The SciPICT called for rigorous evaluation of these innovations to determine their effects and likely benefits for consumers. Field evaluations by several groups demonstrated that IHCs are acceptable to many types of consumers and do have demonstrable benefits, including greater knowledge about their health concerns [20], improved decision making confidence [21], symptom relief [22], and changes in the way consumers access and use health services [2]. Here we summarize three types of IHCs and examine their contribution to empowering consumers and engaging them in healthcare practices: health-related Web sites, experimental Internet-based health services, and integrated clinical information systems access.

Health-Related Web Sites

The advent of the World Wide Web (WWW) created easy access to vast stores of health information. Health-related Web sites appeared almost immediately as the WWW emerged. Health-related Web sites characteristically include factual information about health concerns and how to manage them, advice from health professionals, and communication resources that permit conversations among persons sharing common concerns. Health-related Web sites may be sponsored by professional societies, healthcare providers, and self-help groups. The content ranges from general-purpose health portals that encompass many health problems to highly focused attention to a single disease, syndrome, or concern.

The public health community—government agencies, public interest associations, and activists—employ the Web for a variety of uses. Web sites become gathering places for groups sharing like concerns, enabling unrestricted public dissemination of information and open public debate regarding concerns and community issues. Public Health authorities use the Web to alert citizens of public health concerns and public health warnings [23]. Robust tools such as hyperlinks and discussion groups allow rapid integration of diverse content and easy integration of diverse viewpoints.

Other health-related Web sites provide information related to an individual's experience of health and health care. Healthcare providers, clinicians, and even lay people themselves create Web sites that address the concerns related to specific diseases or conditions and make those sites available to the general public through the Internet. Individuals use network computers to access these health-related Web sites and locate the sites through many pathways—queries initiated from general search engines such as *google.com* or *yahoo.com*, direct referral to the Web site address from colleagues or recommendations of clinicians, or happenstance and browsing.

Consumers report an increased sense of confidence gleaned through obtaining health information from Web sites. Consumers consult health information on the Internet in preparation for visits to their clinicians and report discussing this information with their clinicians. Clinicians vary in their responses to consumer-directed consultation of Internet health sites, with some discussing and clarifying the consumers' information with them and others discouraging this type of exploration.

Some challenge the value of health information on the Internet, noting that consumers may find information that presents inconsistent or confusing results or that simply may be wrong [24]. Others argue that consumers may be only better informed but no more powerful in accessing health services or applying the information in their own care [25]. Some evidence suggests that consumers have difficulty selecting appropriate search terms to locate relevant health information, and coping with differences between "lay language" and professional terminology poses significant challenges for lay people [26]. However, consumers seem undaunted when faced with the multiple results of imprecise searches, demonstrating willingness to sort through a large number of results to find information of interest [27] and showing the ability to discriminate between credible and unworthy information.

Experimental Internet-based Health Services

Although health-related Web sites provided electronic gathering places for persons with like concerns to obtain information and peer support, their use remained limited to motivated individuals who had the technological resources and personal persistence to locate and to access them. Systematic demonstration that Internet-based health services could empower people to act effectively on their own behalf required careful field experimentation with targeted groups.

Experimental Internet-based health services provide a core set of services (e.g., condition- or disease-specific information, communication with peers and professionals, and self-management tools) to a specific sample representing a key population. Key distinctive factors of these initiatives lie in their use of controlled field experimental procedures to determine what effects can be directly attributed to the intervention.

Thus, these experimental innovations are similar in structure to health-related Web sites and can capitalize on their acceptability but, because of the sophisticated experimental design and observation strategies, offer a strong advantage to understanding how these systems are used and greater explanation of the benefits and consequences of the use of IHCs.

Brennan's ComputerLink projects (ca. 1988–1992) and HeartCare initiative (1995–2003), Gustafson's CHESS project (1992–present), and Safran's Baby CareLink stand as exemplars of experimentally tested Internet-based health services designed to complement or augment available healthcare resources. The results of these early experiments were largely positive, demonstrating that providing lay people with access to health-supportive computing resources in the home improved self-care, enhanced well-being, and reduced reliance on traditional health services.

The Projects

Home access to health-related resources predates the World Wide Web. In the late 1980s, Brennan's group designed and deployed ComputerLink, a specialized computer service designed to promote self-care and peer communication among home-bound persons and their family caregivers. Targeting two groups, persons living with AIDS and caregivers of persons with Alzheimer's disease, the two ComputerLinks were similar in design (information, communication, and personal management tools) and were deployed over a 6- to 12-month period with the identified groups [28]. ComputerLink had differential effects on consumers, with the greatest benefit accruing to female caregivers who did not live with the care recipient [29].

Capitalizing on improved technology, Brennan's group developed HeartCare [18], a specialized Web site that included tailored, sequenced information guiding patients through the first 6 months following surgery, private communication with other patients and with a clinical nurse specialist, and a public bulletin board. Patients recovering from coronary artery bypass graft surgery used WebTV® to access HeartCare. A tailoring program, launched when the patient accessed the site, created unique, personalized interfaces and directed the patient to information relevant to his or her point of recovery (Figs. 2.1 and 2.2).

Gustafson and colleagues developed the Computer Enhancement and Social Support (CHESS) system [4] to provide specific assistance to persons facing complex health crises. The system included searchable knowledge bases, text and video presentation of interviews with persons sharing the same condition, and tools for decision assistance and values clarification. Targeting persons with complex, life-threatening problems (persons living with AIDS, women diagnosed with breast cancer, families of children with asthma), the CHESS team deployed the computer tools for information access, social support, self-exploration and values clarification, and decision making assistance.

To support families of children born at a very low birth weight, Safran's team created Baby CareLink [30] (Fig. 2.3). Baby CareLink employed a hospital-based Web site and an interactive video connection between the neonatal intensive care unit and the family's home to provide up-to-date information about the baby and general advice about caring for a prematurely born child. Family members could use the video link from home to visualize the hospitalized child, observe care being provided, and interact with nurses and other care providers. On discharge of the baby, the video linkage allowed in-home conferencing and coaching, supporting the family through the transition from hospitalized care to home management. Major findings of the study included

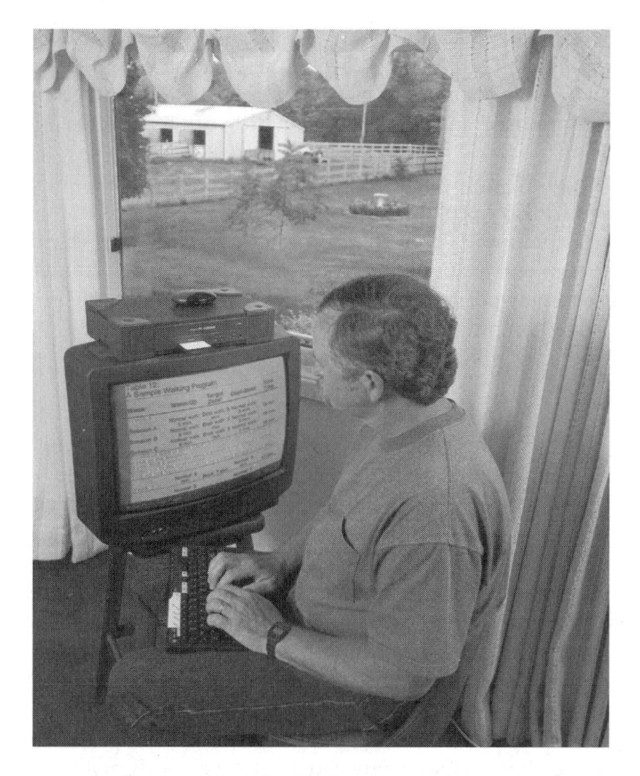

FIGURE 2.1. Web TV Device and Display.

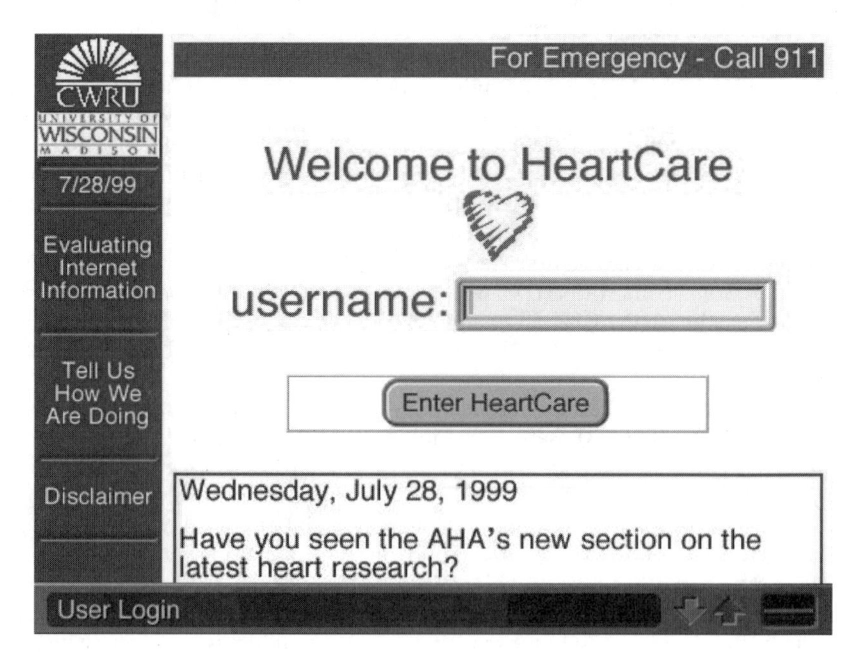

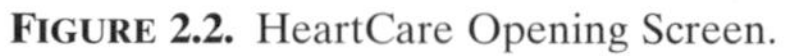

FIGURE 2.2. HeartCare Opening Screen.

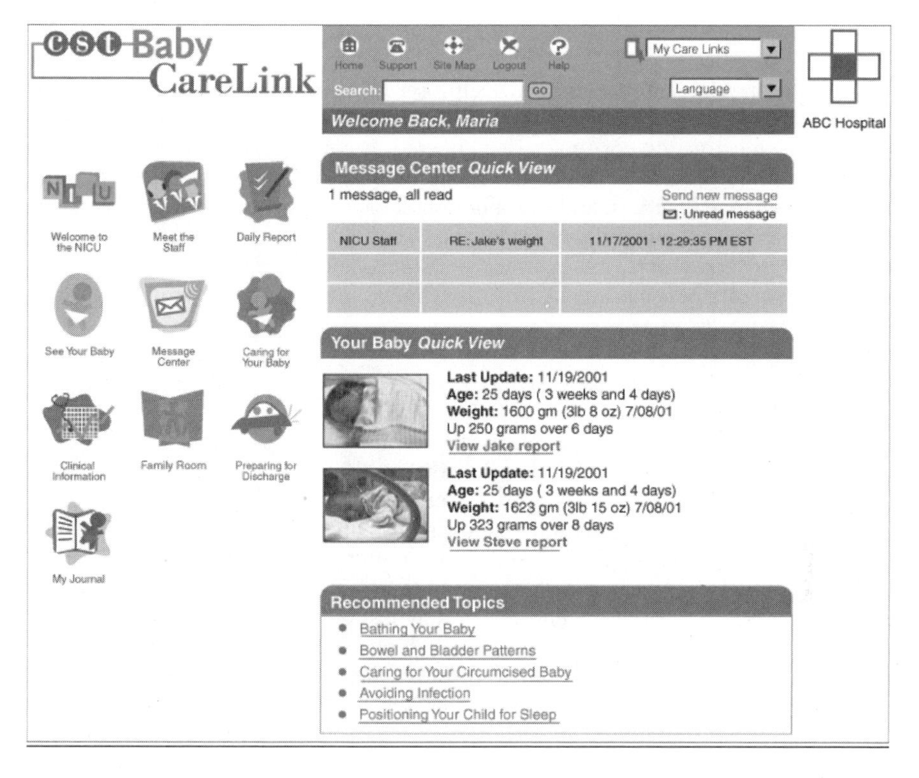

FIGURE 2.3. Baby CareLink opening screen.

improved parent satisfaction with care, greater communication and coordination between the family and the hospital care team, and slightly shortened length of stay for the baby. Today, Baby CareLink operates without the two-way video in 13 hospitals in 8 states [31].

Making self-care information available on the WWW has been shown to be useful to various patient populations in managing their own health concerns. Works of Brennan and colleagues, Gustafson and colleagues, and Safran and colleagues demonstrate that CHI applications are far more complex than simply posting health information on the Web. Brennan's work emphasized self-care and personal management of chronic or acute disease processes. Recently, Brennan's group demonstrated that clinical gains accompany the personal satisfaction and competence experienced by computer network users. Gustafson's CHESS projects provide patients facing health crises with clinical advice, peer experiences, and the opportunity to consult experts. Important successes include reduced negative mood, reduced time spent in health services, and a greater sense of control. Evidence exists that appropriate use of technology decreases health service utilization and promotes timely and appropriate healthcare visits. Problematically, most technology interventions occur independent of, in parallel with, but not integrated within, the clinician–patient relationship. Safran's work stands alone in its demonstration of the application of consumer electronics to extend hospital services directly into the home. Although clinical outcomes of the babies in the Baby CareLink conditions were equivalent to the outcomes of those receiving standard care, families experienced greater satisfaction and confidence in their ability to perform necessary care activities.

The experimental Internet-based health services offer strong support for the concept of technology-empowered patients. These innovations reach underserved persons who have needs not typically addressed in contemporary health care. More importantly, they provide access in the home over long periods of time to the kinds of information, peer support, and skill-building tools that strengthen lay peoples' abilities to participate meaningfully in health care. The full value of these experiments will be available to consumers, the healthcare systems, and lay people when their functional components become linked with the clinical information systems used during formal care services.

Integrated Access to the Clinical Record

With the exception of Baby CareLink, most CHI interventions coexist with, but do not directly integrate with, the formal care delivery resources used by individuals. Healthcare systems and hospitals are now experimenting with providing patients access to their clinical records, to information resources specially screened by the facility, and to care management functions such as secure communication with clinicians or appointment scheduling [32]. An important benefit of these systems is direct access to clinical reports, such as laboratory tests and recent diagnostics.

Columbia Presbyterian Medical Center developed PatCIS, a patient-accessible view into the clinical record [33]. Accessible through standard Web browsers with appropriate encryption and security, PatCIS enables patients to view clinical tests and report self-monitoring information (Fig. 2.4). PatCIS also contains links to relevant health information resources that aid the patient in understanding and interpreting the clinical information. Specialized tools allow some patients, for example, those with diabetes, to chart daily food consumption, home glucose monitoring results, and exercise patterns and to view this information in a manner linked to their clinical records.

Direct access by lay persons to their clinical records aids empowerment in several ways. First, it facilitates balancing of power between patients and clinicians by ensuring that patients and clinicians have access to the same information. Second, it permits patients to review clinically relevant information privately in a circumstance likely to be more conducive to reflection and understanding. It permits disclosure and discussion of the basis for clinical intervention decisions. Finally, by its very existence, consumer-available views on the clinical record demonstrate the commitment by the care-providing facility and the clinician to include the patient as a full partner in clinical decision making (Fig. 2.4).

Discussion

The migration of health care from the clinic to the community, coupled with the rapid diffusion of commercial electronics, contributed to the development of the field now known variously as CHI, e-health, or patient-focused computing. Thus, carefully designed and properly deployed electronic innovations for lay people may enhance the engagement of health professionals and lay persons now well recognized as the optimum environment for health care. Experimental systems and practice innovations in CHI show that lay people can and will use computer tools for health purposes, that this use leads to good health outcomes, and that linking consumers, health information,

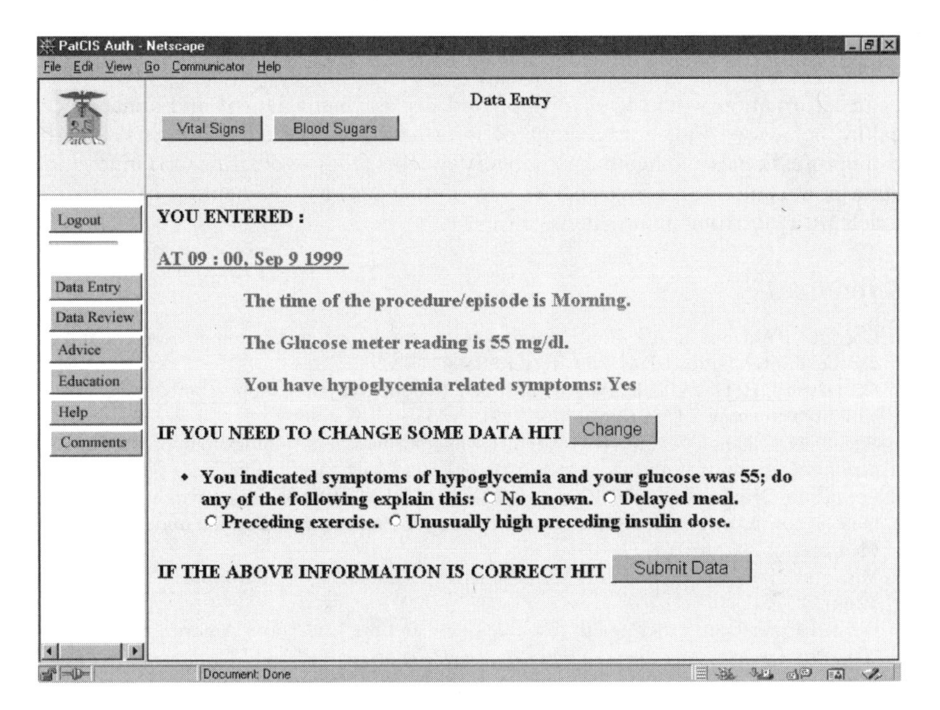

FIGURE 2.4. PatCIS Data Entry Example.

and healthcare providers via systematically deployed CHI innovations facilitates achievement of health and accomplishment of healthcare goals in a way not feasible by the singular efforts of consumers, clinicians, or computers.

It is timely to realign the application of computer tools to patient care in such a way as to ensure that the technologies be systematically applied in a manner most likely to produce desired health outcomes. Philosophies of care provide likely candidates for creating frameworks for the effective deployment of information technology in the service of patients attempting behavioral change or disease management.

The early experiences of lay persons' capturing of the Internet for health purposes persist today—the Internet serves as a vehicle for educating individuals about health problems, linking those coping with complex health problems to others in similar circumstances, facilitating consumer-directed access to up-to-date health knowledge bases and disease management routines, and connecting patients to their clinical records and care providers. What is changing are two things: the underlying technological capacities for ubiquitous access and complex searching and the capacity of clinicians to systematically exploit for clinical care purposes consumers' willingness to use the Internet for personal and public health management.

It is time to move the discussion beyond the feasibility of using emerging technologies to improve lay people's accesses to health information and health communication. Now the challenge to health professionals and medical informatics professionals alike is embedding these emerging technologies into a care system grounded in a philosophy of engagement [34]. Engagement ascribes to the patient–clinician alliance those characteristics that ensure a commitment to joint efforts toward the person's goals of health promotion or disease management.

The quality chasm and emerging healthcare personnel shortage need sophisticated information solutions to replace the naïve view that simply providing WWW-based health information would lead to improved disease management and adherence to healthy behaviors. Full engagement of informed, empowered consumers with the health professionals and healthcare delivery systems requires creating CHI innovations within new clinical care approaches, augmenting and complementing care delivery models with electronic innovations.

References

1. Corrigan PW, Garman AN. Considerations for research on consumer empowerment and psychosocial interventions. Psychiatr Serv 1997;48:347–52.
2. Gustafson DH, Hawkins R, Pingree S, et al. Effect of computer support on younger women with breast cancer. J Gen Intern Med 2001;16:435–45.
3. Weiner M, Callahan CM, Tierney W, et al. Using information technology to improve the health care of older adults. Ann Intern Med 2003;139(5 Pt 2):430–6.
4. Gustafson DH, Hawkins RP, Boberg EW, et al. CHESS: 10 years of research and development in consumer health informatics for broad populations, including the underserved. Int J Med Inform 2002;65:169–77.
5. Venkatesh A. Computers and other interactive technologies for the home. Commun ACM 1996;12:47–54.
6. Fox S, Farmer D. Internet health resources. Pew and the Internet in American Life Project, 2003. *http://www.pewinternet.org/reports/toc.asp?Report=95* (accessed December 15, 2003).
7. Brennan PF, Kwiatkowski K. How do lay people manage health information in the home? In: Marques E, ed. Proceedings of the Eighth International Congress in Nursing Informatics 2003. Philadelphia: Elsevier, 2003.
8. Melville M. Consumerism: do patients have power in health care? Br J Nurs 1997;6:337–40.
9. Gibson CH. A concept analysis of empowerment. J Adv Nurs 1991;16:354–61.
10. Segal L. The importance of patient empowerment in health system reform. Health Policy 1998;44:31–44.
11. Kaplan B, Brennan PF. Consumer informatics supporting patients as co-producers of quality. J Am Med Inform Assoc 2001;8:309–16.
12. Gustafson DH, Hawkins R, Boberg E, et al. Impact of a patient-centered, computer-based health information/support system. Am J Prev Med 1999;16:1–9.
13. Evelyn Kerr Fox.
14. Morris TA, Guard JR, Marine SA, et al. Approaching equity in consumer health information delivery: NetWellness J Am Med Inform Assoc 1997;4:6–13.
15. Simmons JC. Creating portals to quality: how the Internet is changing health care delivery to consumers. Qual Lett Healthc Lead 2001;13:2–10.
16. Balas EA, Jaffrey F, Kuperman GJ, et al. Electronic communication with patients. Evaluation of distance medicine technology. JAMA 1997;278:152–9.
17. Bennett SJ, Hays LM, Embree JL, Arnould M. Heart Messages: a tailored message intervention for improving heart failure outcomes. J Cardiovasc Nurs 2000;14:94–105.
18. Brennan PF, Moore SM, Bjornsdottir G, Jones J, Visovsky C, Rogers M. HeartCare: an Internet-based information and support system for patient home recovery after coronary artery bypass graft (CABG) surgery. J Adv Nurs. 2001;35:699–708.
19. Gustafson DH, Robinson TN, Ansley D, Adler L, Brennan PF. Consumers and evaluation of interactive health communication applications. The Science Panel on Interactive Communication and Health. Am J Prev Med 1999;16:23–9.
20. *http://www.pewinternet.org/index.asp* (accessed December 15, 2003).
21. Brennan PF. Computer network home care demonstration: a randomized trial in persons living with AIDS. Comput Biol Med 1998;28:489–508.
22. Brennan PF, Moore SM, Smyth KA. The effects of a special computer network on caregivers of persons with Alzheimer's disease. Nurs Res 1995;44:166–72.

23. Yasnoff WA, Overhage JM, Humphreys BL, et al. A national agenda for public health informatics. J Public Health Manag Pract 2001;7:1–21.
24. Impicciatore P, Pandolfini C, Casella N, Bonati M. Reliability of health information for the public on the World Wide Web: systematic survey of advice on managing fever in children at home. Br Med J 1997;314:1875–9.
25. Wilkins ST, Navarro FH. Has the Web really empowered health care consumers? The truth is customers may not have changed as much as we think. Mark Health Serv 2001;21:5–9.
26. McCray AT, Dorfman E, Ripple A, et al. Usability issues in developing a Web-based consumer health site. Proc AMIA Symp 2000;556–60.
27. Zeng Q, Kogan S, Ash N, Greenes RA, Boxwala AA. Characteristics of consumer terminology for health information retrieval. Methods Inform Med 2002;41:289–98.
28. Brennan PF. The ComputerLink projects: a decade of experience. Stud Health Technol Inform 1997;46:521–6.
29. Bass DM, McClendon MJ, Brennan PF, McCarthy C. The buffering effect of a computer support network on caregiver strain. J Aging Health 1998;10:20–43.
30. Gray JE, Safran C, Davis RB, et al. Baby CareLink: using the internet and telemedicine to improve care for high-risk infants. Pediatrics 2000;106:1318–24.
31. Goldsmith D, Safran C. Collaborative healthware. In: Nelson R, Ball MJ, eds. Consumer Informatics: Applications and Strategies in Cyber Health Care. New York: Springer-Verlag, 2004.
32. Sands D, Halamka J. *PatientSite.* In: Nelson R, Ball MJ, eds. Consumer Informatics: Applications and Strategies in Cyber Health Care. New York: Springer-Verlag, 2004.
33. Cimino JJ, Patel VL, Kushniruk AW. The patient clinical information system (PatCIS): technical solutions for and experience with giving patients access to their electronic medical records. Int J Med Inform 2002;68:113–27.
34. Essex D. Life line. Consumer informatics has gone beyond patient education on the Web. Healthc Inform 1999;16:119–20, 124, 128–9.

3
Tailored Health Communication

Rita Kukafka

Within the field of public health (PH), much attention has been devoted to using health communication to modify attitudes, shape behavior, and persuade health consumers to better manage and protect their health. However, research indicates that although traditional channels such as newspapers, radio, brochures, and television have been proven capable of reaching and informing large audiences, they are not very effective in changing behavior. Interpersonal channels have been more successful in influencing attitudes and motivating behavior change, although their potential for delivering health communications that reach a large audience in a cost-effective manner is inadequate. The implication of this research is that mass media channels are appropriate for creating awareness, but interpersonal interactions are essential for persuading individuals to change their health behavior [1–3].

In the past few years, advances in technology have led to a new tailored approach to health communication that involves soliciting information from individuals, or alternatively querying information about individuals from existing records, to provide audible and visual feedback tailored to be responsive to the solicited information. This approach is consequential because it combines the potential for delivering cost-effective health communications to reach a large audience combined with the benefits of interpersonal communication. The reason is that communications that are tailored to be responsive to the solicited information can be used to mimic the transactional and response-dependent qualities of interpersonal communication. An interactive cycle of tailored feedback and response can be repeated over and over to facilitate an individual's movement through the persuasive process of motivating health behavior change. Along the way, both source and message factors can be dynamically modified to realize the advantages inherent in interpersonal channels, advantages proven essential for persuading individuals to change their health behavior.

This approach, known as *tailoring*, has been defined as "any combination of information or change strategies *intended to reach one specific person*, based on characteristics that are unique to that person, related to the outcome of interest, and have been *derived from an individual assessment*" [4,5]. This definition highlights the two features of a tailored approach that distinguishes it from other approaches: (1) its collection of messages or strategies is intended for a particular person rather than a group of people and (2) these messages or strategies are based on individual level factors that are related to the health or behavioral outcome of interest.

Although the tailoring approach has notable benefits, it is important to note that not all information needs to be tailored to different individuals [4]. When needs within a population are very similar, the variation between tailored messages will be minimal or nonexistent, and thus tailoring may not be justified. Instead, a targeted approach may be more appropriate to address that need. Targeting involves development of a single intervention approach for a defined population subgroup that takes into account characteristics shared by the subgroup's members. Targeting is based on the advertising principle of market segmentation, which aims to find the right kinds of consumers for a particular product of service. Readers interested in learning more about distinctions between tailoring and targeting are encouraged to review articles by Kreuter and Skinner [6] and others [7,8].

What Is the Rationale for Tailoring?

The rationale for a tailored approach is grounded in theory that explains how people process information. Petty and Cacioppo's (1981) Elaboration Likelihood Model (ELM) provides a theory for understanding this process [9]. They have proposed two routes to attitude formation and change: the *central* and *peripheral* routes. The *central route* involves a cognitive component in which the attitude is formed or revised after much thought. This involves effort on the part of the individual and is more likely to occur when the information is perceived to be personally relevant. Studies have shown that messages processed via the central route leads to more firmly held beliefs and attitudes and results in lasting attitude change. It is therefore considered to be more effective in changing attitudes than general information [10,11]. Subsequently, an attitude is likely to influence behavior [12]. From this theory, the rationale for using a tailored approach can be summarized according to the following logic [13]: (1) by tailoring materials, superfluous information is eliminated; (2) the information that remains is more personally relevant to the message recipient, (3) the message recipient will pay more attention to information he or she perceives to be personally relevant; (4) information that is attended to is more likely to have an effect than that which is not; and (5) when attended to, information that addresses the unique needs of a person will be useful in helping him or her enact and sustain the desired behavior change.

Innovative Uses of Tailoring

Throughout the last decade, tailoring systems have been developed for a very wide variety of applications, providing information for patients at high risk for developing chronic conditions; for patients who already have chronic conditions such as migraines, asthma, and diabetes that require long-term continuing treatment; as well as for patients undergoing more short-term intensive treatment such as for cancer. The goal of these systems have also been diverse, from supporting the patient's role in decisions, providing information to enable management of chronic conditions, and offering health promotion advise and behavior change interventions.

In general, published studies have demonstrated that tailored interventions are effective in changing intentions and behaviors for a number of health behaviors, such as physical activity [14], smoking [15–17], dietary habits [18–22], mammography [23–25], and weight loss [26]. However, it has been difficult to synthesize these studies to better understand the mechanism thought to underlie the tailoring process because studies to date have lacked standardization in data collection methods, theory, variable measurement, and assessment of effectiveness.

One effort to synthesize studies of first-generation tailored print communications (TPC) is provided by Skinner et al. [27]. Thirteen studies of tailored interventions are included in this review. Only 8 of the 13 studies specifically compared tailored and similar but nontailored printed communications. The studies varied by behavior topics (four studied diet, two studied mammography, and one each exercise and smoking cession). The studies also varied by outcomes measured and type of tailoring (i.e., whether tailoring was hidden or whether materials were personalized). However, several themes were noted by the reviewers. First, TPCs were found to be better remembered, read, and perceived as more relevant than nontailored communications. The studies in general provided evidence that in addition to enhanced recall and readership, TPCs are more effective than nontailored communications for influencing health behavior change. However, because some of the studies applied TPCs as only one component of a complex intervention strategy and failed to use a factorial design, it was difficult to isolate the relative contribution of the TPCs to the overall intervention effects. Still, studies in the review did suggest that TPCs can be an important adjunct to other intervention components, for example, self-help manuals and counseling.

Other projects around the world are using natural language generation techniques that enable the delivery of tailored communication via the Web, and thus enable more interactivity. Interactivity is defined as the capability of new communication systems to "talk back" to the user as do individuals participating in a conversation [28]. Although there is interest in producing tailoring systems that enable enhanced interactivity, few studies have been able to demonstrate effectiveness on health behavior. As a result, their usefulness in real-world settings remains uncertain. As an example of a tailoring system with enhanced interactivity, Cawsey and colleagues [29] developed a nutritional tailoring system based on a dialogue with the user centered on practical tips. In this tailoring system the users make a number of simple meal choices and then receive tips for improving the meal. They can respond to each tip in various ways—asking why it is recommended, stating objections to it, or rejecting it outright. The system is based on a simple conversational model emulating aspects of the conversation between human dieticians and advisees. Another example is the PEAS (**P**atient **E**ducation and **A**ctivation **S**ystem) project, which was designed to prepare people to take a more active role in healthcare decisions [30]. The project investigated strategies for helping people to identify their healthcare concerns, to learn what actions they can take on their own, and, if necessary, to be able to verbalize their concerns to healthcare professionals. These strategies combine a multimodal computer interface (including typed text and mouse inputs) with intelligent tutoring and intelligent discourse processing. As PEAS interacts with a patient, it varies the content and pace of the interaction and suggests relevant learning activities.

Bental et al. [31] review many of the projects that have experimented with more advanced techniques for generating tailored patient information. Included in this review is a system called Piglit [32] that uses computational techniques to create tailored information for diabetes patients, given information in their medical record. The goal was to ensure that patients had the information required to understand and manage their conditions. Other projects using similar advanced techniques are Migraine [33], Healthdoc [34], and OPADE [35]. Migraine used computational techniques to generate tailored pages of information for migraine patients. But, rather than use the patient's record for tailoring, an initial tailoring questionnaire was completed. Healthdoc and OPADE use similar techniques again, but to generate leaflets. Healthdoc generates health promotion leaflets, while OPADE creates leaflets to accompany prescriptions. The studies included in Brug's review were similar to those in the Skinner review in that their purpose was to tailor health communication to the needs of the individual; however, the collection of studies reviewed by Brug used tailoring systems that relied on more sophisticated technology and were not limited to generation of tailored print communications.

Developing a Tailoring System

In this next section we look at some of the common issues that emerge when developing any tailored system. As already noted, the goals of tailoring interventions are diverse and the tailoring systems developed vary from simple practical systems being evaluated in realistic context to more experimental systems that push the limits of technology. The more experimental systems, for example, those using software agents and user dialogue models to enhance interactivity, are nevertheless similar to those employing less sophisticated technologies, as when the goal is to change health behavior they both must rely on health behavior models to better understand how attitudes and beliefs inform the generation of tailored communication. Thus, the common ground for tailoring systems to change health behavior has been (1) their reliance on technology and (2) reliance on theory and health communication principles. However, within this common ground, differences exist in the extent to which developers have drawn on these two elements, and this distinction has for the most part varied by the developer's primary discipline. Health communication researchers rooted in the discipline of PH have relied greatly on health behavior models but generally have used simpler technological approaches to generate what has been referred to as *first-generation* TPCs whereas computer science employed more advanced technological approaches but integrated behavior theory to a lesser extent. For this reason, approaches to tailoring are discussed along the lines of these two disciplines.

Approaches to Tailoring in Public Health

Kreuter et al. identifies a five-step approach that is characteristic of the tailoring systems originating by developers from the discipline of PH [36]. Step 1, shown in Fig. 3.1, pertains to identifying the high-level goal that the tailoring system will be developed to influence. As shown, these goals typically have focused on a health behavior such as mammography screening, smoking cessation, or improving nutritional habits. Step 1 also involves analysis of the causal factors, frequently referred to as determinants of that behavior. Behavioral scientists understand that behavior is not caused by a single determinant, and they typically rely on sociocognitive theories to assist in identifying the determinants for a given behavior. In social and behavioral sciences, there are many established and empirically grounded theories and models that help guide the selection of these determinants. Theories such as Health Belief Model [37], Social-Cognitive Theory [38], Theory of Planned Behavior [39], and Transtheoretical Model [40] are examples of the most prominent theories. Examining the research literature for correlates of behavior change in cross-sectional studies and for effective health promotion strategies in intervention studies can provide further information about other determinants. Generally, these theories, combined with empirical data, provide the basis for elucidating the determinants related to a given behavior and it is these determinants that provide the basis for the selection of the tailoring variables.

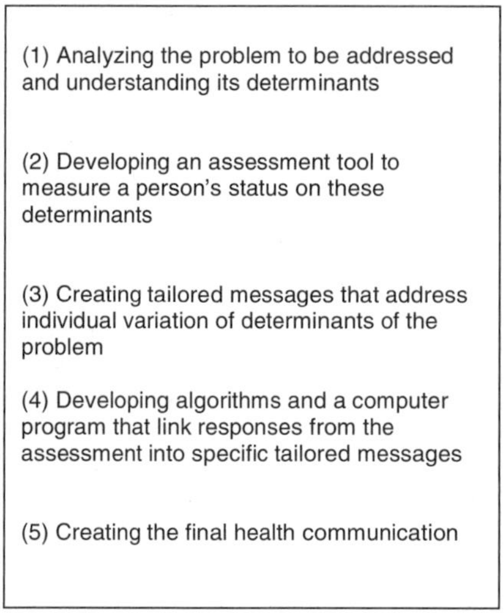

(1) Analyzing the problem to be addressed and understanding its determinants

(2) Developing an assessment tool to measure a person's status on these determinants

(3) Creating tailored messages that address individual variation of determinants of the problem

(4) Developing algorithms and a computer program that link responses from the assessment into specific tailored messages

(5) Creating the final health communication

FIGURE 3.1. The tailoring process in public health.

Step 2 measures each individual's status on the tailoring variables. In most cases a tailoring questionnaire must be developed to assess each person's status on the tailoring variables [13,41]. The tailoring questionnaire requires that the developer predetermine a limited set of questions and response options that are most optimal to assessing each person's status on the tailoring variables. In Step 3, text and other content that may include visuals are developed for each question and possible response option in the tailoring questionnaire. Although this step is straightforward in principle, it requires that an extremely large number of bits and pieces of text be authored: each piece of text expressed in each possible way that is appropriate in content to a particular user. Next in this process (Step 4) is assembling these text chunks into a final health communication document (Step 5). Tailoring algorithms, usually developed by domain experts, are used to formalize the logic, or decision rules that link response options to the appropriate piece of authored content.

This process for tailoring is perhaps the simplest kind of tailoring and can be achieved using straightforward tools available with popular database, word processor, and multimedia authoring packages. Mail merge features available with most word processors or similar tools have been successfully used in most of the systems developed in PH to date that aim to produce tailored written materials. However, only limited kinds of tailoring are possible. Usually it is possible to fill in blanks in some template using information from a database, and include, or not, a chunk of text according to some criteria.

Furthermore, the developer of a tailoring system using this process faces two additional challenging requirements: (1) acquiring the expert knowledge needed to author the content, that is, the bits and pieces of text that the system uses to generate the tailored communication and (2) the task of assembling the bits and pieces of text into a structured health communication document that is coherent, cohesive, and effectively persuasive.

PH has employed the most obvious method of acquiring expert knowledge for message content by directly asking experts to write it. The experts (e.g., health educators, behavioral scientists, health communication specialists, etc.) write the content used for tailoring informed by a variety of cognitive and sociobehavioral theories, for example, Health Belief Model [42], Social–Cognitive Theory [43], Theory of Planned Behavior [44], and Transtheoretical Model [45]. To provide an illustration of how theory can inform the expert in writing content, we draw on Fishbein's guidance for applying the Integrative Model of Behavioral Prediction, which was developed to inform health communications that are intended to change behavioral intentions:

> If strong intentions to perform the behavior in question have not been formed, the model suggests that there are three primary determinants of intention: the attitude toward performing the behavior, perceived norms concerning performing the behavior, and one's self efficacy with respect to performing the behavior. It is important to recognize that the relative importance of these three psychosocial variables as determinants of intention will depend upon both the behavior and the population being considered. Thus, for example, one behavior may be primarily determined by attitudinal considerations while another may be primarily influenced by feelings of self-efficacy. Similarly, a behavior that is attitudinally driven in one population or culture may be normatively driven in another. Thus, before developing communications to change intentions, it is important to first determine the degree to which that intention is under attitudinal, normative, or self efficacy control in the population in question [46].

Thus, the theory informs the expert whose goal is to influence intention in a given population, or in the case of tailoring to a specific individual, to focus their writing on the three determinants of intention: the attitude toward performing the behavior, perceived norms concerning performing the behavior, and one's self-efficacy with respect to performing the behavior. Knowing which construct to focus on is dependent on both the behavior and the population or individual being considered. The empirically derived data from cross-sectional studies and behavior change intervention research provide further guidance regarding these latter issues.

Beyond this the PH literature is disappointingly scant in providing guidance on writing content for tailoring system. As stated, expert authoring typically relies on behavior change theories as well as empirically derived principles. However, this assumes that experts have the ability to integrate their theoretical knowledge with their actual practice. Findings from one of the few publications in the PH literature that examined this assumption raise concern. Kline [47] examined the extent to which theoretical knowledge is integrated in communications that focus on breast self-examination (BSE). The study was to quantify and describe the inclusion of four message variables: severity, susceptibility, response efficacy, and self-efficacy. Inclusion of these constructs, which are from the Health Belief Model, was an indicator used to measure the potential strength of the persuasive arguments in BSE pamphlets. The study found that messages rarely included communication that addressed these constructs and thus the persuasive arguments for BSE in these pamphlets were determined to be very weak.

However, even beyond acquiring knowledge to inform the content of the message, a second knowledge source necessary in any tailoring technique is that which could guide the assembly of message fragments, that is, chunks of text into a structured and cohesive document. Structure in this regard refers to optimally combining the chunks of text into paragraphs and to sentence structures. Simply pasting pieces of text together is unlikely to result in a coherent smooth document, unless the author painstakingly ensures that every possible combination of texts is coherent and smooth. Even when the author engages in this laborious task, the issue of persuasiveness remains. Communication studies emphasize the role that structure plays, because although the understanding of a message decreases smoothly as the same semantic information is presented in a less and less structured way, the persuasive effects vanish rapidly [48].

To guide the structure of assembling these chunks of text into a final document, one needs also a theory that would describe how messages could be put together in a coherent sequence and explains why certain multiargument structures are more persuasive than others. Although such theories are not considered in the PH five-step tailoring process, they have been prominent to the tailoring process employed among computer science researchers.

Approaches to Tailoring in Computer Science

Because of the limitations of existing tools and techniques, several of the more experimental projects attempt to use more complex techniques, taking ideas from computer science. Most of these projects have built their systems using Natural Language Generation (NLG) methods. Natural language generation systems are computer software systems that produce texts in English and other human languages, often from nonlinguistic input data [49]. NLG systems, like most linguistic systems, need substantial amounts of knowledge. The basic idea in most of these systems is to represent explicitly information about the patient (as a "user model"); to represent general rules about communication, such as "use simple language if patient has low educational level"; and to automatically "generate" text from some database of health-related information, given the rules and user model. Achieving this, with only limited knowledge of how humans tailor their communications (required for developing the user dialogue model), has proven to be very difficult, and in practice even the systems that have this approach as their goal have lacked access to a knowledge base that contains specific information about the determinants of the selected behavior in general (acquired using health behavior theory), and thus information about each user's status on these determinants specific to that behavior. Because of the complexity of this process, approaches in NLG that incorporate tailoring on determinants of health behavior have been limited and have been focused more on tailoring to factual information and medical history rather than the behavioral determinants that are elucidated using the sociocognitive theories previously discussed.

More frequently the tailoring systems developed using NLG draw on theories of argumentation to inform the structure of persuasive arguments that are fitting to the goal of promoting behavior change. The NLG community has fully embraced the understanding that the same semantic information can be conveyed through a variety of text, paragraph, and sentence structures, and that a multiargument structure is critical to developing communications in a domain as complex as health behavior change.

Two types of knowledge acquisition (KA) techniques are based on (1) working with experts in a structured fashion, such as structured interviews, think-aloud protocols, sorting, and laddered grids [50,51] and (2) learning from data sets of correct solutions (such as text corpora); the latter are currently very popular in natural language processing and used for many different types of knowledge, ranging from grammar rules to discourse models (for an overview, see [52]). There are of course other possible KA techniques as well, including the approach used in the PH tailoring process which is to simply ask experts how to write the texts in question.

Reiter et al. [53] used this direct approach in preliminary stages of developing the STOP, an NLG system to tailor smoking cessation letters based on the Stages of Change Model [22]. When experts (three doctors, one psychologist specializing in health behavior, one nurse) were asked to write example smoking cessation letters based on a Stages-of-Change tailoring questionnaire, they found that the specific example letters produced had a different structure from the "general" structure that the experts had initially proposed. The investigators pointed out this fact to the experts, and the experts subsequently attempted to revise the general structure to more closely conform to the example letter that they had actually written; in other words, to combine their "theoretical" and "practitioner" knowledge. It was relatively straightforward for the experts to state theoretical knowledge, or to use their practitioner knowledge to produce example letters, but attempting to integrate the two types of knowledge was far more difficult. This is a common finding in knowledge acquisition, and it is partially due to the fact that it is difficult for experts to examine introspectively the knowledge they use in practice [54].

Thus rather than relying on acquiring expert knowledge directly as a sole method, computational tailoring systems have given prominent attention to argumentation theories, which focus on persuading people to change their beliefs and desires. Mainly, the interest is on the rhetorical structure of arguments, and as a consequence, in the structure of rhetorical argumentative discourse. Several researchers have attempted to improve the construction of rhetorical discourse or persuasive argument through the use of formal representations. Stephen Toulmin pioneered this direction in 1958, creating a model of argumentation with a notation for depicting arguments graphically [55]. Perelman and Olbrechts-Tyteca further developed this approach in 1969, resulting in what has been termed the New Rhetoric, which provides a comprehensive typology of argument schemes [56]. Anscombre and Ducrot in 1983 developed a set of argumentative rules (called topoi) that capture common sense relationships between sections of text (primarily in French) [57]. Rhetorical structure theory (RST) developed a general set of functional relationships for understanding the structure of discourse. While RST covers much of the structures used in previous approaches to argumentation, Marcu has shown that it is inadequate as a model of persuasive argumentation [58,59]. Further work is required for notations and formal rules that can capture the structures employed in tailored health messages.

Future Directions

Applying persuasive argumentation theories to communication for behavioral change has been complex. Research in argumentation has been concerned only with the structure of single arguments, and likewise, NLG systems that provide explanation and advice do not explore the planning mechanisms that would account for the generation of text that consist of multiple arguments. To generate persuasive arguments, one needs also a theory that would describe how arguments could be put together in a coherent sequence and explains why certain multiargument structures are more persuasive than others [39].

Some of the computational tailoring systems (e.g., Daphne) have attempted to combine theories of argumentation with behavioral theories, realizing that if the aim of an intervention is to induce people to modify their behavior, specific theories of how and why people change behavior to guide the advising process is necessary. These interventions have used Stages of Change and the Health Belief Model in addition to linguistic and argumentation theories to develop their tailoring systems [60]. However, all of these systems have been difficult to move into real-world environments primarily because of the complexity of using NLG techniques to generate multiargument structures in domains as complex as health behavior. In addition, there is very little in

Table 3.1. Merging social–cognitive, linguistic, and argumentation theories for a next generation tailoring system.

	Public health (content)	Computer science (form)	Next generation system (content + form)
Theory (KR)	Social–cognitive models (e.g., HBM)	Discourse structure (e.g., RST)	Persuasive strategies
Methods (KA)	Empirically derived principles	Linguistic analysis	Empirically derived principles, linguistic analysis

the way of reusable NLG resources (software, grammars, lexicons, etc.), which means that most NLG developers still have to more or less start from scratch.

The nonlinguistic ("PH") tailoring approach has other limitations. This approach is done via manipulating character strings; the user writes a program that includes statements such as "include X if condition Y is true, and Z otherwise." The key difference between this approach and NLG is there is no attempt to represent the text in any deeper way, at either the syntactic or "text-planning" level.

It is conceivable that the integration of both PH and computer science approaches is important for developing tailored messages. To design a system whose ultimate aim is to try and influence the user's behavior, very diverse sources of knowledge have to be integrated. Knowledge about the specific domain, about how individual behavior is influenced by beliefs and attitudes, and about how argumentation techniques can be used all have a crucial role in producing effective and persuasive messages.

Table 3.1 proposes such an integrated approach that merges the theoretical perspective, thematic views and experiences from both PH and computer science communities. Knowledge about the specific domain and about how individual behavior is influenced by beliefs, attitudes, and knowledge is best gleamed from sociocognitive theories and empirically derived principles of health communication. Theories of argumentation and persuasive structure are best gleamed from linguistic and argumentation theories. Using this combined approach is perhaps what is needed to build on and extend current tailoring research, with a view to moving toward the next generation of tailoring studies.

In addition, one can anticipate that in the future, additional types of tailoring variables will be experimented with. Theory must inform the most parsimonious strategies that will enhance outcomes without omitting essential mechanisms or including redundant element. This will require the adoption of a common language and standard measures of the basic mechanism and processes thought to underlie tailored interventions.

For integration to occur between the more sophisticated technologies, theory and real-world applications, opportunities for multidisciplinary and collaborative basic research are needed. As such, it remains to be seen whether the advances in our understanding of the tailoring process en masse will deliver the tailored health communication approaches sufficient to engineer an impact on improved decision making, patient health behavior, and chronic disease management in a cost-effective manner.

References

1. Chaffee SH. Mass media and interpersonal channels: competitive, convergent, or complementary? In: Gumpert G, Cathart R, eds. Interlmedia: Interpersonal Communication in a Media World. New York: Oxford University Press, 1982, pp. 57–77.

2. Valente TW, Poppe PR, Merritt AP. Mass media generated interpersonal communication as sources of information about family planning. J Health Commun 1996;1:259–73.
3. Hornik RC. Channel effectiveness in development communication programs. In: Rice RE, Atkin CK, eds. Public Communication Campaigns. Newbury Park, CA: Sage, 1989.
4. Kreuter M, Strecher V, Glassman B. One size does not fit all: the case for tailoring print materials. Ann Behav Med 1999;21:1–9.
5. Kreuter M, Farrell D, Olevitch L, Brennan L. Tailoring health messages: customizing communication with computer technology. Mahwah, NJ: Lawrence Erlbaum, 1999.
6. Kreuter MW, Skinner CS. Tailoring: what's in a name? Health Educ Res 2000;15:1–4.
7. Rimer BK. Response to Kreuter and Skinner. Health Educ Res 2000;15:503.
8. Kreuter MW, Wray RJ. Tailored and targeted health communication: strategies for enhancing information relevance. Am J Health Behav 2003;27(Suppl 3):S227–32.
9. Petty RT, Cacioppo JT. Attitudes and Persuasion: Classic and Contemporary Approaches. Dubuque, IA: Wm C. Brown, 1981.
10. Brug J, Steenhuis I, van Assema P, de Vries H. The impact of a computer-tailored nutrition intervention. Prev Med 1996;25:236–42.
11. Dijkstra A, DeVries H. The development of computer-generated tailored interventions. Patient Educ Couns 1999;36:193–203.
12. Eagly AH, Chaiken S. The Psychology of Attitudes. New York: Harcourt, Brace, Jovanovich, 1993.
13. Kreuter MW, Farrell D, Olevitch L, Brennan L. Tailoring Health Messages: Customizing Communication Using Computer Technology. Mahwah, NJ: Lawrence Erlbaum, 1999.
14. Bull FC, Kreuter MW, Scharff DP. Effects of tailored, personalized, and general health messages on physical activity. Patient Educ Couns 1999;36:181–92.
15. Strecher VJ, Kreuter M, Den Boer DJ, Kobrin S, Hospers HJ, Skinner CS. The effect of computer-tailored smoking cessation messages in family practice settings. J Fam Pract 1994; 39:262–8.
16. Dijkstra A, De Vries H, Roijackers J. Long-term effectiveness of computer-generated tailored feedback in smoking cessation. Health Educ Res 1998;13:207–14.
17. Dijkstra A, De Vries H, Roijackers J, van Breukelen G. Tailored interventions to communicate stage-matched information to smokers in different motivational stages. J Consult Clin Psychol 1998;66:549–57.
18. Campbell MK, DeVellis BM, Strecher VJ, Ammerman AS, DeVellis RF, Sandler RS. Improving dietary behavior: the effectiveness of tailored messages in primary care settings. Am J Public Health 1994;84:783–87.
19. De Bourdeaudhuij I, Brug J, Vandelanotte C, Van Oost P. Differences in impact between a family- versus an individual-based tailored intervention to reduce fat intake. Health Educ Res 2002;17:435–49.
20. Brug J, Steenhuis I, van Assema P, de Vries H. The impact of a computer-tailored nutrition intervention. Prev Med 1996;25:236–42.
21. Brug J, Glanz K, Van Assema P, Kok G, van Breukelen GJ. The impact of computer-tailored feedback and iterative feedback on fat, fruit, and vegetable intake. Health Educ Behav 1998;25:517–31.
22. Brug J, Campbell M, van Assema P. The application and impact of computer-generated personalized nutrition education: a review of the literature. Patient Educ Couns 1999;36:145–56.
23. Skinner CS, Strecher VJ, Hospers H. Physicians' recommendations for mammography: do tailored messages make a difference? Am J Public Health 1994;84:43–9.
24. Lauver DR, Settersten L, Kane JH, Henriques JB. Tailored messages, external barriers, and women's utilization of professional breast cancer screening over time. Cancer 2003;97: 2724–35.
25. Rakowski W, Ehrich B, Goldstein MG, et al. Increasing mammography among women aged 40–74 by use of a stage-matched, tailored intervention. Prev Med 1998;27:748–56.
26. Kreuter MW, Bull FC, Clark EM, Oswald DL. Understanding how people process health information: a comparison of tailored and nontailored weight-loss materials. Health Psychol 1999;18:487–94.

27. Skinner CS, Campbell MK, Rimer BK, Curry S, Prochaska JO. How effective is tailored print communication? Ann Behav Med 1999;21:290–8.
28. Rogers EM. Communication Technology: The New Media in Society. New York: The Free Press, 1986.
29. Cawsey A, Grasso F, Jones RB. A conversational model for health promotion on the World Wide Web. Artificial intelligence in medicine. In: Proceedings of the Joint European Conference on Artificial Intelligence in Medicine and Medical Decision Making, AIMDM'99, Aalborg, Denmark, June 20–24, 1999.
30. McRoy SW, Liu-Perez A, Ali SS. Interactive computerized health care education. J Am Med Inform Assoc 1998;5:347–56.
31. Bental D, Cawsey A, Jones R. Patient information systems that tailor to the individual. Patient Educ Couns 1999;36:171–80.
32. Binstead K, Cawsey A, Jones R. Generated personalized patient information using the medical record. In: Barahona P, Stefanelli M, Wyatt J, eds. Proceedings of the Fifth Conference on Artificial Intelligence and Medicine Europe (AIME-1995). Heidelberg: Springer-Verlag, pp. 29–41.
33. Carenini G, Mittal VO, Moore JD. Generating patient specific interactive natural language explanations. Proc Annu Symp Comput Appl Med Care 1994:5–9.
34. Hirst G, DiMarco C, Hovy E. Authoring and generating health education documents that are tailored to the needs of the individual patient. In: Proceedings of the Sixth International Conference on User Modeling, Sardinia, Italy, 1997.
35. De Carolis B, de Rosis F, Grass F. Generating recipient centered explanations about drug prescription. Artific Intell Med 1996;8(2):123–45.
36. Kreuter M, Farrell D, Olevich L, et al. Tailoring Health Messages: Customizing Communication with Computer Technology. Mahwah, NJ: Lawrence Erlbaum, 2000.
37. Rosenstock IM. Historical origins of the health belief model. Health Educ Monogr 1974;2: 328–35.
38. Bandura A. Social Foundations of Thought and Action: A Social Cognitive Theory. Englewood Cliffs, NJ: Prentice-Hall, 1986.
39. Ajzen I. The theory of planned behavior. Organ Behav Hum Decis Proces 1991;50:179–211.
40. Prochaska JP, Diclemente CC. Measuring process of change: applications to the cessation of smoking. J Consult Clin Psychol 1998;56:520–8.
41. Rimer BR, Glassman B. Tailoring communications for primary care settings. Methods Inform Med 1998;37:171–8.
42. Rosenstock IM. Historical origins of the health belief model. Health Educ Monogr 1974;2: 328–35.
43. Bandura A. Social Foundations of Thought and Action: A Social Cognitive Theory. Englewood Cliffs, NJ: Prentice-Hall, 1986.
44. Ajzen I. Theory of planned behavior. Organ Behav Hum Decis Process 1991;179–211.
45. Prochaska JP, Diclemente CC. Measuring process of change: applications to the cessation of smoking. J Consult Clin Psychol 1988;56:520–8.
46. Fishbein M. Using theory to design effective health behavior interventions. Commun Theory 2003;13:164–83.
47. Kline KN, Mattson M. Breast self-examination pamphlets: a content analysis grounded in fear appeal research. Health Commun 2000;12:1–21.
48. Bettinghaus EP, Cody MJ. Persuasive Communication. New York: Holt, Rinehart and Winston, 1987.
49. Reiter E, Sripanda S. Acquiring correct knowledge from natural language generation. J Artif Intell Res 2003;18:491–516.
50. Scott A, Clayton J, Gibson E. A Practical Guide to Knowledge Acquisition. Reading, MA: Addison-Wesley, 1991.
51. Provost FJ, Buchanan BG, Clearwater SH, Lee Y. Machine learning in the service of exploratory science and engineering: a case study of the RL induction program. Technical Report ISL-93-6, Intelligent Systems Laboratory, Computer Science Department, University of Pittsburgh, Pittsburgh, PA, 1993.

52. Jurafsky D, Martin JH. Speech and Language Processing. Upper Saddle River, NJ: Prentice-Hall, 2000.
53. Reiter E, Cawsey A, Osman L, Roff Y. Knowledge acquisiton for content selection. In: Proceedings of the 1997 European Workshop on Natural Language Generation, Duisberg, Germany, pp. 117–26.
54. Anderson J. Cognitive Science and Its Implications, Fourth Edition. New York: W.H. Freeman, 1995.
55. Toulmin S. The Uses of Argument. New York: Cambridge University Press, 1959.
56. Perelman C, Olbrechts-Tyteca L. The New Rhetoric: A Treatise on Argumentation. Notre Dame, In: Notre Dame Press, 1969.
57. Anscombre JC, Ducrot O. Philosophie et langage. Volume: L'argumentation dans la langue. Bruxelles: Pierre Mardaga, 1983.
58. Marcu D. The Conceptual and Linguistic Facets of Persuasive Arguments. In: Proceedings of the ECAI-96 Workshop, Gaps and Bridges: New Directions in Planning and Natural Language Generation, Budapest, Hungary, August 1996, pp. 43–46.
59. Marcu D. Perlocutions: the Achilles' heel of speech act theory. J Pragmat 2000;32: 1719–41.
60. Grasso F. Exciting avocados and dull pears: combining behavioral and argumentative theory for producing effective advice. In: Proceedings of the 20th Annual Meeting of the Cognitive Science Society, Madison, WI, 1–4:436–41.

4
Design and Evaluation of Consumer Health Information Web Sites

GUNTHER EYSENBACH

The World Wide Web has become an important (if not *the* most important) medium for providing health information to consumers [1,2]. Even cancer patients, who are not in the typical demographic group of Internet users, often name the Internet as the second most important source for cancer information after health professionals [3,4,5], and people are more satisfied with information they receive from the Web than from other media [6].

The aim of this chapter is to give an overview of best practices for developing and providing consumer health information on the Web and to provide a framework for best practices, quality criteria, and methods for quality assurance and evaluation.

Developers and health information providers are faced with "everyday" practical questions such as how to ensure, monitor, and continuously improve the quality of the information they publish. End-users (consumers) are also interested in "quality criteria" and best practices, as they wish to have "markers" (attributes of a Web site or Web page or a health information provider) that can be used to predict the "quality" in order to select "trustworthy" health information. The issue of quality criteria is also important for third-party expert evaluators working for gateways or portals, or other intermediaries such as librarians or healthcare workers putting together lists of "recommended" health Web sites, because they need to specify and apply selection criteria for the sites they endorse. Similarly, organizations that are in the business of Web site certification need to have a checklist of quality criteria to justify their decisions to certify a Web site. Finally, policy makers are interested in the subject of what makes a good (or bad) health Web site, especially in the context of making regulatory and legislative policy decisions.

There has been considerable debate and research on the variable quality of health Web sites [7] and how to best evaluate health information Web sites. One reason for the controversy is that "quality" is an elusive concept and implies subjectivity. Quality can be broadly defined as the "totality of characteristics of a product or service that satisfy stated or implied needs of the user" [8,9]. This definition stresses that "quality" is determined by the concordance (or gap) between individual user needs and the actual attributes of the service or product. *Perceived* quality (or satisfaction) is further confounded by the users' prior expectations, which also vary individually. In other words, certain aspects of quality seem to be in the eye of the beholder, and can be measured only by the gap between user needs and attributes of the Web site or service [10]. This apparent subjectivity has led to a pessimistic view that quality of Web sites cannot be measured or evaluated, at least not by third parties [11].

The fact that we are talking about "health information" makes the issue even more problematic, as in medicine there are often "gray" areas with no clear black-or-white answer. If the evidence is poor or conflicting, it may be impossible to determine a "gold standard" or to determine "the truth" [12] (at least without conducting a systematic review of the literature). Even in the presence of clinical guidelines, these standards for medical practice often vary regionally, which is yet another problem on a global medium. Moreover, conflicting views and standards exist on how (and how much) medical information should be provided to consumers (e.g., to what degree and how should things be simplified; how risks should be communicated). Quality of content can be determined only if we have a clear answer to a medical question and if we have an evidence base that tells us how best to convey this information to consumers, but both elements are often absent.

Thus, it has been argued or implied that quality of consumer health information on the Web cannot be measured in an objective, reliable, and valid way, and that efforts to do so are going into a questionable direction [11,13]. On the other hand, abandoning any efforts to evaluate a Web site and to determine "quality" because it is hard to avoid a debate on the reliability and validity of these criteria would mean "throwing out the baby with the bath water." There are many reasons why quality assurance on the Web is a must, and perhaps even more important than in offline media [14]. One of these reasons is that consumers retrieve information on the Web typically "just in time," that is, when they need it and are much more likely to act on it. In terms of consumer protection one has just to invent new informatics methodologies rather than transferring offline methods such as static trustmarks (also found on food, furniture, etc.) into the online world (see Chapter 18, this volume). From a developer's point of view, continuous evaluation of a consumer health Web site should be an integral part of any (iterative) development process of a health Web site (hence the word "design" in the chapter title). To shy back from evaluating Web site attributes because some have argued that these criteria are not "validated" (whatever this means in our context) or because there is "no evidence" that instruments and checklists containing such criteria "should exist in the first place" [13] would be a mistake. This debate is akin to a humorous piece published in the Christmas edition of the *British Medical Journal* in which the authors did a (fruitless) systematic review on randomized trials on the benefits of "parachutes for gravitational challenges" to prevent injuries—does lack of evidence mean that we should jump out of the plane without parachutes [15]?

In fact, apart from ascertaining face validity (by asking aspects), the criteria and processes presented here are difficult or perhaps impossible to "validate" in terms of showing construct or criterion validity, that is, predicting beneficial health outcomes (the same is true for quality criteria for patient leaflets). Most of the instruments which exist today have "face validity" because the criteria in them are based on a broad (ethical) consensus of stakeholders or they are based on experience.

A multitude of methods and instruments are in fact available that can be used to measure the "quality" or impact of a health Web site. The field is still emerging and in its infancy, but in the decades to come we will learn much more about what makes a good consumer health Web site and perhaps also be able to present more hard data on which processes or Web site attributes predict quality or a successful consumer health Web site. The beauty of the Web is that in theory it allows rapid testing, for example, of alternate presentation formats with rapid feedback [16], and provides developers with a much richer dataset than, for example, a printed patient pamphlet, which—once distributed—cannot be varied easily and provide little feedback to developers.

We also have to realize that creating an engaging and instructional consumer health Web site is as much an art as it is a science, much as creating a good book or a great movie. Thus, certain aspects of evaluating a health Web site, especially when conducted by third-party evaluators, are a matter of taste and inherently lead to a high interobserver variability. However, low reliability does not automatically mean that these reviews are useless. The analogy here is a movie review or a peer-review report of an academic paper. To conclude that because of this low interrater reliability it is impossible to assess the quality of a movie or an academic paper (or not worth reporting results) would again mean throwing out the baby with the bath water. Although certain evaluations may be subjective, taken together, movie reviews help consumers to make up their minds about which movie to go to, and peer-review reports help editors to decide whether an academic paper is valid and helps authors to improve it. On the same level, Web site evaluations—whether conducted by the developer himself or by third parties—help developers to improve their sites. Even if reviews of a Web site are not reliable in a sense that different people spot different flaws (i.e., low interobserver reliability), evaluation may be useful to educate developers and users what to look at and help them to improve sites—in analogy to the function of an art critic, for which many say the task is not to judge art, but to educate the public on what to look for.

Another aspect frequently missed in the current debate in the literature is that when speaking about evaluation and quality criteria we have to take into account the very different perspectives of developers, third-party evaluators, researchers, and users. In this chapter we will, starting on pg. 45, take into account the different perspectives of different stakeholders on "quality", which may avoid some of the ambiguities and confusions frequently associated with this topic if people talk about best practices for quality evaluation without being clear who the audience is.

Underlying Ethical Principles for Providing Health Information

Although different stakeholders (developers, end-users, third-party evaluators, researchers, and policy makers) will "operationalize" quality criteria in different ways, and put different weights on certain quality criteria, some criteria can be seen as being based on a common set of overarching ethical principles. A number of organizations have provided ethical codes or high-level ethical guidelines for provision of consumer health information on the Web. These codes refer mostly to the way the information should be presented and the meta-information that should be provided. The most well known ethical codes are discussed in the following sections.

HONcode

The "HONcode" [17] was developed under the umbrella of the Health on the Net Foundation, a small nonprofit organization founded out of a 1995 international conference on the use of the Internet and World Wide Web for telematics in health care. Webmasters can indicate their commitment to stick to the code by publishing the HONcode logo on their Web sites. The code originally consisted of eight broad principles for medical Webmasters (each basically consisting of just one or two sentences), without going into much detail on how each of these overarching principles shall be achieved. For example, in the principle on "confidentiality," Webmasters pledged to "respect confidentiality of data relating to individual patients and visitors," without defining exactly what this means or being held accountable for implementing the processes that lead to fulfillment of this pledge. Other principles of the code are concerned with how clearly the source of both data and funding for a site can be determined as well as whether advertising policies are available. Although the original idea was mere self-commitment and dissemination of the code as "best practice" (with Webmasters being able to publish the HON logo without any external control, whether or not they actually stick to the principles), HON has stepwise taken a more active approach in actually "reviewing" and "verifying" applications. For this purpose, some minimal operational definitions of the principles have been added. HON stresses, however, that accuracy and appropriateness of content are not part of the review process. Thus, a HON- approved Web site can still present inaccurate content. Indeed, it has been shown several times that adherence to the HON criteria (including Silbergs accountability criteria, see pg. 39) does not necessarily predict content quality (e.g., accuracy) [18,19]. It is also an open question whether sites reviewed by HON are actually doing a better job in sticking to these ethical principles than sites not carrying the HONcode logo. There is some evidence that this might not be the case: In one study, investigators reviewed the compliance with quality criteria on "HONoured" sites (approved by HON) versus sites found on a general search engine. Among 19 tested quality criteria, there was no difference between HONoured sites and sites from the general search engine, and for 8 quality criteria sites found on the general search engine were even more likely than "HONoured" sites to stick to these criteria [20]! These results suggest that sites displaying a HONcode are not necessarily "better" than those that do not, and the presence of a HONcode logo neither predicts content quality nor signifies that the site is more likely to comply with these criteria. It should be stressed, however, that even if these criteria do not predict accuracy, it should not be concluded that these are "invalid" quality criteria, because ethical behavior is a quality criterion per se [21].

eHealth Code of Ethics

The eHealth Code of Ethics [22] was developed on an international workshop convened and sponsored by the Internet Healthcare Coalition [23], another nonprofit organization with a broader membership than HON. This is a more elaborated code than the HON Code. The eight guiding principles are candor ("Disclose information that if known by consumers would likely affect consumers' understanding or use of the site or purchase or use of a product or service"); honesty; quality ("Provide health information that is accurate, easy to understand, and up-to-date; and provide the information users need to make their own judgments about the health information, products, or services provided by the site"); informed consent; privacy; professionalism in online health care ("Respect fundamental ethical obligations to patients and clients and inform and educate patients and clients about the limitations of online health care"); responsible partnering ("Ensure that organizations and sites with which they affiliate are trustworthy"); and accountability ("Provide meaningful opportunity for users to give feedback to the site and monitor their compliance with the eHealth Code of Ethics").

HI-Ethics Code of Conduct

The Hi-Ethics Code of Conduct [24], consisting of 14 principles, was developed by a group of leading for-profit consumer health information Web sites, drafted with the assistance of the Washington, DC law firm of Hogan and Hartson. According to Baur and Deering [25], the initiative is an attempt to prove the viability of industry self-regulation in lieu of U.S. federal legislative remedies such as regulatory measures by the Federal Trade Commission (FTC) and other federal agencies such as the Food and Drug Administration (FDA). Hi-Ethics members, who pay a $6000 annual membership fee, use a third party, URAC's Health Web Site Accreditation Program, to demonstrate adherence to their quality standards.

AMA

The AMA Code of the American Medical Association [26] was developed by a committee of the American Medical Association, primarily for use by AMA Web sites, but also intended to help Webmasters of non-AMA Web sites.

E-Europe Criteria

In 2002, the European Commission published a communication called "Quality Criteria for Health related Web sites" [27], based on a workshop in Brussels that brought together representatives of the key initiatives mentioned earlier and key academic projects such as DISCERN or MedCERTAIN/MedCIRCLE (see Chapter 18, this volume). The broad headings for quality criteria mentioned in the communication include Transparency and Honesty, Authority, Privacy and data protection, Updating of information, Accountability, Responsible partnering, Editorial policy, and Accessibility. The document also makes various references to EU legislation (directives).

Comparison of Ethical Codes

An excellent comparison of the first four codes has been published by Baur and Deering [25]. It should be stressed that these ethical codes are all "high-level" guidelines that should not be mistaken as "quality checklists," "rating instruments," or "scoring systems." The Codes contain few "practical" hints for developers on how the principles contained therein should be implemented. Therefore, these codes cannot be simply taken by a third party as an evaluation template; rather they have to develop their own checklist (possibly based on these criteria). For example, the broad ethical tenets of "privacy" or "accuracy " need to be translated into checklists with finer granularity, actually spelling out what this means for specific applications or topic domains. Similarly, for developers it is not enough to "commit themselves" to one of these codes, but they must think about (and spell out in an institutional quality manual) how these principles will be operationalized in the institution.

HSWG Quality Criteria for Health Web Sites

As mentioned earlier, the ethical codes mentioned in the preceding sections are only broad principles. Further documents exist that compile more specific quality criteria with a more operational focus. One of the earliest attempts to compile quality criteria for health Web sites is a policy paper of the Health Summit Working Group (HSWG) [28]. The group held three Health Summit Meetings over a period of 18 months (November 1996–May 1998). Broad input and outside review of these criteria were solicited at a number of medical and scientific meetings, and an interim white paper was posted on the Web for comment. The resulting policy paper was in turn endorsed or adopted by the Institute of Electrical and Electronics Engineers (IEEE) [29] as well the American Public Health Association (APHA) [30] and influenced many other publications about quality of health Web sites. The second and third Health Summit Meetings centered on implementing these criteria into a Web-based, interactive tool, the IQ-Tool (see later). The HSWG criteria are abbreviated as follows:

- **Credibility**: includes the source, currency, relevance/utility, and editorial review process for the information.
- **Content**: must be accurate and complete, and an appropriate disclaimer provided.
- **Disclosure**: includes informing the user of the purpose of the site, as well as any profiling or collection of information associated with using the site.
- **Links**: evaluated according to selection, architecture, content, and back linkages.
- **Design**: encompasses accessibility, logical organization (navigability), and internal search capability.
- **Interactivity**: includes feedback mechanisms and means for exchange of information among users.
- **Caveats**: clarification of whether site function is to market products and services or is a primary information content provider.

Silberg's Criteria

The most often cited quality criteria—perhaps due to their simplicity—are four criteria mentioned by Bill Silberg, then editor at JAMA, in an influential article in 1997. These four criteria are a subset of the criteria mentioned in the HSWG document (and virtually all "ethical" codes), and were meant to be those core "accountability" criteria a critical reader should look at when making up their mind on the trustworthiness of a Web site [31]. These are:

- **Authorship:** Authors and contributors, their affiliations, and relevant credentials should be provided.
- **Attribution:** References and sources for all content should be listed clearly, and all relevant copyright information noted.
- **Disclosure:** Web site "ownership" should be prominently and fully disclosed, as should any sponsorship, advertising, underwriting, commercial funding arrangements or support, or potential conflicts of interest. This includes arrangements in which links to other sites are posted as a result of financial considerations. Similar standards should hold in discussion forums.
- **Currency:** Dates that content was posted and updated should be indicated.

As with the HONcode, a number of investigators attempted to investigate the predictive properties of these "technical" criteria for content quality (e.g., by correlating a "Silberg-Score" with a content score [19]), but no study so far has shown a convincing correlation between these technical criteria and content criteria (accuracy, completeness) [1,7] although some trends for narrow topics have been established. For example, for drug information about St. John's wort, two criteria (citation of scientific sources and absence of financial interest) have been found to be indicators of reliable information, while the other two, date of publication and provision of individual author names were less predictive for content quality [32]. This is not surprising, as, for example, large organizations such as government sites or pharmaceutical companies often do not provide individual author names, despite providing usually reliable and internally peer-reviewed information, often because reference material has not been created by a single author. "Ownership disclosure" is also a bad discriminator, as 99% of all Web sites fulfill this quality criterion at any rate [7]. Based on these findings, the CREDIBLE criteria were developed, which may have a better predictive value for content accuracy [21,32].

Thus, although the Silberg criteria have face validity in a sense that many agree that they should be fulfilled, attempts to use these criteria as a basis for a scoring algorithm to predict content quality and thus to "validate" these criteria are misguided and fail to recognize that these criteria are ethical criteria that are quality criteria per se even if they do not have predictive value for content quality.

Systematic Reviews of Quality Criteria

Two important systematic reviews compiling quality criteria for health Web sites should be mentioned. One review by Kim et al. [33] gathered quality criteria from 29 rating tools or publications such as the ethical codes mentioned earlier or other theoretical articles where authors discuss quality criteria. Kim et al. compiled a total of 165 criteria mentioned in rating tools and articles. However, as these criteria come from theoretical articles, not all of these criteria actually can be, should be, and have been used by external evaluators.

A more recent review by Eysenbach and colleagues [7] compiled quality criteria from 79 different studies in which authors have actually "operationalized" these criteria to evaluate health Web sites and reported evaluation results. The 15-page appendix to this review (Online Table B) lists 88 categories of actually implemented quality criteria. In this framework, the authors discriminate content criteria (content accuracy, completeness) from "technical" criteria (including disclosures), design criteria, and readability criteria (the latter being at the intersection between content and technical).

Another notable taxonomy of quality criteria is the framework developed in the MedCERTAIN project, funded under the Action Plan for Safer Use of the Internet by the European Commission [10] (see Chapter 18, this volume). One of the deliverables of this "semantic web" project was to develop a standardized framework in form of a metadata vocabulary, so that gateways describing, annotating, or evaluating health Web sites could be interoperable, addressing the problem of ambiguity of terminology and lack of consensus on terms and definitions, as noted by Baur et al. [25]. Each vocabulary element from this framework—which is based on the abovementioned systematic reviews—consists of a definition of a quality-related concept (a Web site or health information provider attribute), a standardized question (to be answered by the health information provider or a third party to obtain the value for this attribute), and the definition of a controlled vocabulary or a scale to answer the question (i.e., a definition of possible values for each attribute). The metadata vocabulary is also known as HIDDEL and is available at *http://www.hiddel.org*.

Privacy Principles

In the year 2000, the California HealthCare Foundation published a report on privacy policies and practices of 21 consumer health Web sites [34]. This report provides a methodology on how "outsiders" can evaluate the privacy practice of a Web site without actually going into the organization. Investigated were whether a privacy policy was published, what this privacy policy said, and whether the actual practices of the Web site seem to match what the company said in its privacy policy. Not surprisingly, the researchers discovered several shortcomings, such as not providing adequate notice, failing to give users some control over their information, and not holding business partners to the same privacy standards. Most surprisingly, however, was that the researchers discovered that in several instances Web sites did not stick to their own privacy policies. For example, on a number of sites information was collected through the use of cookies and banner advertisements by third parties without the host sites disclosing this practice. There were also instances in which personally identified data was transferred to third parties in direct violation of stated privacy policies.

In the United States, the Federal Trade Commission (FTC) has promoted Fair Information Practice Principles as a standard for privacy protection in e-commerce and advocates industry adherence to these Principles [35]. Other countries have very similar e-commerce principles or data protection legislation.

According to these principles, consumer-oriented commercial Web sites that collect personal identifying information (non–health-related—for health-related information additional rules come into play; see later) from or about consumers online would be required to comply with the four widely accepted fair information principles which can be summarized as "notice," "choice," "access," and "security":

- "Notice" means that Web sites should provide clear and conspicuous notice of their information practices, including what information they collect, how they collect it (e.g., directly or through nonobvious means such as "cookies"), how they use it, how they provide choice, access, and security to consumers, whether they disclose the information collected to other entities, and whether other entities are collecting information through the site. This is typically done in a privacy statement that is easily accessible from the home page and from all points of data collection.
- "Choice" means that Web sites should offer consumers choices as to how their personal identifying information is used beyond the use for which the information was provided (e.g., to consummate a transaction). Such choice would encompass both internal secondary uses (such as marketing back to consumers) and external secondary uses (such as disclosing data to other entities). Typically this is implemented by opt-in checkboxes within the form used to gather personal information.
- "Access" means that Web sites should offer consumers reasonable access to the information a Web site has collected about them, including a reasonable opportunity to review information and to correct inaccuracies or delete information.
- "Security" means that Web sites should take reasonable steps to protect the security of the information they collect from consumers.

European counterparts of these principles are, for example, the Data Protection directives (Directives 95/46/EC and 2002/58/EC), regulating Information to be Given to the Data Subject, The Data Subject's Right of Access to Data, The Data Subject's Right to Object, and Confidentiality and Security of Processing.

While the aforementioned general guidelines are generic guidelines for any personal information (e.g., name and address of a consumer in an e-commerce transaction), special regulations exist for exchanging and protecting *health information*. In the United States, the Privacy Rule of the Health Insurance Portability and Accountability Act of 1996 (HIPAA) creates a set of requirements and restrictions for the handling of so-called Protected Health Information (PHI). PHI is defined as a subset of individually identifiable health information (IIHI). IIHI in turn is defined as health information that is "maintained or transmitted in any form, including oral, that is created or received by a health care provider, relates to the past, present or future physical or mental condition of an individual; provision of health care to an individual; or payment for that health care; and identifies or could be used to identify the individual". "Protected health information" refers to individually identifiable health information that "is or has been electronically maintained or electronically transmitted by a covered entity, as well as such information when it takes any other form." For example, protected health information would remain protected after it is read from a computer screen and discussed orally, printed onto paper or other media, photographed, or otherwise duplicated. HIPAA restricts access to protected health information by anyone not involved in treatment, payment, or healthcare operations without the patient's permission. Under HIPAA, consumers also have the right to request a restriction on certain uses and disclosures of PHI, to inspect and obtain a copy of PHI, request an amendment of PHI, receive an accounting of disclosures of PHI, and request communications of PHI by alternative means or at alternative locations.

Again, similar regulations exist in other countries. For example, the Health Information Protection Act of 2003 in Canada sets regulations that require that personal health information be kept confidential and secure, ensure that people know how their information will be used, give people the right to access their own personal health information and the right to request a correction of any inaccurate or incomplete personal health information in their files, and set out who can act on another person's behalf with respect to personal health information and in what circumstances.

The American Health Information Management Association (AHIMA) also has published "Recommendations to Ensure Privacy and Quality of Personal Health Information on the Internet" [36]. These recommendations are based on an E-Health Consumer Conference in which AHIMA brought together representatives from national consumer advocate groups to identify concerns and opportunities that face consumers when their personal health information is on the Internet. A task force then developed 39 fundamental principles and tenets on e-health privacy.

Accessibility

"Access" to information is another major issue often discussed in the context of consumer health informatics. On a macro level (policy level) "access" mostly refers to physical access to the Web. On a meso and micro level, "accessibility" of information is also often quoted as a "quality criterion" for health Web sites, but there is a great deal of confusion about what is actually meant by this, and even in the context of a Web site different people often mean different things when talking about access. In fact, it can refer to issues such as findability of information (influenced by such factors as availability of meta-data and quality of search engines) or readability. An "access barrier" in this wider sense can really be anything preventing the user to access, find, make use of, or even grasp the meaning of a document on the Internet.

Taking into account that accessibility issues can arise at many different steps in the pathway of accessing health information, the following levels of access barriers can be proposed:

Level 1 Accessibility: Physical accessibility
Level 2 Accessibility: Findability
Level 3 Accessibility: Readability, comprehendability
Level 4 Accessibility: Usability

Whether or not one of these accessibility issues becomes a problem also depends on the individual experience, literacy, skills, knowledge, and education of the end-user. For example, an individual may well have a computer at home, but may lack the skill to operate it, creating a physical accessibility barrier (Fig. 4.1).

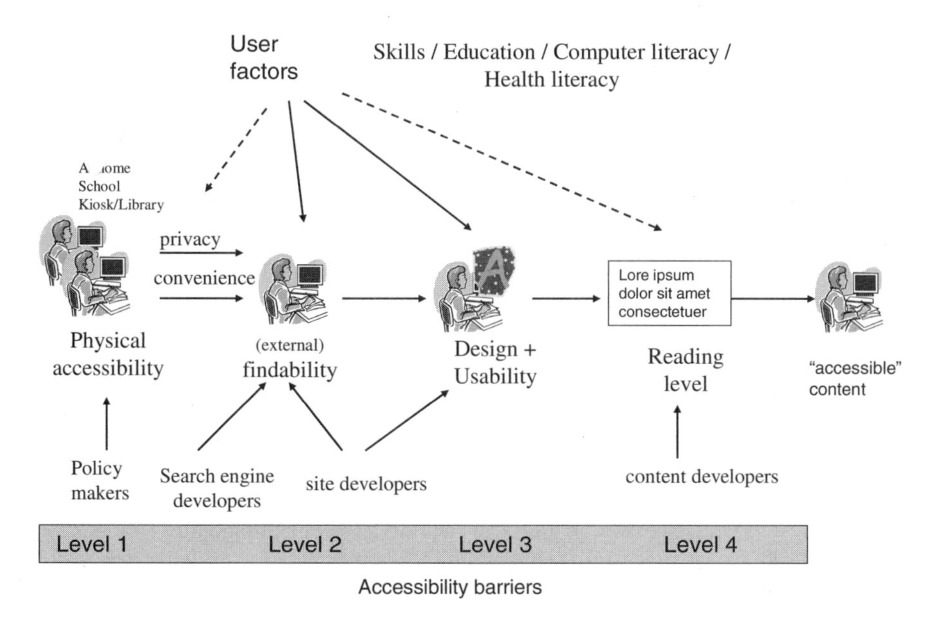

FIGURE 4.1. Levels of accessibility barriers.

Level 1: Physical Accessibility

A discussion at the macro level on barriers that prevent people from accessing the Internet in the first place is beyond the scope of this chapter, and readers are referred to the "digital divide" literature. However, two observations, which are frequently missed in the debate around physical accessibility, should be made. First, no standardized metric on what constitutes "access" exists, and although some surveys count, for example, the number of households having a computer with Internet access, other survey data count people who say they have used the Internet in the past *x* months, and so forth. It is therefore dangerous to compare different surveys across countries or time periods without knowing the methodology. Second, access is not a binary variable, but rather a (qualitative) continuum [37] (hence our difficulty to come up with an agreed-on operational definition). In the years to come, in which Internet statistics may suggest that virtually everyone in the Western world has "access" to the Internet (be it only through Internet cafes or public libraries), qualitative factors along this continuum, that is, the *conditions* of access, will play an increasingly important role. It must be taken into account, for example, that it does make a difference whether the Internet is accessible from home, or only from a library or school, in terms of convenience, privacy, filters, and costs. For example, a recent article of Richardson and colleagues [38] provides evidence that current filtering software, often installed in public libraries and schools, may be poor in discriminating pornographic Web sites from health Web sites. This is relevant in the context of this chapter, because while overcoming the digital divide in a sense of creating Internet access points is a responsibility of policy makers, it is in the hands of (and a responsibility of) health information providers to prevent false-positive blockings—by labeling their health Web site with an appropriate metadata vocabulary [39].

Level 2: Findability

With "findability" we address the situation in which people cannot find the relevant information that may be somewhere "out there" on the Web. This refers mainly to an appropriate listing in search engines and directories and cross-linking from relevant Web sites, so that users become aware of the Web site (external findability). However, it also refers to findability of a certain piece of information within a Web site (internal findability). Although it is an essential quality criterion from the developer's view, external findability is often overlooked as a quality criterion, because most of the ethical codes do not mention it and it is not a criterion for third-party certification (e.g., URAC). As people generally click on only the first 1 to 10 links displayed in a search engine and do not go beyond the first results page [40], findability is directly related to the ranking within a search engine. Findability can be increased by various search engine optimization techniques. The first rule is to use appropriate keywords on all Web pages. (These may be hidden in the text, not visible to users. It should be pointed out that many search engines do not make use of the meta-tags, that is, these keywords should be hidden in the page body.) Keywords should match terms users would use (e.g., "cancer cure," not just "cancer therapy"), and also include frequent misspelling ("prostrate," etc.). Various keyword suggestion tools exist, for example on Google AdWords.

The words in the title of the Web page, even the filename and most importantly the domain name, are important factors in the ranking algorithm of Google, so the most important keywords should be included there. Google also factors in the number of inbound links to a domain, so that sometimes it is better to host an academic Web project on the university server (which is by far better "linked" than a new domain). If this is not possible or desirable, ask colleagues from universities to put links to your site. Google not only counts the raw inbound links, but also weights each link according to how often the linking site is in turn linked by others, and so on. Receiving links from highly linked organizations such as universities will boost the ranking in Google. Initial marketing efforts should focus on getting as many links as possible—the visitor will follow.

Level 3: Readability

Numerous studies have suggested that information on the Web is not "accessible" in a sense of being written on a too-high readability level, as tested with various readability formulas [7]. (It should be stressed that by readability we do not mean "technical" readability or "legibility" determined by font size, font, and colors—this kind of "readability" would fall under usability issues.) The readability problem is not confined to the Web, as a number of studies have documented that most patient education material and informed consent forms used "offline" are written at a language level too complex for most people to understand. The problems regarding illiteracy and the various methods to test literacy of target populations and readability of materials are addressed in Chapter 6.

Level 4: Usability

Usability can be thought of as a dimension (i.e., a potential barrier) of accessibility. Usability is determined by the way the information is grouped and presented, by how the user navigates through the information, and by the amount of help the system gives (the best systems are those that are intuitive enough so that the user does not have to look up help files) [41]. Usability can and should be tested throughout the development process.

Another dimension of usability is accessibility for special user groups such as seniors or disabled users. In fact, the W3C's definition of "accessibility" is "content is accessible when it may be used by someone with a disability" (*http://www.w3.org/wai*; see also Chapter 11, this volume). Available standards and guidelines for "accessibility" in that sense include the W3C's Web Content Accessibility Guidelines (WCAG), the US government's Section 508, and the UK's Disability Discrimination Act.

Dozens of evaluation tools (which perform an analysis of pages or sites regarding their accessibility and return a report or a rating) and repair tools (which not only identify accessibility issues but also assist the author in making the pages more accessible) are available (see *http://www.w3.org/WAI/ER/existingtools.html*). Among the available tools is, for example, Bobby (*http://bobby.watchfire.com/*). A "Bobby Approved" kitemark indicates compliance with accessibility standards.

Different Perspectives on Quality Criteria and Evaluation

As mentioned earlier, there are literally hundreds of criteria that can be evaluated, and the number of different approaches to evaluation as well as the number of guidelines and publications dealing with "quality of health information on Web sites" is overwhelming. Critical in selecting a method (or methods) and criteria is that one has to be clear about the purpose of the Web site as well as the purpose of the evaluation, and select the evaluation method as well as the criteria according to the purpose and possibilities. "Quality criteria" or "evaluation methods" should not be discussed without consideration of questions such as "quality—for whom?" or "evaluation—for what purpose and in what context?" As indicated previously, there are several different types of stakeholders (developers, end-users, third-party experts, and policy makers) who could be interested in "evaluating" a health Web site, and all of them have a slightly different angle on quality, because they have different rationales to evaluate:

- *Developers* are primarily interested in continuously improving their service and Web sites and to benchmark the performance of their sites compared to other sites.
- *Researchers* are interested in generating evidence to inform users, developers, and policy makers. Some of the studies are aimed at describing and analyzing the "epidemiology of information" or "infodemiology" (determinants, predictors, and effects of good/bad health information) [21]. Some of the studies are designed to identify knowledge translation gaps and areas where fraud is highly prevalent. Some studies try to evaluate the impact of individual Web sites on health and behavioral outcomes.
- *Third-parties* such as librarians, gateways, portals, certifiers, or health professionals want to guide users to trusted health information.
- *End-users* (consumers) are interested in being able to evaluate a health Web site in order to separate the wheat from the chaff.

Some examples on how views and approaches may differ according to a particular perspective are the following: (1) From the point of view of a commercial health information provider "comprehensiveness" of the content is an important quality criterion, as the user should be prevented from leaving the Web site ("stickiness" and "pageviews per visitor" are important metrics from the business perspective). On the other hand, from the point of view of the end-user or a public health researcher, completeness of a single Web site within the universe of information on the Internet is less important, as long as the information can be easily found on other Web sites. From the end-user/consumer point of view, there is nothing wrong with a Web site that deals with one narrow topic in depth (e.g., treatment options) rather than providing "comprehensive" information, for example, providing the full information spectrum about a disease (epidemiology, diagnosis, prognosis, treatment). An expert evaluator evaluating completeness on a Web site or Web page level fails to recognize that people typically gather information from various sites and that complementing information is often only a mouse-click away [7]. (2) A randomized trial is an excellent evaluation method for researchers, but expensive and complex to conduct—obviously an unsuitable evaluation method for end-users or even third parties such as gateways. It will also not be a routine method for developers. (3) Developers have a wider array of possibilities to evaluate internal structures and processes and have access to more data (e.g., log-file data) than, for example, third-party evaluators (gateways, libraries), who often can evaluate a health Web site only by looking at the end result (the Web site).

In the following, we focus on the developer's view, with some additional remarks at the end of the chapter for other types of evaluations.

Developer's View: Best Practices for Site Developers

While the aforementioned ethical codes and quality criteria documents all contain criteria of the final product (the Web site), the following is an attempt to compile some "best practices" on the process of creating a high-quality consumer health information Web site in order to achieve a high-quality consumer health site. As surprisingly not much literature is available on how to develop a consumer health information Web site, this is mainly based on the experiences of the author and on the generic literature. Best practices on development and evaluation are *not* expanded on in most ethical codes [25].

Formative versus Summative Evaluation

For developers, creating a quality consumer health Web site starts with a thorough planning and needs assessment process, followed by a user-centered design process that involves repetitive testing with consumers throughout the (iterative) development (prototype–testing–refined prototype–testing . . . , etc.). Any evaluation that takes place during the development (formation) of the project is called *formative evaluation*. If the core development is considered completed and the Web site is running successfully, a *continuous quality assurance program* should kick in, allowing developers to monitor their performance continuously (this can still be considered formative). In addition, some developers may (e.g., in the research context, at the end of a funded project) want to investigate whether the set goals are achieved, which is called "*summative evaluation*." Given that in many cases a Web site development is a lifelong project, and that it is always iterative and formative (permanently under construction), the distinction between formative and summative evaluation is blurred and may be less useful in our context. According to evaluation theorist Bob Stake, the difference between formative evaluation and summative evaluation is: "When the cook tastes the soup, that's formative; when the guests taste the soup, that's summative." In the consumer health informatics kitchen, the chef should cater guests throughout the cooking process, encourage them to give feedback, and qualitatively analyze their comments. After the soup is cooked with input from the guests, continuous quality assurance means to constantly monitor the number and satisfaction of the guests and periodically invite gourmets (experts) to taste the soup and compare it against others. Summative evaluation would then mean to either look back and count the number of guests and analyze their satisfaction scores over a certain period of time, or to do a prospective study to test the impact of the soup on relevant outcome measures such as giving tips and recommending the restaurant to others or even on health outcomes, such as the number of food poisoning incidents.

Initial Design Considerations and Development Process

The following typical development process of a consumer health Web site is for the sake of clarity presented in a sequential manner; however, in practice, many of these tasks are conducted simultaneously or in an iterative manner, rather than step-by-step. To start the development process, most organizations faced with developing content for a Web site will set up a **web committee** (or development team) consisting of content experts, educators, consumers (representatives of the target group), and members with a technical background. The committee first discusses and agrees upon the **purpose and the target audience** of the Web site. It should, for example, be clarified whether the primary aim of the Web site should be information dissemination, education/training, e-commerce, entertainment, or communication (e.g., the Web can be an interface for one-to-one communication), or for building communities (see Chapter 8). While a Web site can have several of these elements, priorities should be defined [42]. To set down a broad mission statement can help guide future development, although developers should be prepared to amend the mission statement based on user feedback. To have clear aims is a prerequisite for evaluation, because a Web site is best evaluated in relation to its objectives.

To define, refine, or validate the mission statement, a **needs assessment** [43] should be conducted, to clarify what consumers (or the target audience) expect or wish to see. A thorough needs assessment should include multiple methodologies to "triangulate" the information by collecting it from different sources, including a **literature and Internet review** (e.g., What are the described information needs of consumers with a certain disease e.g., from surveys?) and **focus groups** [44] or in-depth interviews with consumers and other stakeholders (using separate sessions for each group). By "Internet review" we mean, for example, a systematic review of what the target audience discusses in Internet communities, for example, collecting consumers' information needs and preferences from mailing lists. It is important that this is done in an ethical manner [45]. Another way to use the Internet to gather information on what people need is to analyze search terms entered into search engines (one possible method is described in [46]). Another possible method is to use keyword suggestion tools such Google Adwords or the 7search keyword suggestion tool (*http://conversion.7search.com/scripts/advertisertools/keywordsuggestion.aspx*), which provide statistics on how often a certain keywords and other searches containing that keyword have been conducted.

In order to determine the gap between needs and resources already available, an *information needs matrix* (see Fig. 4.2) can be developed, spelling out for each topic what the "needs" are, what information is already available, and—resulting from the gap of these—what the Web site could focus on.

Once the purpose and target audience have been defined and a requirement (gap) analysis has been conducted, the **content** is broadly compiled by gathering key messages and describing the scope and depth of the content in a content outline. During the development of the content outline one can already gather ideas for how the content is best conveyed and which content can be and should be "tailored." Text is

Topic: …………………	**What the literature (incl. Internet) says**	**What experts/health professionals say** (focus groups, interviews)	**What consumers say** (focus groups, interviews)
Information needs and common misunderstandings			
What is already out there / commonly known			
Gap-Analysis: Focus of content to be developed, key messages			

FIGURE 4.2. A template for a "needs analysis matrix" for consumer health information, to determine information needs and the focus of a Web site. Topics or themes that are candidate topics to be covered by the Web site are identified from the literature and through interviews with health professionals and consumers. For each topic, a matrix is used, compiling needs (what is required) and status quo (what is already there), which will help to identify the focus of the content.

not always the best medium—graphics, multimedia, and streaming video and audio (talking heads) and interactive Macromedia Flash or Shockwave presentations are viable alternative presentation formats. Additional focus groups may be necessary to iteratively refine an initial content outline and to identify the most suitable presentation format as well as the site structure (which content should be displayed first and which content should be deeper buried in the site structure). The next step is to develop a **site map**, that is, the navigational tree structure with key crosslinks between the sections. A consumer health Web site should always have an "About us" menu point (describing who behind the Web site is, including credentials of the authors, internal quality assurance procedures and editorial policies, advertising and privacy policies), and a menu point for consumer feedback, for example, a proprietary feedback form or—better—a link to a validated and standardized feedback form, which allows one to measure user satisfaction and allows comparisons between Web sites, for example, the SUSHI-Questionnaire (see pg. 54). The next step is to develop a **rapid prototype or a nonfunctional mock-up version** (e.g., showing just the menu structure, either on paper or on the screen), which is presented to additional **focus groups**. Using feedback from the focus groups, the prototype or mock-up is iteratively refined and presented to further focus groups, until no major new issues are brought up (saturation). After a **functional prototype** has been developed, additional focus groups and **usability studies** should be conducted. Usability studies can take on the form of a heuristic evaluation by a usability expert, who reviews the prototype against a set of design rules based on experience, or they can consist of studies testing the system with actual users [41]. To achieve a user-centric design it is important to involve users as early as possible and continuously throughout the development process, rather than waiting to test the "final" system with real users at the very end. Often at that stage developers are reluctant to make any major changes. Before the site can be launched (goes "live"), it is important that the organization first develops and agrees upon some **internal policies** and procedures related to running a consumer health Web site (see later). Even after the site goes live, the development process should not be considered "finished"—developers should implement a **continuous quality improvement program**, for example, gathering systematically user feedback and respond to the issues and suggestions flagged by users.

Textbox: Specific Design Considerations

When developing the content for a consumer health Web site, site developers should take into account the following considerations:

- When considering topic to be covered, developers should focus on the development of original content, rather than repeating what is already out there. Does it really make sense to set up yet another Web site on melanoma prevention?
- When deciding which content should be produced, consider the organization's unique strengths and special expertise (access to experts or other resources and information), together with what consumers need.
- Do not necessarily strive for comprehensiveness or completeness. Although "completeness" is a quality criterion often used by researchers determining the quality of a Web site (and most Web sites have been shown to provide "incomplete" information when compared against key facts provided in medical guidelines) [2], complementing information is only a mouse click away.
- If you do not strive for completeness, make clear that further information is available and link to other organizations that may complement the information.
- A Web site is a fundamentally different medium than paper. Resist the temptation to simply put existing patient pamphlets as PDFs or converted to HTML on the Web without adapting it for this medium.
- Enrich text information with graphics and multimedia (audio, video) where appropriate.
- Do not provide too much text. Consumers scan content on the Web rather than reading it. Consider to offer each document in two versions: one document with bullet points for skimming and reading on screen, another downloadable and printable file for detailed information.
- Consider whether content can be tailored for specific target audiences, and whether different version for different audiences should be produced.
- Do not assume that users always come through the "front door" (homepage). Many (in fact most) visitors will come from a search engine such as Google and end up directly on a Web page without seeing the homepage first. It is important that each Web page allows visitors to orient themselves quickly and provides a quick glimpse of who is behind the information and whom the information is for.
- Consider using metadata (e.g., HIDDEL) to describe the target audience, site owner, and so forth (see Chapter 18), so that applications (search engines, browser plug-ins) can support consumers in making informed choices.

Formative Evaluation Methods

As noted earlier, the most important evaluation methods during the "formation" of a health Web site involving consumers are focus groups and usability tests. These methods can also be used as "summative evaluation."

Focus groups are a qualitative research method with a long tradition in the social and marketing sciences [47]. A group of stakeholders, for example, consumers, are brought together and, facilitated by a skilled moderator, encouraged to talk about certain issues broadly defined a priori in an interview guide. Participants could, for example, be asked to discuss what information they expect on a Web site with a certain topic, or they could be asked to react to a mock-up or prototype version of a Web site. Typically, focus group discussions are audio-recorded and transcribed, and emerging themes coded. Focus groups are increasingly recognized as an integral and essential methodology in all phases of developing a health Web site, from initial needs assessment to continuous quality improvement.

Usability tests are another qualitative research method in which participants in a usability lab are placed in front of a computer with the Web site or application in front of them. Participants are then given a task or scenario, for example, they are asked to find a certain piece of information on the Web site (see [48] for a published usability study of a consumer health Web site). The actions (sometimes also the facial expressions) of the participants are recorded on video, and keystrokes and screen content are captured by software. For high-end usability studies, eye-tracking hard- and software can be used to identify and quantify screen areas that are fixated by the participant. Sometimes participants are also asked to "think aloud" in order to give some insights into cognitive processes. Usually, researchers afterwards interview the participant and recapitulate some of the actions of the participant, soliciting suggestions for improvements, and collect themes for usability issues. Although a professional usability lab environment (Fig. 4.3) is ideal, the costs for renting such a lab are often prohibitive. However, an improvised lab with a consumer grade video camera also fulfills the purpose. Any testing is better than no testing!

Usability tests with actual participants can also be preceded or complemented by a heuristic usability evaluation, that is, a review of the site by a human factors expert.

Policies Development

Often neglected in the planning stages is the fact that developing a consumer health information Web site entails more than "just" developing content and publishing

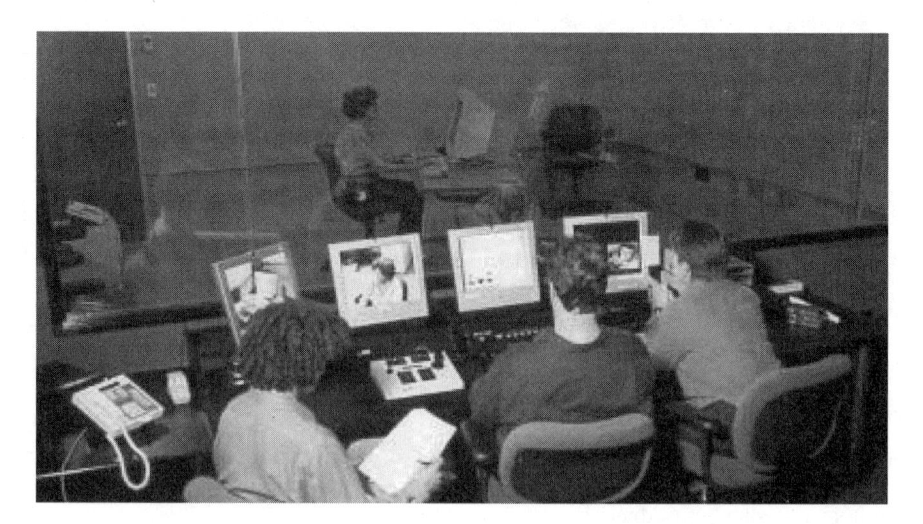

FIGURE 4.3. A high-end usability lab (Source: Sun Microsystems, *http://www.sun.com/usability/*).

HTML pages, in analogy to producing a printed patient leaflet. Running a health Web site also means that internal policies and processes need to be defined, for example, a privacy policy, an editorial policy, and—if applicable—an advertising policy (defining, e.g., acceptable and inacceptable products). Also, responsible persons for privacy (Privacy Officer), content/site quality (editor in chief or "chief quality officer"), technical fixes (Webmaster or chief developer), and staff members responding to subject-related e-mail requests (administrative staff, librarian, junior medical doctor) need to be named. Often forgotten is also the fact that Internet information is not and should not be static—content development does not end with the initial release of a Web site but is an ongoing process, and information needs to be reviewed and updated regularly. Internal policies need to spell out who is responsible for maintaining and updating the information.

All policies and responsibilities should be compiled in writing in an internal "Quality Assurance Manual." This manual should contain a description of the general workflow for publishing/updating information, the workflow to respond to e-mail requests, complaints, and so forth. It should be stressed that any organization that publishes health information will also get e-mails with personal medical questions, whether they are invited or discouraged, and whether an e-mail address for feedback is published or not. Such e-mails sometimes include questions that are clearly inappropriate for answering by e-mail, such as how to treat or diagnose a disease. In one study, 61.8% of e-mail requests were "medical," while 20.6% were classified as "technical." In another study, 28% of all unsolicited e-mails sent to a consumer health Web site that contained a health information request would have required a health professional to answer, and 27% of e-mails would have required a face-to-face consultation and examination, that is, should not be answered via e-mail [49]. A standard disclaimer such as stressing that individual consultations cannot be provided via e-mail may reduce the number of such e-mails, but is unlikely to eliminate individual health-related questions completely. Although health information providers should always respond to user e-mails (be it only with an automatic response), health information providers have to be careful not to cross the boundary to giving personal advice in health-related matters that can be misconstrued as offering a medical consultation, as liability issues arise [50–52]. Internal guidelines should address issues such as what constitutes inappropriate requests and how to respond to them. They can be based on other previously published guidelines [53]. Systematically analyzing comments or other feedback about the content (including frequent misunderstandings) should be a routine measure for continuous quality assurance [54].

Establishing Credibility

As illustrated in Figure 4.4, users will surf away or not act on the content if the Web site does not appear credible or trustworthy, even if the content is judged excellent by experts. Although in focus groups and surveys people often claim that the source of the information is their primary yardstick when evaluating credibility [40,55], direct observational research in a usability lab setting has shown that health consumers actually rarely look at the "about us" section in order to make decisions on whether or not to trust a Web site [40]. Rather, the study concludes that in reality consumers are more impressed by surface credibility markers, such as the Web site design (Does it appear "professional"?). Some consumers even use markers such as the picture of the site owner [40]. This is consistent with a model proposed by Wathen and Burkell [56] and research conducted by the Stanford Persuasive Technology Lab [57]. As a result, the

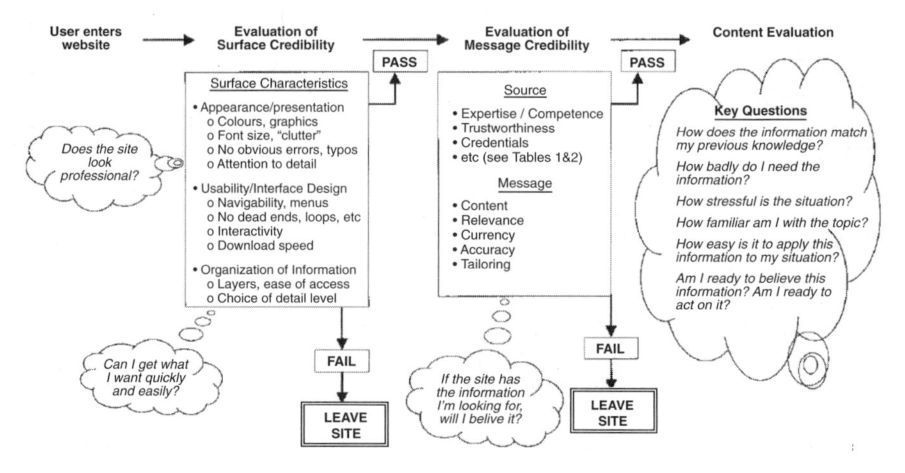

FIGURE 4.4. Proposed model for how users judge the credibility of online information [56].

Stanford investigators have produced a set of 10 guidelines for developers on how to "boost a Web site's credibility" (*http://www.webcredibility.org/guidelines/*). Among these guidelines are the following suggestions:

- Make it easy to check the accuracy of the information on the site. In the consumer health field, this could, for example, mean providing links to references (e.g., in *pubmed.gov*) or other trusted sources (e.g., government sites) that confirm certain key messages.
- Show that there is a real organization (or person) behind the site. (Consumer health Web sites could, for example, show the picture of the author—and if he or she wears a white coat this will boost credibility even more . . . !)
- Use a professional design that is appropriate to the content of the site. (Sometimes, a "too-professional" look can also negatively affect credibility. A fancy Web site with flash animation and videos run by a small self-support group may make people believe that a pharmaceutical company is sponsoring the content.)
- Avoid typos and broken links. Even a single typo can make people conclude that internal quality management processes are insufficient.
- Make the site easy to use.
- Use restraint with promotional content (ads, offers).

We find few criteria here that are not already mentioned in the context of "ethical codes," such as showing credentials, providing a feedback mechanism, providing information on the last update, showing references—so that ethical conduct should have a positive impact on credibility.

Whether or not third-party seals (kitemarks, trustmarks) enhance trustworthiness and credibility is an open question. Although some consumers say it would enhance their confidence in a Web site [40], some experimental research suggests that they do not make a difference [58]. However, in this particular study researchers used a fictional seal. It is more likely that the actual effect on trustworthiness depends on how trusted the endorsing organization creating the trustmark is—if the seal contains a well-known respected brand name, a respected nonprofit or educational organization (e.g., university) or a government organization, and if the consumer is aware of the evaluation processes needed to get the trustmark, it is likely that this could boost the credibility of a Web site.

Marketing a Site

As noted previously, the "findability" of a site (i.e., the ability of people to find your consumer health Web site) is an import "accessibility" criterion. Findability is mainly dependent on search engine listing and ranking.

If an appropriate search engine ranking is not (yet) achieved, active advertising and marketing a Web site online and offline should be considered. One of the most effective online advertising strategies is keyword-triggered advertising in search engines, for example, Google AdWords, the world's largest search advertising program. In AdWords developers can choose keywords to precisely target ad delivery to Web users seeking information about a particular disease, symptom, product, or service. The program is based on cost-per-click (CPC) pricing, so advertisers pay only when an ad is clicked on. Referral costs (e.g., each click) can be as low as 8 cents per click-through, but the cost also depends on the "competitiveness" of the chosen topic (it becomes more expensive if many other advertisers compete for the same keyword). Advertisers can also geographically target their ad by choosing who should see the ad from among 250+ countries and 14 languages. It is even possible to restrict it to individual US states. On average, 0.5% to 1% of visitors in Google will click on an ad. For example, an advertisement triggered with the keyword "cancer" (searched on Google about 240,000 times per day) would lead to approximately 1200 click-throughs (visitors), requiring a budget of at least $96 per day. Other topics may have far fewer searches. Advertisers can also set a fixed budget, for example, determine that they want to spend only $10 per day.

Other typical Internet marketing strategies include so-called viral marketing strategies (recommend-a-friend functionality on the Web site allows people to make others aware of the Web site).

"Guerilla marketing" techniques, such as announcing a Web site in special-interest communities, which constitute the target audience of the site, can be very effective, but should be used only if the developer is part of the community; otherwise they are often seen as an unwelcome intrusion and "spam."

Continuous Quality Improvement and Summative Evaluation

As mentioned earlier, an integral part of quality assurance is analyzing user feedback continuously, for example, analyzing unsolicited e-mails and other feedback received from users. In addition to this qualitative method, online surveys can help to gather feedback and suggestions for improvement in a more structured and quantitative manner. Rapid "online polls" (e.g., page ratings) displayed on the bottom of every Web page that invite visitors to rate the usefulness of the article (Fig. 4.5) can also help to identify weak areas of the site or trends over time.

Owing to selection bias (volunteer bias), responses to online surveys are never representative for all users. Only those very dissatisfied (or very satisfied) will volunteer to fill in a survey, and survey results should never be extrapolated to the visitor population. Thus, online surveys have limited role as a sole summative evaluation method unless the responses can be compared with another Web sites (e.g., using the SUSHI-Q instrument). A statement in the results section of a report or academic paper such as "95% of all respondents thought the Web site was 'good' or 'very good'" is meaningful only if the response rate is proven to be high (which is never the case in online

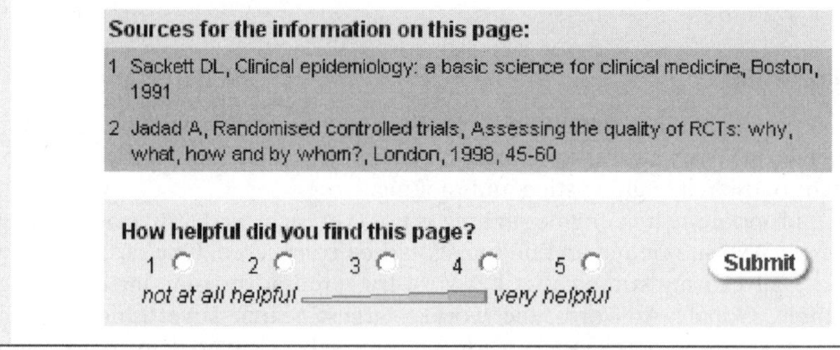

FIGURE 4.5. Example footer of a Web page (from *http://www.besttreatments.org*, a Web site of the BMJ Publishing Group). Apart from illustrating several elements from ethical codes that every Web page should have, including references, a disclaimer, the origin of the information, and a "last update" date, each Web page also has a rapid feedback (polling) form, allowing users to rate each page.

surveys, unless the survey is mandatory) or if it can be compared against something (e.g., another site or an initial survey). Various techniques exist to administer surveys so that multiple entries from the same user can be detected and fake entries can be eliminated [59].

SUSHI-Q

One particular instrument and tool for developer is SUSHI-Q (Standardized Usability and Satisfaction with Health Information Questionnaire) (*http://www.sushi-q.org*). The aim of the SUSHI-Q project is to develop and validate an electronic questionnaire instrument that can be used as standardized feedback form, scorecard, and quality monitoring instrument for developers of health information Web sites. The instrument is intended to measure the user's experience with a health Web site along several dimensions including overall satisfaction and usability. SUSHI-Q offers developers a login area where they can compare their score against those of other similar sites. The SUSHI-Q score can be used by developers to measure progress when iteratively refining their Web site. SUSHI-Q is an essential tool for health information providers to achieve user-centered design based on their feedback, to measure progress when iteratively refining their Web site, to benchmark their site against other Web sites, and to continuously monitor user feedback.

Log-File Analysis

Log-file analysis can give developers important information on visitors (geographical location, domain names, Web browsers, operating systems), access statistics (most requested Web pages, page views per day, unique visitors per day, most popular hour per day, etc.), site stickiness (total visitor stay length, site entry and exit pages), and referrer pages (referring domains and pages, search engine keywords used, etc.). Powerful log-file analysis software exists that allows one to track and to visually illustrate the path of visitors with specific attributes through the Web site (Fig. 4.6).

Outcomes Evaluation

Studies evaluating the impact of a Web site on individual health-related or social outcomes are often proposed in the research context and certainly not a routine evaluation method. To discuss all possible research methods is beyond the scope of the chapter, but the most important methods used in the context of evaluating health Web sites should be mentioned. The easiest studies to conduct are before-and-after studies (with one pretest and one posttest questionnaire after the intervention) or interrupted times series (with several measurement points before and after the intervention). If in such a study design the outcome (e.g., knowledge) increases, it can be a piece of evidence suggesting that this is attributable to the Web site intervention. However, all sorts of other factors can affect the outcome measures and lead to false-positive results, for example, maturation, regression to the mean, learning effect from the pretest, and so forth, so that it is better to include a control group (e.g., people who are *not* using the Web site). If the change score in the intervention group is significantly higher than the change score in the control group it can be concluded that the effect is the result of the intervention. Choosing an appropriate control group can be a challenge, and even results from controlled studies are wide open to criticism as all sorts of biases can lead to false-positive (or false-negative) results. Selection bias can lead to systematic group differences, which in turn affect results.

The only research design that avoids problems of potential systematic group differences is the randomized trial. However, Web-based randomized trials, in which one group is randomized to the intervention (e.g., gets access to the Web site) and the control group either receives "dummy pages" (not containing the full material to be

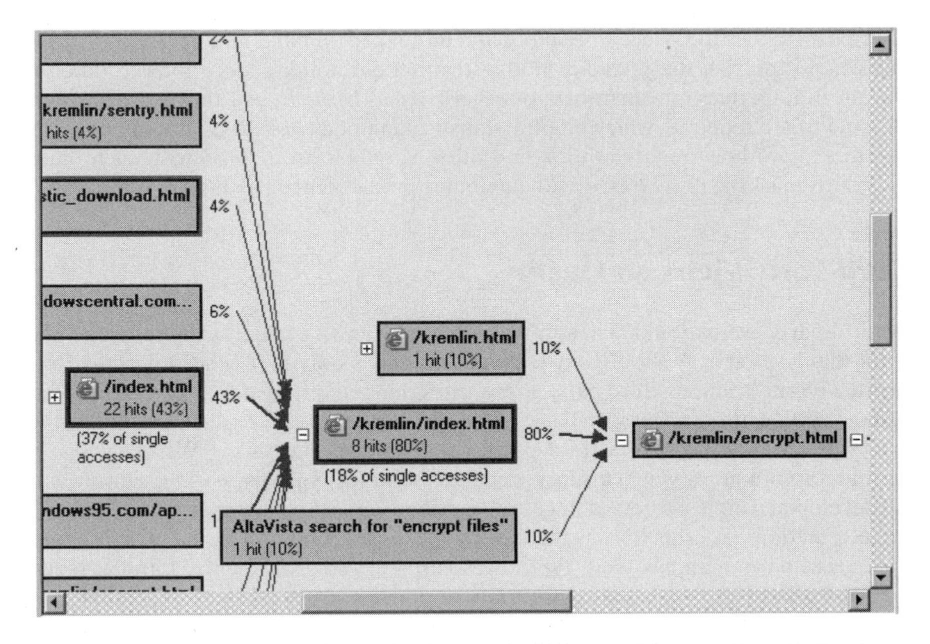

FIGURE 4.6. Visualization of visitor paths through the Web site with a log-file analysis software (M5 Analyzer).

tested) or no access to the Web site at all, are also a methodological challenge. In particular, most researchers see very high dropout rates (people randomized into the intervention group who are not using the Web site or who are lost to follow-up), and contamination, as the control group often can obtain similar information from other Web sites [60]. An intention-to-treat analysis (including all consumers who have been randomized into the intervention group, even if they are not using the system or are lost to follow-up) is required, but the high number of drop outs increases the risk of false-negative results.

Researchers' Views on Quality

Consumer health informatics researchers are usually either interested in assisting developers in evaluating a single Web site (see earlier), or they have been taking a "bird's eye view" (public health perspective) and attempted to assess the quality of health Web sites on the Web. This emerging area—the study of the determinants and distribution of health information and misinformation on the Web—has been called information epidemiology, or "infodemiology" [21].

The first infodemiological study was published in 1996 [61], but this type of research became widely known only with a subsequent publication in a prominent journal [62], leading to dozens of "me-too" publications. A recent review identified 79 infodemiological studies [7], and as of today hundreds of such articles have been published. Most of the early studies were descriptive, reporting the percentage of Web sites that had inaccurate imperfect health information [7]. Although in the late 1990s such studies may have been useful to draw the attention of researchers and policy makers to the emerging issue that information on the Web is highly "variable" and that systems are needed to guide consumers to trustworthy information, the value of these purely descriptive studies today becomes more and more questionable, and in fact many journals will not publish these studies if investigators did nothing more than to describe how much imperfect information is out there. It has been argued that more "analytical" studies are required, which employ statistical methods such as multivariate regression to explore how quality criteria and other variables are related with each other, and which markers, processes, or site attributes predict outcomes [5,21].

Third-Party Views on Quality

By third-party evaluation of a health Web site we mean an evaluation by someone who is not the developer. A third party sees and evaluates only the finished product (e.g., health Web site). Among third party approaches, one can distinguish a "review process" from a "certification process" [64].

In a *certification* process, a third party (the certifier) checks the Web site (or the health information provider) against predefined criteria, typically working closely with the developer, who is interested in getting certified, and who may grant access to internal information not otherwise available (log files, inspection of internal processes and quality assurance manuals, etc.). Typically, a certifier also gives feedback to the developer and gives him or her the opportunity to address issues to become compliant. A number of third-party certification programs, awarding seals, kitemarks, or trustmarks are available, awarding, for example, privacy seals (TRUSTe, BBBOnLine, PrivacyBot), accessibility seals (Bobby), Internet pharmacy seals (VIPPS), and seals for health Web sites (URAC). Kitemarks are so controversial because at the end of this process they call for collapsing the multiple dimensions and aspects of quality into a binary yes/no (recommended/not recommended) decision. In contrast, the MedCERTAIN project, often misrepresented as yet another certification seal, tried to overcome the limitations of traditional yes/no trustmarks, and is in fact more an infrastructure for decentralized self- and third-party rating and disseminating meta-information (information about information). MedCERTAIN is now called MedCIRCLE and advocates the use of richer metadata to describe detailed evaluation results rather than just the (binary) end result (see Chapter 18). Whether or not to trust a Web site can be determined only by the user, who should be able to define himself the cutoff points on the evaluation scales of the various dimensions.

In contrast to certification, in a *review* process, a third party evaluates a product or service (e.g., a health Web site) without the developer's cooperation. Usually the reviewer has limited or no access to internal data such as log files and site statistics and no possibility to evaluate internal processes of the organizations providing the information, other than what is stated on the Web site. Site reviews are, for example, conducted by gateways, libraries, or portals, which have to make a decision on whether or not to endorse/list a site. Approaches are very different and range from subjective ad hoc decisions, to using checklists and scoring systems, to evaluating primarily the trustworthiness of the source (e.g., Medline Plus lists only government sites).

End-User View on Quality

As mentioned previously, no universal checklist or scoring system for consumers exists that could enable them to discriminate trustworthy from untrustworthy or incorrect information. The tools and questionnaires that exist are all primarily educational tools in that they try to teach consumers what to look for. Such tools are, for example, the IQ-Tool (*http://hitiweb.mitretek.org/iq/default.asp*), or DISCERN (*http://www.discern.org.uk/*). The latter is specifically for *treatment* information, and—although originally developed for printed material—is also advocated by their developers for Web-based information (a modified version for Web-based information is also under development). Although it is often described as a "valid and reliable instrument," it should be stressed that validity refers to face validity (thus, it is not more or less valid than all other instruments, which were developed on the basis of a broad consensus), and the reliability metrics when used by consumers are not impressive ($\kappa = 0.3$) [64].

Another educational tool, used in the context of an Internet school for patients, is the CREDIBLE mnemonic, developed to remind patients what they should look for at a trustworthy Web site [21], namely:

- ***C***urrent and frequently updated
- ***R***eferences cited
- ***E***xplicit purpose and intentions of the site
- ***D***isclosure of sponsors
- ***I***nterests declared and no conflicts of interests
- ***B***alanced content, lists advantages and disadvantages
- ***L***evel of ***E***vidence indicated

Another strategy, particularly for obtaining cancer information, is to tell patients to watch out for "red flags" indicating questionable information [65], for example:

- Are "patient testimonials" available?
- Is the treatment described as a "cancer cure"?
- Is the treatment described as "having no side effects"?
- Is online purchasing permitted?

References

1. Baker L, Wagner TH, Singer S, Bundorf MK. Use of the Internet and e-mail for health care information: results from a national survey. JAMA 2003;289:2400–6.
2. Eysenbach G Consumer health informatics. BMJ 2000;320:1713–16.
3. Satterlund MJ, McCaul KD, Sandgren AK. Information Gathering Over Time by Breast Cancer Patients. J Med Internet Res 2003;5:e15.
4. Peterson MW, Fretz PC. Patient use of the internet for information in a lung cancer clinic. Chest 2003;123:452–7.
5. Eysenbach G. The impact of the Internet on cancer outcomes. CA Cancer J Clin 2003;53:356–71.
6. Raupach JC, Hiller JE. Information and support for women following the primary treatment of breast cancer. Health Expect 2002;5:289–301.
7. Eysenbach G, Powell J, Kuss O, Sa ER. Empirical studies assessing the quality of health information for consumers on the world wide web: a systematic review. JAMA 2002;287:2691–700.
8. Eysenbach G, Diepgen TL. Towards quality management of medical information on the internet: evaluation, labelling, and filtering of information. BMJ 1998;317:1496–500.
9. International Organization for Standardization, Technical Committee ISO/TC 176. ISO 8402: Quality management and quality assurance—Vocabulary. 2nd ed. Geneva: International Organization for Standardization, 1994.
10. Eysenbach G. Final MedCERTAIN Project Report (Part 1). *http://www.medcertain.org/Deliverables/aks-final-report5.zip* . Heidelberg:University of Heidelberg, 2002.
11. Delamothe T. Quality of websites: kitemarking the west wind. Br Med J 2000;321:843–4.
12. Heidelberg Consensus Recommendations on Trustmarks. J Med Internet Res 2000;2:e12.
13. Jadad AR, Gagliardi A. Rating health information on the Internet: navigating to knowledge or to Babel? JAMA 1998;279:611–4.
14. Eysenbach G. An ontology of quality initiatives and a model for decentralized, collaborative quality management on the (semantic) world-wide-web. J Med Internet Res 2001;3:E34.
15. Smith GC, Pell JP. Parachute use to prevent death and major trauma related to gravitational challenge:systematic review of randomised controlled trials. Br Med J 2003;327:1459–61.
16. Bader JL, Strickman-Stein N. Evaluation of new multimedia formats for cancer communications. J Med Internet Res 2003;5:e16.
17. Boyer C, Selby M, Scherrer JR, Appel RD. The Health On the Net Code of Conduct for medical and health Websites. Comput Biol Med 1998;28:603–10.
18. Hardwick JC, MacKenzie FM. Information contained in miscarriage-related websites and the predictive value of website scoring systems. Eur J Obstet Gynecol Reprod Biol 2003;106:60–3.
19. Griffiths KM, Christensen H. Quality of web based information on treatment of depression: cross sectional survey. Br Med J 2000;321:1511–5.
20. Shon J, Musen MA. The low availability of metadata elements for evaluating the quality of medical information on the World Wide Web. Proc AMIA Symp 1999, pp. 945–9.
21. Eysenbach G. Infodemiology: the epidemiology of (mis)information. Am J Med 2002;113:763–5.
22. e-Health Ethics Initiative. e-Health Code of Ethics. J Med Internet Res 2000;2:e9.
23. Mack J. The Internet Healthcare Coalition. J Med Internet Res 2000;2:e3.
24. Hi-Ethics Group. Health Internet ethics: ethical principles for offering Internet healthservices to consumers. HIETHICS (accessed December 3, 2000).
25. Baur C, Deering MJ. Proposed frameworks to improve the quality of health Web sites: review. MedGenMed 2000;2.

26. Winker MA, Flanagin A, Chi-Lum B, et al. Guidelines for medical and health information sites on the Internet. JAMA 2000;283:1600–6.
27. Commission of the European Communities. eEurope 2002: quality criteria for health related Websites. J Med Internet Res 2002;4:e15.
28. Rippen H. Criteria for assessing the quality of health information on the Internet. *hitiweb.mitretek.org/docs/policy.pdf*. 1998.
29. IEEE-USA Board of Directors. Quality of health information on the Internet. *http://www.ieeeusa.org/forum/POSITIONS/healthnet.html*. 1999.
30. APHA Interim Policy Statement 99-LB-2: criteria for assessing the quality of health information on the Internet. Am J Public Health 2000;90:489–90.
31. Silberg WM, Lundberg GD, Musacchio RA. Assessing, controlling, and assuring the quality of medical information on the Internet: caveat lector et viewor—let the reader and viewer beware [editorial]. JAMA 1997; 277:1244–5.
32. Martin-Fecklam M, Kostrzewa M, Schubert F, Gasse C, Haefeli W. Quality markers of drug information on the Internet: an evaluation of sites about St. John's wort. Am J Med 2002.
33. Kim P, Eng TR, Deering MJ, Maxfield A. Published criteria for evaluating health related web sites: review. Br Med J 1999;318:647–9.
34. Goldman J, Hudson Z, Smith RM. Privacy—report on the privacy policies and practices of health web sites. Oakland, CA: California HealthCare Foundation, 2000.
35. Federal Trade Commission. Privacy online: fair information practices in the electronic mjarketplace. A Report to Congress. *http://www.ftc.gov/reports/privacy2000/privacy2000.pdf.* 2000.
36. Fuller B, Hughes G, Fox L, et al. AHIMA's Recommendations to Ensure Privacy and Quality of Personal Health Information on the Internet. *http://www.ahima.org/infocenter/guidelines/tenets.html.* 2000.
37. Skinner H, Biscope S, Poland B. Quality of internet access: barrier behind Internet use statistics. Soc Sci Med 2003;57:875–80.
38. Richardson CR, Resnick PJ, Hansen DL, Derry HA, Rideout VJ. Does pornography-blocking software block access to health information on the Internet? JAMA 2002;288:2887–94.
39. Eysenbach G, Diepgen TL. Labeling and filtering of medical information on the Internet. Methods Inform Med 1999;38:80–8.
40. Eysenbach G, Köhler C. How do consumers search for and appraise health information on the World-Wide-Web? Qualitative study using focus groups, usability tests and in-depth interviews. Br Med J 2002;324:573–7.
41. Nielsen J. Usability Engineering. San Diego: Morgan Kaufmann, 1993.
42. Williams P, Nicholas D, Huntington P, McLean F. Surfing for health: user evaluation of a health information website. Part one: Background and literature review. Health Inform Libr J 2002;19:98–108.
43. Kinzie MB, Cohn WF, Julian MF, Knaus WA. A user-centered model for Web site design: needs assessment, user interface design, and rapid prototyping. J Am Med Inform Assoc 2002;9: 320–30.
44. Barbour RS. The use of focus groups to define patient needs. J Pediatr Gastroenterol Nutr 1999;28:S19–S22.
45. Eysenbach G, Till JE. Ethical issues in qualitative research on internet communities. Br Med J 2001;323:1103–5.
46. Eysenbach G, Kohler C. What is the prevalence of health-related searches on the World Wide Web? Qualitative and quantitative analysis of search engine queries on the Internet. Proc AMIA Annu Fall Symp 2003, pp. 225–9.
47. Kitzinger J. Qualitative research. Introducing focus groups. Br Med J 1995;311:299–302.
48. Williams P, Nicholas D, Huntington P, McLean F. Surfing for health: user evaluation of a health information website. Part two: Fieldwork. Health Inform Libr J 2002;19:214–25.
49. Eysenbach G, Diepgen TL. Patients looking for information on the Internet and seeking teleadvice: motivation, expectations, and misconceptions as expressed in e-mails sent to physicians. Arch Dermatol 1999;135:151–6.
50. Eysenbach G, Diepgen TL. Responses to unsolicited patient e-mail requests for medical advice on the World Wide Web. JAMA 1998;280:1333–5.

51. Kuszler PC. A question of duty: common law legal issues resulting from physician response to unsolicited patient email inquiries. J Med Internet Res 2000;2:E17.
52. Smith JJ, Berlin L. E-mail consultation. AJR Am J Roentgenol 2002;179:1133–6.
53. Eysenbach G. Towards ethical guidelines for dealing with unsolicited patient emails and giving teleadvice in the absence of a pre-existing patient-physician relationship —systematic review and expert survey. J Med Internet Res 2000;2:e1.
54. D'Alessandro DM, Qian F, D'Alessandro MP, et al. Performing continuous quality improvement for a digital health sciences library through an electronic mail analysis. Bull Med Libr Assoc 1998;86:594–601.
55. Fox S, Rainee L. The online health care revolution: how the Web helps Americans take better care of themselves. Washington, DC: The Pew Internet and American Life Project, 2000.
56. Wathen CN, Burkell J. Believe it or not: factors influencing credibility on the Web. JASIS 2002;53:134–44.
57. Fogg BJ. Stanford-Makovsky Web Credibility Study 2002: investigating what makes Web sites credible today. Research Report by the Stanford Persuasive Technology Lab and Makovsky & Company, 2002.
58. Shon J, Marshall J, Musen MA. The impact of displayed awards on the credibility and retention of Web site information. Proc AMIA Annu Fall Symp 2000, pp. 794–8.
59. Eysenbach G, Wyatt J. Using the Internet for surveys and health research. J Med Internet Res 2002;4:e13.
60. Eysenbach G. Issues in evaluating health websites in an Internet-based randomized controlled trial. J Med Internet Res 2002;4:e17.
61. Davison K. The quality of dietary information on the World Wide Web. J Can Diet Assoc 1996;57:137–41.
62. Impicciatore P, Pandolfini C, Casella N, Bonati M. Reliability of health information for the public on the World Wide Web: systematic survey of advice on managing fever in children at home. Br Med J 1997;314:1875–9.
63. Lampe K, Cross P, Brickley D, Kohler C, Roine R, Eysenbach G. Societal dimensions of third-party evaluation of Internet health content. Stud Health Technol Inform 2003;95:661–6.
64. Charnock D, Shepperd S, Needham G, Gann R. DISCERN: an instrument for judging the quality of written consumer health information on treatment choices. J Epidemiol Community Health 1999;53:105–11.
65. Matthews SC, Camacho A, Mills PJ, Dimsdale JE. The Internet for medical information about cancer: help or hindrance? Psychosomatics 2003;44:100–3.

5
Information Delivery Methods

JAMES H. HARRISON, JR.

Individuals who use online health-related information resources have a variety of goals. Some users may wish to find reference information on a particular topic. Others may wish to monitor a particular topic or related topics over time. Still others may need answers to particular questions or to become members of a community that can provide ongoing information and support. It is a reflection of the diversity and success of the Internet as a general information resource that all of these needs can be met reasonably effectively with current technology.

Information delivery methods can be characterized in several ways. Perhaps the simplest approach classifies methods as either "push" or "pull" based on whether the user specifically requests the information that is delivered [1]. In "push" systems, the user may initially join the system, but subsequently the user receives information without the need to request it further. (Information is "pushed" to the user.) E-mail mailing lists that are focused on a particular topic as well as various types of instant messaging, pop-up notification systems, and indicators embedded in World Wide Web pages are examples of this strategy. The "pull" approach is exemplified by the standard World Wide Web (without pop-ups) or Usenet news, where resources are available for users to search or browse and the user must take specific action (e.g., clicking a link) to retrieve an information resource.

A key feature in the push/pull concept is that information "pushed" to the user is assumed to be filtered so that it is of interest to the user and the user will wish to view most items, whereas information that is "pulled" comes from large data sets and only a small fraction of the data, which is identified by the user as of definite interest, is retrieved for viewing. "Push" systems tend to require less work from users because they replace the necessity to search for information explicitly, but their effectiveness is dependent on the ability of the system to select relevant content for its users, which can be difficult in settings where users vary in interests, needs, and goals.

To some extent, the pull/push classification is arbitrary, and modern information delivery systems may offer components of both. Systems can be alternatively classified by whether they function primarily for *information distribution* from a central repository or whether they in addition support *human–human communications and community building.* In this chapter we review delivery methods from this perspective and then briefly discuss several network communications, alternative hardware, and open source software issues that impact all delivery systems.

Information Distribution Systems

File Repositories

The simplest information distribution system is a document repository that allows file download via either File Transfer Protocol (ftp, [2]) or Hypertext Transfer Protocol (http, [3]). FTP is an efficient protocol designed for transfer of large files over the Internet. It is managed by an ftp server on a central computer containing the file repository and it is accessible using free or low-cost client software; most Web browsers also support ftp. HTTP is the native communications protocol of the World Wide Web and it can also be used for file download from the Web server. Links to file repositories within ftp or http servers can be embedded in Web pages that organize and describe the contents of the files and allow them to be downloaded with a click.

File repositories have some disadvantages. Text files encoded as ASCII (the American Standard for Computer Information Interchange) are very compact and can be read by most types of computers, but provide no formatting other than block text. Certain characters (e.g., "curly quotes") that are not part of the standard ASCII character set may appear as different characters on different types of computers. The endings of lines are marked with different characters on Windows, Macintosh, and Unix computers, leading to potential line-wrapping problems or the appearance of extraneous characters. These problems are being solved by the introduction of broader character encoding standards such as UTF-8 [4] and Unicode [5]. Currently, systems are in transition with respect to these broader character coding schemes and thus older systems may not support them until they are replaced over the next several years.

Word processor files offer more formatting choices and may solve character coding issues in settings where the same vendor's word processor is available on multiple platforms. However, users who do not own the particular world processor may not be able to use the files. This situation is partially mitigated if word processor files use Rich Text Format (rtf, [6]), a standard word processor format developed some years ago by Microsoft. Most word processors can read and write rtf and it supports basic text formatting, although support for placing images in text or the use of tables is limited. Word processor files also contain references to specific fonts (typefaces) that may not be installed on a user's machine. When a particular font is unavailable, systems can substitute fonts, but that may disrupt the intended page layout and appearance. Finally, word processor files that support multiple undo steps or change tracking may allow users to view interim drafts of a document, which may not be desirable. Similar considerations apply to spreadsheets, presentations, and other files of proprietary programs.

For these reasons, Adobe's Portable Document Format (PDF, [7]) is currently the leading technology for creating and distributing formatted reference documents by electronic means. PDF files carry font and other required display information with them and render accurately across multiple display devices. Adobe distributes free reader software for displaying the files, third-party readers are available, and some operating systems are shipped with reader software included. Simple PDF files can be created from word processor files using inexpensive or free utilities. More complex PDF files require Adobe's Acrobat product (or on Macintosh OSX machines, PDF files can be produced directly from any program).

File repositories have an additional disadvantage in that they are difficult to index for searching. It is possible to do so, but this increases the complexity of the repository system considerably. Thus it is generally best to use repositories for large complex documents related to a specific topic, such as brochures or narratives that are intended to be printed for reading. These documents can then be linked to brief descriptive material on Web pages which will then be found using a typical search.

Electronic Mail

E-mail [8] can be an effective way to distribute information, either in the body of e-mail messages or as e-mail attachments. An e-mail system consists of a central mail server and associated mail clients on users' machines. This system may be used either to respond individually to requests for information that arrive by e-mail or other means, or the e-mail client can be used to store a small list of e-mail addresses who will all receive copies of a message and its attachments. For larger groups, a mailing list manager [9] is generally used in combination with the mail server. The manager maintains the list of members and their e-mail preferences. One of the widely used early mailing list managers was named "Listserv," and for this reason mailing lists are sometimes called Listservs. Today there are a number of commonly used mailing list manager programs with varying features.

Depending on its configuration, a mailing list may be essentially one way (an information distribution system) or it can allow replies and discussion as described in the next section. As configured for information distribution, a mailing list would receive a message from the person coordinating the list and re-mail it and any attachments to all members of the list. The list members would not be able to respond directly to the list, although they could control certain aspects of the list's operation with respect to their account using commands sent to the list by e-mail at a special address [10]. For example, users may use these commands to join or leave mailing lists and control whether they receive individual messages or a single message digest per day containing all messages.

Information may be represented in e-mail messages in several ways. The body of the message may contain block-formatted plain text, which all e-mail clients will accept. Some e-mail clients also accept Hypertext Markup Language (HTML) formatted text that may contain embedded images and active links. This information is shown in a display resembling a Web browser. This can provide a more attractive display that resembles a newsletter or a brochure, but it may not display at all in some e-mail clients and may display inaccurately in others. Pages such as this may also fail to display if the user's computer is not connected to the Internet at the time of display (to allow images and other elements to be downloaded) whereas a text-only display is self contained. E-mail messages may contain attached files of the types mentioned earlier under file repositories. Because this is merely an alternative approach to distributing the files to the users, all the considerations mentioned earlier with respect to particular file types apply here as well.

Mailing lists function like the "push" systems described earlier. Once a user has joined, messages and documents flow without further action into the user's inbox for review. Assuming that the mailing list does a good job of filtering to include content of interest to the user, it can be quite convenient. However, mailing lists and e-mail in general have some weaknesses. Information sent to the user through e-mail must be actively saved into logical locations on the user's system if the user wishes to find it again. Many e-mail systems and local clients do not have intrinsic archiving features meant to organize information for later retrieval, although some clients do allow e-mail to be sorted easily for saving, and some users will use this feature. Some mailing list managers do provide a Web display of previous messages, but in a busy mailing list finding previous individual messages can be challenging. Furthermore, the prevalence of unwanted e-mail ("spam") and malicious software that interacts with the Microsoft Windows e-mail framework has made the use of e-mail and e-mail attachments problematic in some settings.

The World Wide Web

At the most basic level, the Web consists of http servers and Web browsers. The servers contain text documents that include HTML [11] in addition to the document content. Browsers can request these documents and display them using the HTML instructions. HTML text documents are best developed with text editors or HTML-enhanced text editors, but can also be created using HTML editors that hide the HTML with a browser-like display or by exporting files as HTML from word processing or spreadsheet programs.

HTML documents may contain links to images, sound files, videos, and other media that are downloaded separately and inserted into the documents by the browsers at display time. HTML documents can also contain links to other documents, allowing easy traversal through a group of documents and creation of a context for documents. These capabilities allow substantial flexibility in laying out collections of documents that can effectively communicate healthcare concepts. Web documents persist at their locations and can be "bookmarked," allowing future reference; their contained text can be indexed for searching locally and by large-scale search engines. Because Web pages can contain (and Web browsers can process) links to files on ftp servers and links containing e-mail addresses, Web pages integrate relatively well with other Internet systems. In general, Web pages are easily readable and, depending on their design, can also be effective when printed. These features make the Web an excellent presentation system for quick-lookup reference information related to health care, particularly in settings in which multimedia enhances the effectiveness of presentation.

The Web does have some weaknesses. Web browsers are not identical in their display of HTML and its associated standards. There is currently a core set of standards recommended by the World Wide Web Consortium (*http://www.w3.org*) that essentially all browsers support. Designers operating within reasonable limits using these standards can expect good behavior across multiple platforms and browsers. Certain additional or alternative features that are available in some browsers may not be available in others and designers who are not aware of this situation may create pages that have limited browser scope.

Although the Web is searchable based on free text, the degree of page linkage (Google, *http://www.google.com*) and other characteristics, it does not have the kind of structure required for precise or complete searches; useful information may be missed. Improvements related to the expression of concepts within pages and the relationships between pages are part of what makes up the Semantic Web effort, discussed elsewhere in this book.

The Web is also the prototypical "pull" [1] strategy in information delivery. This means that users must know a Web resource is present, find it, and then find the appropriate section within it that addresses their needs. This can work well if the Web resources are well designed, but it does require effort from the user. Candidate Web pages for review are frequently located through large-scale Web search engines, which are useful but, as noted earlier, can miss desirable resources. This may not be an issue for local users who are familiar with a Web site, but alerting users to an interesting update can be problematic, even locally. One effective hybrid approach has been to maintain primary information documents on the Web while also supporting a mailing list that alerts users to updates on the Web sites with a brief note.

Communications and Community

The systems discussed in the preceding section are primarily designed to provide information to users for reference purposes. Although they may include some interactivity (an e-mail requesting a document or access to a mailing list, entry of parameters defining a search), the primary purpose of those systems is to provide their preexisting contents to users, not to support person-to-person communications or user development of new content. As discussed previously in this book, patient-to-patient and patient-to-provider communication are important needs in community-based health care. Internet communities that form around topics of interest, including health care, are well known [12]. Essentially all of the content of these communities is created by the members and facilitated by software as the community develops. This software is well known, generally available, and often open source [13]. Evidence indicates that a similar coalescence of interest communities can and does occur related to healthcare issues [14].

Discussion Lists

E-mail mailing lists were mentioned earlier as a method for distributing information to list members. Discussion lists extend this function by allowing members to comment on issues raised on the list. Replies to list messages go back to the mailing list manager and are distributed to all list members. Over time, issues and replies are listed chronologically in a member's e-mail inbox (or ideally in a separate e-mail folder the user has dedicated to the mailing list). Mailing lists can be relatively quiet or quite active (up to hundreds of messages a day) and they may or may not be moderated. Unmoderated lists allow all member postings to be distributed immediately. Moderated lists return all member postings to one or more list moderators for review, who may then post the message to the list for distribution or delete it. Moderation helps avoid inappropriate postings and keeps the list discussions on topic.

The primary benefit of a mailing list is that messages are processed through e-mail software. If the list member spends a good bit of time with e-mail normally, having the messages arrive in the inbox can be convenient. It is also convenient to take a thread of conversation off the list by e-mailing a responder directly (rather than replying back to the list) without needing to change programs. File attachments can be handled in the usual ways.

Discussion lists also have some downsides for community communication. E-mail is not inherently secure (it is not encrypted) and thus contents of e-mail messages may be accessible to others unless an encrypted e-mail system is used. Even with an encrypted system, a mailing list of any size will go outside of the local system and messages sent to outside systems will not be encrypted. There are additional issues specifically related to patient–provider communications by e-mail that have been reviewed in previous chapters.

Topic discussions are associated in a mailing list merely by the title of the message, and messages are usually sorted in reverse chronology. If the title is changed or a message is delayed in the system, some members may miss it. Discussions often quote previous notes in the body of the message in an attempt to provide context, but in an avid discussion, multiple responses may come back that quote various combinations of previous messages, and responses to those produce simultaneous messages with varying histories. Thus it can be difficult to confirm that all important contributions to an issue have been reviewed. Passing e-mail messages through multiple e-mail clients often leads to formatting oddities that intensify the problem of reviewing previous material. Finally, the lack of an inherent archive capability can be a limitation as previously mentioned, although this feature is provided by some mailing list managers (e.g., [15]). Even in systems that do archive, finding previous conversations in a busy list among the archived messages can be challenging.

Usenet News

The Usenet system [16] is generally referred to simply as "Newsgroups." It includes a world-wide network of bulletin board servers accessible through the Internet or by direct dialup. The system contains many thousands of active discussion groups covering a wide variety of topics, including many healthcare topics. Newsgroup servers use their own communications protocol and client software, but many modern e-mail clients incorporate the newsgroup protocol and provide a display of newsgroups that is similar to an e-mail message display. Newsgroup messages are plain text, similar to plain text e-mail messages, and can have file attachments. The main advantage of the newsgroup system is that the server enforces "threading" of messages—a reply to a message is marked as a reply to that message—and messages are maintained on the server and temporarily downloaded into the client for reading. Thus there is one canonical version of the newsgroup history that can serve both as an archive and a reference of the complete listing of all postings in the correct order. Newsgroups may be moderated or unmoderated.

Newsgroup servers are efficient and provide a useful foundation for an Internet community. They are still widely and avidly used, particularly by software developers. However, for general-purpose community sites, they have been largely superseded by the Web-based discussion and community sites described in the following paragraphs.

Web-Based Discussion Groups

In addition to providing a flexible system for distributing documents, the Web provides a limited facility for data entry that includes text boxes, drop-down menus, and other interface elements displayed within Web pages. These data entry "forms" can be used to enable text entry by users and also to select documents for uploading. The text and attached documents can be processed on the server, stored in a database, and displayed or linked from a dynamic Web page. Because all content is maintained within the discussion group system on the server and accessed through a Web browser, communications with the system can be encrypted and reasonable security for the content can be provided.

Most Web discussion systems allow entry of a title, name, and e-mail address, topic or keyword categorization, brief summary, optional body text, and an optional document attachment; the system will add a time stamp on submission. The main page of the discussion group will typically list a set of initial postings with brief summaries in reverse chronology. The number of replies may be noted but the replies themselves are not generally shown on the main page. Clicking on a posting will display that posting and its follow-up replies on a single page in chronological or reverse-chronological order for easy reading and/or printing. Thus simultaneous discussions on multiple topics are displayed in compact form on the top page and the full discussions on each topic are displayed only when that topic is opened. This has advantages over the complete display of all original postings and replies that are standard for mailing lists and Usenet groups.

Web-based discussion forums can be embedded in a Web site and designed to be stylistically similar to other Web pages on the site. In addition, because data entry occurs through a form within a Web page, the data entry page can have associated graphics, instructions, links to other locations, and help. Because the text of the postings and replies is contained in a database, all entries are fully searchable. Some systems incorporate an e-mail notification option that will alert members to new postings. Thus Web-based discussion forums can provide functionality similar to that of Usenet newsgroups with a more attractive and functional presentation and built-in alerting. Most Web-based discussion systems support optional moderation by presenting a preview for review by an administrator before an entry is released for general viewing.

The prototypical Web discussion forum is Slashdot [17], a discussion group for software developers and others with a technical orientation. Similar groups have been established related to health care [18] and many other special interests. A substantial number of software packages for managing Web-based discussion groups are available, including both commercial and high-quality open-source offerings.

Several related types of software provide similar capabilities. Weblogs ("blogs," [19]) are similar to Web-based discussion groups except that the primary postings are usually all written by the same person. Thus blogs are not typically designed to allow many different users to add initial postings or to be moderated, as are Web discussion groups. Blogs do allow replies to postings but do not typically allow document uploading. In normal use, the primary content of Web-based discussion groups is often in the replies and counter-replies, whereas the primary content of blogs is usually in the initial postings and the follow-up comments are brief. Good quality commercial and open source blog software is available.

Web-based issue-tracking systems are also closely related to Web-based discussion groups. Issue trackers developed from software bug-tracking systems and project management systems. Essentially, issue trackers support an initial categorization and descriptive posting with multiple follow-ups. The display may be similar to Web discussion postings and replies, and document attachments are often supported. The two additional capabilities that these systems offer are a status indicator for each conversation (open, on hold, completed successfully, dropped, etc.) and the option to assign particular issues to particular members of a work group. This type of software would be most useful in discussion settings with a strong problem-solving orientation. Commercial and open source issue tracking systems are available.

Web Community Software

A number of software packages combine the features of the systems described in the preceding section to provide a comprehensive framework for building Internet communities. Systems such as this that aggregate and present resources for a particular purpose are sometimes called Web portals. These packages include features for managing users/members, regular static Web pages, database-driven pages, Web-based discussion groups with notification, document repositories, announcement management, calendar management, and other features. They are generally products built on existing application servers, which are extensive software toolkits for creating Web applications. Examples of this class of software include PHP-Nuke [20] and Drupal [21], built on PHP [22]; Moveable Type [23], built with the Perl programming language; and Plone [24], built on Zope [25]. These systems are open source and widely used. Commercial systems are also available.

Additional Software and Hardware Considerations

Network Speed

Most home users of the Internet in the United States dial in on phone networks using modems, although broadband (DSL and cable TV networking) continue to increase market share. Current modems communicate at a nominal 56 kilobits per second, although actual connections are typically 40 to 48 Kbits/s. Files sizes are generally measured in kilobytes (8 bits = 1 byte). Thus modems would be expected to support data transfer rates approaching 6 Kbytes/s (generally a bit less including error correction). A typical HTML page of text might contain about 3500 characters or just under 3.5 Kbytes. Compressed images may contain from 1 K to 15 K bytes or more depending on their size and other characteristics. Thus a few images in a page can substantially increase modem download times. Images and other large multimedia files can contribute much to a document but should be used sparingly if they are to be transferred across modems.

Mailing lists and file downloads can be more convenient than a Web presentation if large files are used with a slow connection, because e-mail and file transfers can be carried out while doing other tasks or the computer can be left to allow the job to complete. Web sites, in contrast, are designed to be viewed page-by-page, and larger than necessary files with long download times can make a site very frustrating to use.

Broadband connections improve download speeds substantially. For example, basic rate ISDN (two-channel) can yield 12 to 14 Kbytes/s and cable modems can reach up to 300 Kbytes/s or more, comparable to Ethernet local area networks. DSL connections are generally between those values depending on the type of connection available. Wireless networks are roughly similar to cable modems. However, the speed of the local network may not be an indication of the speed of connection to the Internet. For example, a local Ethernet network (300 Kbytes/s) connected to the Internet via a T1 line (60 to 70 Kbytes/s) would be limited to the T1 speed in accessing Internet resources. Increased network or Internet traffic could slow the process further. Thus limiting files sizes to the extent that is reasonable is always a good idea.

Alternative User Hardware

For the foreseeable future, standard computers are likely to remain the primary tool for accessing online healthcare information. For researching healthcare topics, it is beneficial to have a large enough display so that reading is comfortable and information can be placed into context. The multimedia capabilities of the Web are also more effectively applied with a reasonable screen size and processor speed. Cost is likely not to be an issue: computer hardware continues to decrease in price, and with the development of open source software there is a good chance that the cost of quality standard software will also decrease. Thus a basic full-size computer with reasonable performance for Web access is likely to sell for less than a mid-range Personal Digital Assistant (PDA) in the future. PDAs and Web-enabled phones may be useful in displaying specific data elements such as test results, or capturing temperature or glucose level values that may be measured in the home. They also may be useful for healthcare providers who need to check specific reference information. However, it is unlikely that in their current form they will be useful for consumers who are researching and critiquing health information and who benefit from well-designed images and diagrams as well as appropriate context. There is potential for systems such as WebTV, but so far it has not had a substantial impact and consumers appear to prefer to use standard computers for information gathering. Small computers dedicated to e-mail and Web use also have not attracted consumers to any great extent, although there is a possibility that such a device, if available with good performance and a good display, might be attractive in the future.

It is likely that alternative hardware will appear to allow individuals with disabilities to interact more effectively with online systems. For example, implementation of read-aloud and Braille terminals for vision-impaired individuals is ongoing. These types of devices are not well suited by the current features of the Web and Web design styles, and they generally require special pages for effective use. Future Web design based on Extensible Markup Language (XML) and Extensible Style Language (XSL) stylesheets (see [26]) will allow content to be developed once and then used with multiple stylesheets to drive multiple-output devices.

Open Source Software

Open source software is copyrighted software that is licensed for use at no cost. In addition, the source code is freely available for inspection and modification by users. Open source software is typically developed and maintained by teams of volunteer programmers. Documentation is available through the Web and often from local bookstores, and vendors are available if commercial support is necessary. The open source effort has expanded considerable over the past 10 years, and many open source projects are regarded as similar to or exceeding the quality of comparable commercial software. Many widely used Internet communications packages, including Web servers and application server frameworks, are open source as noted earlier. More information on open source and a listing of open source licenses is available at the Open Source Initiative [27].

Conclusion

The Internet has proven to be a remarkable medium for the dissemination of information and the spontaneous generation of collaborative interest groups over a period of more than 20 years. The technologies that have formed the basis for these strengths of the Internet—and the offspring of these technologies—can also support the development of useful and accessible online healthcare resources, healthcare interest groups, and "caring communities" focused on sharing knowledge and support. The best features of past Internet systems have found their way into current community portal software built on industrial strength open source application servers. These software packages offer a locally customizable framework containing all the tools necessary to provide multimedia reference information and secured interactive communications in a healthcare setting.

References

1. Hermans B. Desperately seeking: helping hands and human touch. Cap Gemini white paper, section 3.1.2, 2000. *http://www.hermans.org/agents2/ch3_1_2.htm* (accessed April 20, 2004).
2. Wikipedia. File Transfer Protocol. *http://en.wikipedia.org/wiki/File_transfer_protocol* (accessed April 21, 2004).
3. Wikipedia. HTTP. *http://en.wikipedia.org/wiki/http* (accessed April 21, 2004).
4. Wikipedia. UTF-8. *http://en.wikipedia.org/wiki/UTF* (accessed April 21, 2004).
5. Wikipedia. Unicode. *http://en.wikipedia.org/wiki/UTF-8* (accessed 4/21/042).
6. (accessed 4/21/04).
7. Wikipedia. RTF. *http://en.wikipedia.org/wiki/Rich_Text_Format* (accessed April 21, 2004).
8. Adobe Systems Inc. What is Adobe PDF? *http://www.adobe.com/products/acrobat/adobepdf.html* (accessed April 21, 2004).
9. Wikipedia. E-mail. *http://en.wikipedia.org/wiki/E-mail* (accessed April 21, 2004).
10. Wikipedia. Electronic mailing list. *http://en.wikipedia.org/wiki/Electronic_mailing_list* (accessed April 21, 2004).
11. Milles J. Discussion lists: mailing list manager commands. Case Western Reserve University Law Library, 1997. *http://learn.ouhk.edu.hk/~u123/unit2/mirror2/mailser.html* (accessed April 21, 2004).
12. Wikipedia. HTML. *http://en.wikipedia.org/wiki/Html* (accessed April 21, 2004).
13. US Dept of State. Global issues: Internet communities 5(3), 2000; *http://usinfo.state.gov/journals/itgic/1100/ijge/ijge1100.htm* (accessed April 20, 2004).
14. Udell, J. Practical Internet Groupware. Sebastopol, CA: Oreilly and Associates, 1999.
15. Eisenbach G, Till JE. Ethical issues in qualitative research on Internet communities. Br Med J 2001;323:1103–5.
16. Mailman. *http://www.list.org/* (accessed April 20, 2004).
17. Wikipedia. Usenet. *http://en.wikipedia.org/wiki/USENET* (accessed April 21, 2004).
18. Slashdot. *http://slashdot.org/* (accessed April 20, 2004).
19. LinuxMedNews. *http://www.linuxmednews.com/* (accessed April 20, 2004).
20. Wikipedia. Weblogs. *http://en.wikipedia.org/wiki/Blog* (accessed April 21, 2004).
21. PHP-Nuke. *http://phpnuke.org/* (accessed April 20, 2004).
22. Drupal. *http://drupal.org/* (accessed April 20, 2004).
23. PHP. *http://www.php.net/* (accessed April 20, 2004).
24. Moveable Type. *http://www.movabletype.org/* (accessed April 20, 2004).
25. Plone. *http://plone.org/* (accessed April 20, 2004).
26. Zope. *http://www.zope.org/* (accessed April 20, 2004).
27. The World Wide Web Consortium. *http://www.w3.org/* (accessed April 21, 2004).
28. The Open Source Initiative. *http://www.opensource.org/* (accessed April 20, 2004).

6 Delivery of Online Learning for Healthcare Consumers

Deborah Lewis

Well-informed healthcare consumers are better able to make decisions and become active participants in the process of care. Providing adequate information that is personally meaningful is a major challenge for healthcare providers. It is important that we understand how informatics can best be used to support the process of online consumer health education. Chapter 4 describes the design and evaluation of Web sites for healthcare consumers. This chapter focuses on online consumer health education and barriers to success in the delivery of technology innovations for consumer health education.

Emotional distress, physical discomfort, limited privacy, and limited time with healthcare providers can all contribute to the ineffectiveness of the healthcare setting as a learning environment. Information technologies provide new opportunities for consumer health education and the information sharing process. Consumers and healthcare providers can come together to share information, engage in healthcare education processes, and form online groups for learning and social support all at a time that is most convenient for them. Information gathered from the Internet can improve comprehension and recall of information provided during the healthcare visit. The individualization of content and reinforcement of learning, which can occur in online learning environments, ensure prolonged retention of information and facilitate knowledge attainment [1–3].

Online learning environments are particularly useful for clients with special needs. Clients with low literacy skills benefit from the individualized pace of instruction and the multisensory learning experience. Elderly clients with very little prior computer experience have successfully learned computer-based material and reported high satisfaction with online information and learning [1–3].

As a leading resource for consumer health information and education the Internet also generates concerns about information quality, misunderstandings of information complexity, and information volume. These concerns and the unique needs of the target audience must all be considered by those who are designing online consumer health education programs [1–3].

The Process of Developing Online Consumer Health Education

The delivery of consumer health education and information is a process rather than a product. The focus of the process is providing consumers with the knowledge they need to make the best healthcare choices; this involves the effective union of consumer health information, healthcare education theory, and information technology. The online learning environment should move the healthcare consumer through the process of information discovery to the transformation of information to knowledge. Development of healthcare educational materials for online learning are best accomplished by a team of multidisciplinary experts each contributing their specialized expertise. Content experts lend their knowledge of the specific content and context for the learning materials, education specialists frame the learning content for delivery and devise the evaluation strategy, and instructional designers develop the learning material using the appropriate multimedia design. Each member of the development team should remain actively involved in all phases of the design, development, delivery, and evaluation of the learning materials. It is also important to receive ongoing feedback from healthcare consumers.

Understanding the learning preferences, learning needs, and learning goals of the target audience is essential to the process of developing effective consumer-directed healthcare education. The design of online consumer health education resources should be based on feedback from consumer focus groups that represent the target population. While this is discussed at length in Chapter 4, it will be mentioned briefly here. Focus group feedback provides the education designers with an opportunity to understand the consumer groups' cognitive abilities including reading ability. The consumer group's cultural values, socioeconomic status, and beliefs about the health problem are also important in informing the process of educational material development. Most chronic diseases are so prevalent that few healthcare consumers come to the diagnosis without preconceived notions and most have had personal experience with family members or loved ones who have the same disease.

Effective Learning Objectives

Consumer health education should be based on measurable outcome goals. Learning objectives provide outcome goals that can be used to measure the success of online education. Objectives identify the expected level of achievement and provide criteria for evaluation. Well-defined learning objectives provide a mechanism to measure the extent of learning or knowledge acquisition that has occurred. Learning objectives may be written to measure individual or program outcome achievement. In this chapter we are concerned with the individual healthcare consumer as learner.

Learning objectives specify what behavior a learner must demonstrate or perform in order for the healthcare educator to conclude that learning took place. A learning objective describes an intended learning outcome and contains three parts: the *situation* under which the behavior is to be performed or demonstrated, a *verb* that defines the behavior itself, and the measurable target goal (*outcome criteria*) for learner achievement [5]. The following textbox describes the components of a learning objective.

Textbox: Developing Learning Objectives

The Situation

The situation specifies the circumstances or directions that the learner is given to initiate the learning process. Learning objectives usually begin with a simple declarative statement (situation) such as:

Upon completion of the learning activity the healthcare consumer will . . .
After reviewing module one the learner will . . .

The Verb

The verb is an action word that describes an observable behavior. Bloom's Taxonomy represents a hierarchy of educational objectives that divides cognitive behaviors into six subdivisions ranging from the simplest to the complex. It is used frequently by health educators as they develop learning objectives. Verb examples that represent intellectual activity on each level of Bloom's Taxonomy are listed here.

Knowledge

Knowledge is defined as the recall of previously learned material. Knowledge represents the lowest level of cognitive learning outcomes. **Knowledge verbs include: arrange, name, order, define, duplicate, label, list, memorize, recognize, repeat, and reproduce.**

Comprehension

Comprehension is the ability to understand the meaning of information. Comprehensive learning outcomes extend the simple recall of material to a basic level of understanding. **Comprehension verbs include: discuss, explain, identify, indicate, locate, recognize, classify, describe, restate, and review.**

Application

Application reflects the learner's ability to use the newly learned material in realistic situations. Learning outcomes require a higher understanding than those under comprehension. **Application verbs include: apply, demonstrate, illustrate, interpret, practice, and use.**

Analysis

Analysis represents higher cognitive skills than comprehension and application because it requires a systematic examination of both the content and the context of the information. **Analysis verbs include: analyze, categorize, contrast, criticize, compare, differentiate, discriminate, distinguish, examine, and test.**

Synthesis

Synthesis refers to the ability to combine different ideas and processes to create a new understanding. **Synthesis verbs include: arrange, assemble, collect, construct, create, design, develop, formulate, prepare, and propose.**

Evaluation

Evaluation is concerned with examining something in order to judge its value, quality, or importance. Evaluation learning outcomes are highest in the cognitive hierarchy because this category contains elements of the others, plus systematic judgments based on explicit criteria. **Evaluation verbs include: appraise, argue, assess, attach, defend, judge, predict, value, compare, and evaluate.**

The Outcome Criterion

The outcome criterion of a learning objective is a statement that describes the measurable level of completion necessary to satisfy the intention of the learning objective. The following are examples of complete learning objectives that include all three components (situation, verb, and outcome criterion):

Continued

At the conclusion of this interactive diabetes education program the learner will (situation) formulate (synthesis level verb) a plan for sick day management that includes four strategies (outcome criteria).

Upon completing the online learning module on asthma medication (situation) the healthcare consumer will demonstrate (application level verb) the ability to correctly administer his inhaler medication (outcome criterion).

Adapted from: B.S. Bloom [4]

Strategies for the Development of Educational Materials

Once the learning objectives have been established, you will need to decide what online learning approach to use. Because healthcare consumers understand information in different ways, individual learners will have preferences for the style of presentation or format of the information. These preferences depend on many things: who we are, where we live, and our prior knowledge and experience. There is a shortage of research relating learning styles and online education; however, researchers have found that individuals learn best when information is presented in ways that are consistent with their preferred learning styles [6]. To improve the design of instructional materials, educators should integrate knowledge about individual learning styles into the process. Although it would be difficult to assess the learning styles of an entire target population, it is possible to assess a representative sample (healthcare consumer focus group) of your target group. This healthcare consumer focus group should provide insights into the target population's unique preferences for learning. Tailoring of consumer health learning environments is discussed more fully by Dr. Kukafka in Chapter 3.

Although there are a number of learning styles inventories, one of the most popular and one that is used often in research is the Kolb Learning Style Inventory [7]. Kolb identified four types of learning styles based on the experiential theory of learning:

- **Convergers** value abstract concepts over concrete experience and are active learners. Their forte is the practical application of ideas. They learn conceptually and are less likely to learn in a personal interaction. Because online learning requires independent learning skills, healthcare consumers who are active learners are better suited to the online format.
- **Divergers** value concrete experience and reflective observation. They view concrete experiences from a variety of perspectives. People with higher scores on concrete experience tend to be more reflective and expressive with others. They may benefit from more interaction with healthcare educators.
- **Assimilators** value abstract conceptualization and reflective observation and hence have the ability to formulate theories. They have strong inductive reasoning abilities and prefer abstract concepts to personal interaction. This more abstract approach favors success in online learning.
- **Accommodators** value concrete experience and active experimentation. Their strength is the ability to adapt to immediate circumstances. Accommodators are at

ease with interpersonal interaction and may be suited to online education that is interactive and reinforces the learning that occurs in the healthcare setting [8].

Other Factors to Assess

In addition to a Learning Style Assessment, it is important to identify the unique characteristics of your target population. Socioeconomic factors, age, culture, and racial identity should always be considered. If resources allow, it is also beneficial to understand specific psychosocial factors that are related to the disease or health issue to be addressed in the online learning environment. These factors may include stress or anxiety known to be associated with the particular healthcare issue. There are numerous instruments to measure psychosocial variables and they are best identified by the content experts and clinicians who are working with the design team. You will not be able to assess every member of your target population; however, iterative evaluation with a representative focus group will inform the ongoing design.

Learning Theories

Another aspect to consider when developing online learning environments is the way that learners learn. Learning theories guide developers by providing a framework for the learning programs. Most online learning materials are based on multiple theories of learning. Clinical experts and healthcare educators are the lead players in selecting content and redesigning (editing) existing educational materials for online learning environments. Members of the target population focus group should also be included to validate understanding and readability of the selected content.

The following learning theories are most often connected to online learning, in part because they are learner-centered and focus on the unique needs of the learner. It is important to note that we are not discussing developmental theories in this chapter, as the focus is primarily on development of online consumer health learning for the adult population. The reader is encouraged to review theories of growth and development for additional insights into age-appropriate development of educational materials for children [9].

Adult Learning Theory (Androgogy)

Adults have unique needs as learners. Adult learning theory was pioneered by Malcolm Knowles [10], who identified the following characteristics of adult learners that should be considered when designing learning materials:

- Adults are autonomous and self-directed. They respond best when they are free to direct themselves.
- Adults have accumulated a foundation of life experiences and knowledge.
- Adults are goal oriented. They usually know what goal they want to attain. They value learning material that is organized and has clearly defined elements.
- Adults are relevancy oriented. They must see a reason for learning something.
- Adults are practical, focusing on the aspects of learning that are most useful.
- Adults need to be shown respect. Education designers must acknowledge the experiences of the target population.

Health educators should incorporate the principles of adult learning in the design of online learning.

Constructivism

Constructivism is founded on the principle that, by reflecting on personal experiences, we construct our own knowledge [11]. Learning becomes the process of changing one's ways of thinking in order to accommodate new experiences. The learning process focuses on conceptualizing knowledge and personalizing the meaning of the concepts. Constructivism promotes using information and education concepts that are customized to the learners' prior knowledge. Problem solving is an important component of this learning approach. Health educators who utilize constructivist theory in the design of online learning tailor the educational material to the needs of the learner. This theory is well suited to the development of adaptive learning programs.

Multiple Intelligences

The theory of multiple intelligence, developed by psychologist Howard Gardner [12], suggests there are at least seven ways that people perceive and understand the world. Gardner defines an "intelligence" as a collection of capabilities that has a core of information-processing operations embedded within the stages of human development. The seven intelligences are:

- Verbal–linguistic: the ability to use language and words
- Logical–mathematical: the capability for analytic thinking and reasoning, as well as pattern recognition
- Visual–spatial: the ability to imagine objects and dimensions in space, and create internal images and pictures
- Body–kinesthetic: the ability to control physical movement
- Musical–rhythmic: the ability to distinguish musical patterns and sounds, and a sensitivity to rhythms
- Interpersonal: the capacity for person-to-person communication and relationships
- Intrapersonal: spiritual awareness and self-reflection

Health educators integrate multiple multimedia modalities into their educational materials to meet the needs of multiple intelligences. This theory is well suited to the development of interactive multimedia learning programs.

Online Learning Strategies

The considerable assortment of software tools available for design, planning, and problem solving enables healthcare educators to create complex healthcare learning tools to meet their target audience's specific learning needs. Multimedia may be the most effective teaching method because it adapts easily to and satisfies more types of individual learning styles than does a text-based or verbal presentation. Research suggests that specific types of multimedia are better suited to help people learn certain kinds of information. These advantages result from how certain multimedia combinations support the differing ways in which people understand, organize, and access information [13].

Najjar [13] reviewed studies that provide suggestions on selecting the appropriate media for the types of information to be learned:

- Procedural information: explanatory text with diagrams or animation
- Problem-solving information: animation and explanatory verbal narration
- Recognition information: graphics
- Spatial information: graphics
- Small amounts of verbal information for a short time: audio
- Story details: video with a soundtrack (or text with supportive illustrations) (p. 138)

Media Selection

Selection of media types is often driven by the budget of the project. Multimedia learning resources can be quite expensive to develop; program costs of $100,000.00 or more are not uncommon. These projects require careful planning and administrative support if they are to be successful. A development plan that includes a realistic budget may be the first hurdle. If funding is secured then the work of design and development can begin.

Understanding your target populations computer access and connectivity is an important factor to consider when deciding what types of media to use. If healthcare consumers have computers at home they might be accessing online health information by dialing-in or by using higher bandwidth connections. If some healthcare consumers do not own computers, they may be using public resources, such as public libraries or health education libraries in healthcare settings. Knowing the target populations access to computers and the available connection speed will determine the type of media you can use to develop the online learning environment. For example, full-motion video is appropriate only if the target population has access to fast network connections. If access and increased bandwidth are needed and are not generally available to your target population, will you have the necessary funds to provide and sustain the consumer's access to your online learning environment?

The Design

The iterative process of design is described by Dr. Eysenbach in Chapter 4. In this section we will focus on a brief overview of designing online learning environments for consumers. As Dr. Eysenbach noted, good designs require a team approach. An experienced designer is an essential member of the team. The following are broad suggestions for supporting the process of effective educational material design. The reader is encouraged to review the work of Dr. Jakob Nielsen [14], who has written extensively on the topic of user-centered design.

To reduce the likelihood of the healthcare consumer getting "lost in cyberspace," it is recommended that a clear and systematic organization scheme be created for the educational materials. The information should be developed in a modular fashion within a well-structured hierarchy and the main points should be obvious to the learner. Design teams often begin with a content outline and then progress to a storyboard or paper-based graphic representation of the online learning resource before actually beginning to write the program for the selected media. This level of attention to detail will allow for an iterative process of both user and design team feedback and will ensure that the design is appropriate for the content to be presented and that it will meet the needs of the target population. The following diagrams provide one approach for the representation of online learning content in the early stages of design.

Step One: Content Outline Example: Hierarchy

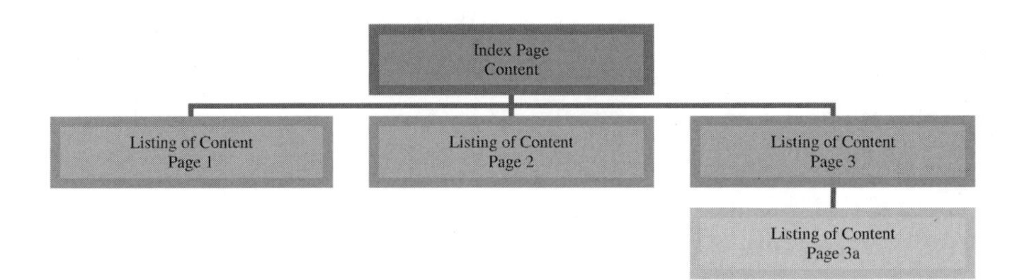

The Content Outline is a structured list of the content that will be represented in the online learning environment. Only the text is listed. It helps the design team structure the text and provides insight into relationships between key content elements. This outline may take a number of configurations. It may be hierarchical (as depicted here), it may be linear, or it may take the form of a simple outline.

Step Two: The Storyboard Template

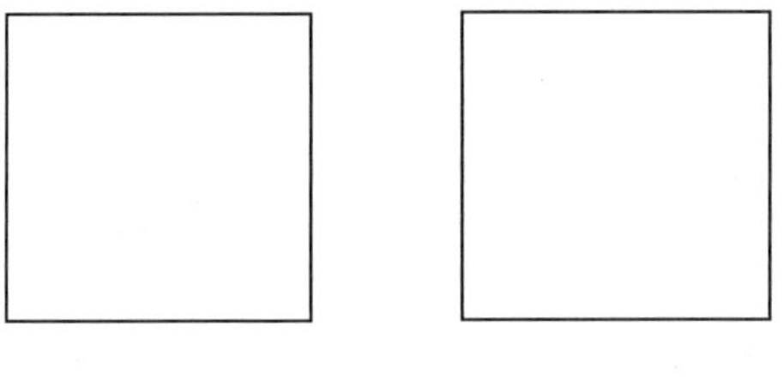

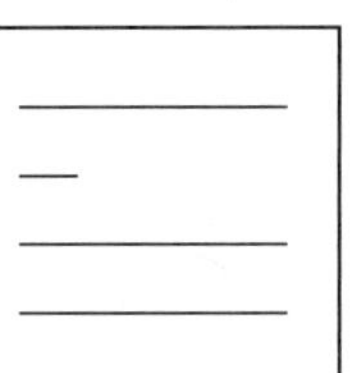

Text and graphic representation of the Content Outline are displayed in a series of boxes (the Storyboard). Only one concept or Web page is developed in a Storyboard box.

The associated lined box is used to annotate the graphics and text in the Storyboard box.

Developing the Storyboard demonstrates the fit of the Content to the online learning environment.

Taking time to complete this step will assist the Content Experts in editing content and the design team in graphic selection and text layout.

The following guidelines serve as a reminder of the importance of simplicity and attention to principles of good design:

- Leave white space and avoid clutter.
- Consider colors carefully, as some are visually displeasing.
- Use an appropriate size and type font (those older than age 40 might benefit from larger font sizes).
- Limit the use of animation.
- Use graphics to illustrate your point (a picture may be worth a thousand words).
- Always include a navigation bar or site map so that your user will be able to move easily through the information and educational content.
- Ensure that your Web page conforms to quality standards and is accessible for those with disabilities.

- Most Web site users do not read for detail but rather scan for information. Keep all written material short (paragraphs should be fewer than 75 words).
- Maintaining consistency in design across all the pages of the Web site is important.

Outcomes Evaluation

Evaluation of educational program outcomes may consist of a variety of strategies including post-test, observation, skill performance, and learner verification interviews. You may also use physiologic parameters such as Hgb A_{1c}, blood pressure, or cholesterol values to evaluate the clinical success of your online consumer health education program. Whatever strategy you choose it is most important to ensure that you are evaluating the expected learning outcomes described in your initial learning goals and objectives. Your evaluation will tell you if your outcomes were expected or unexpected. If your outcomes were unexpected then a follow-up assessment and perhaps new goal setting needs to occur. Be aware of the common mistakes made when providing consumer health education, including failing to negotiate goals, providing too much information at once, or the use of inappropriate educational material. Careful planning and attention to detail in design should significantly reduce project failures. Keeping your target population and content experts involved at every stage of design and development should ensure success.

Right Content + Right Audience + Right Design + Right Media = Success

Summary of Stages in the Design of Online Learning Environments

Stage 1: Identify the learning needs of your target population. Understanding the unique needs of the target population will help to ensure that your design is indeed user-centered.

Stage 2: Define the theoretical approach you will use to design the learning materials. The design team should work together to develop the framework for the online learning environment. Multiple learning approaches may be combined, staying user-centered is the priority.

Stage 3: Select the content. This stage should be led by content experts and clinicians who have expertise in healthcare education. Members of your consumer target population may contribute valuable content suggestions.

Stage 4: Organize the learning content to meet the needs of your target population. Once the learning content has been identified, content outlines and storyboarding will help to ensure that the content is realistically structured for the online learning environment.

Stage 5: Select the final design. All members of the design team work together to select a final design that conveys the intended message and is within budget for the project. Consumer (end-user) testing is essential at this point.

Stage 6: Develop the instructional materials. The instructional designers and developers use the appropriate media to develop the online learning environment.

Stage 7: Evaluate and revise. Design of learning materials is an iterative process; evaluation should occur at each stage of the process. Creativity can keep you in budget and on time.

Barriers to Online Education

Although online consumer health education holds many advantages and promises, it is not well suited or even available for all healthcare consumers. Research is varied regarding access to computer use among healthcare consumers. Several studies have reported that urban populations are more likely to have Internet access at home. Other studies report that Internet access remains limited for the economically disadvantaged in both rural and urban settings [3].

The "digital divide" usually refers to disparities in access to information technology that occur as a result of inequities regarding race, education, or economic status. The United States is becoming an increasingly diverse country. The traditional demographics of "majority" and "minority" are rapidly changing. Healthcare providers need to be sensitive to the needs of all healthcare consumers and provide information and education based on broad multicultural perspectives. Content should be sensitive, accurate, and nonbiased.

A variety of diverse racial, cultural, gender, and social-class groups should be used to illustrate key concepts. More and more health-related Web sites are being developed for bilingual audiences, which is one important aspect. Others factors may be equally important but are often overlooked.

As an example, consider the newly diagnosed person with diabetes. He or she will be asked to control his or her diet and will often be given diet programs or information sheets. Those information sheets frequently ignore cultural or religious practices pertaining to food selection. The healthcare consumer may be uncomfortable asking the healthcare provider to adjust the food information sheets so he or she goes home and continues his or her normal diet. In this example, online tailored health education might be particularly useful in delivering consumer-centered information that is provided in the appropriate language, with illustrations to reinforce difficult concepts. Because multiple food lists can be maintained in the program database, food preferences could be tailored to meet ethnic or religious preferences. The personal characteristics of the actors can be changed to represent the target population's racial identity.

A few studies have addressed the issues of diversity and economic disadvantage in computer-based healthcare learning environments [15–20]. Winzelberg and colleagues [21] found no significant differences in access across racial demographics in their study of Caucasian, African-American, Asian, or Hispanic young women with eating disorders who utilized an Internet-based educational program. Finkelstein et al. [22] assessed inner city healthcare consumers' use of a home asthma telemonitoring system that collects spirometry data and symptom reports and then transmits these data and reports to a medical center's clinical information system. Although most of these healthcare consumers had no prior computer experience, they indicated that performing the spirometry test and working with the palm-top computer was "not difficult at all." In a study of young women with breast cancer, Gustafson et al. [23,24] noted that the benefits of Computer Enhancement and Social Support (CHESS) appeared to be greater for healthcare consumers who are economically disadvantaged.

Physical disabilities may also exist that prevent or reduce access. Disability informatics is discussed in depth by Dr. Appleyard in Chapter 11. The reminder of this chapter focuses on the problem of health literacy. Health literacy is often overlooked and this can render healthcare education programs ineffective for those who need them most.

Health Literacy

Nutbeam [25], Rudd [26,27], and Kickbush [28,29] all describe the problem of health literacy as a complex process that includes reading ability, comprehension, and the ability to apply the new knowledge to improve health outcomes. Ninety million American adults (45% of the US population) have limited health literacy skills. About one half (40 to 44 million) read at or below a fifth-grade level, if at all. The remainder (50 million) are marginally illiterate and unable to perform tasks that require them to synthesize information from complex and lengthy texts [30]. For some healthcare consumers the problem goes beyond reading skills. It is not that they do not know how to read; they don't understand what they read and as a consequence may be unable to think critically and make complex healthcare decisions.

Poor health literacy skills have profound economic consequences. Healthcare costs related to low health literacy were estimated at $73 billion in 1998. Seventy-five percent of American healthcare consumers are either functionally or marginally illiterate, contributing to increased hospitalizations and longer lengths of stay [30,31]. In addition, poor health literacy contributes to ineffective communication between providers and consumers, which may result in errors caused by misunderstandings about the plan of care [32,33].

Persons with low health literacy are more likely to be economically disadvantaged and are less likely to seek preventive health services [32,34]. Evidence associates low health literacy, independent of socioeconomic factors, with increased incidence of chronic disease, decreased adherence, poor health outcomes, and early death [34–41]. Researchers have indicated that the literacy skills of consumers with diabetes, hypertension, and asthma are strong correlates of their knowledge about their illness and disease management skills [36,37].

Assessment of Literacy and Readability

Traditional healthcare information (prescription labels, health education materials, insurance forms, informed consents) are often provided to consumers as text-based print information. This text-based printed material is frequently written at the 10+ grade levels [32,42–45], well beyond the reading ability of a large number of healthcare consumers. A national survey of 10% of all US hospitals examined surgical and medical procedure informed consents for readability. The average grade level required to read the consents was 12.6 (+/–3.1) [46]. In another national study, online text-based information provided by Institutional Review Boards was found to be as much as 2.8 grade levels higher than their own accepted standards [47].

Evaluating readability of text can be accomplished with a variety of formulas: Flesch–Kincaid Grade Level, Fry Graph, FOG, SMOG, and FORCAST are commonly used. These instruments provide a score that reflects the grade level a person would need to achieve to be able to read the text. Consumer health material should be available for readers at or below the fifth-grade level [42].

A number of instruments exist to measure the literacy of healthcare consumers and the readability of the information and educational material provided. The Rapid Estimation of Adult Literacy in Medicine (REALM), Wide Range Achievement Test (WRAT), and the Test of Functional Health Literacy in Adults (TOFHLA) are used most often. The CLOZE technique, which is contained in the TOFHLA, is a measure of comprehension that asks subjects to interpret information gleaned from reading a passage of text.

Technology-Based Interventions to Support Low-Literacy Delivery of Health Information

The method of presenting information to healthcare consumers is as important as the information itself. Multimedia can provide dynamic illustrations (animations and video) that support comprehension [48]. Healthcare consumers with varied reading skills can use multimedia presentation to develop mental models, reducing reliance on reading as the primary means of learning. Conversely, multimedia and graphics that are too complex may be as confusing as difficult text.

Pernotto et al. [49] reported that the use of graphics and audio sound made an interactive program for healthcare consumers undergoing endoscopic procedures more understandable by people with limited reading ability. In another study, Liao et al. [50] found that healthcare consumers who had little education benefited most from an interactive video program. In contrast, Graber et al. [51] found that much of Web-based material was "too difficult" for most consumers and not readable by those with low literacy levels.

References

1. Lewis D. Computer-based approaches to patient education: a review of the literature. J Am Med Informatics Assoc 1999;6:272–82.
2. Lewis D. Computers in patient education. Comput Inform Nurs 2003;21:88–96.
3. Lewis D, Behana K. The role of the Internet in managing the chronic disease population: patient perspective. Dis Manag Health Outcomes 2001;9:241–7.
4. Bloom BS. Taxonomy of Educational Objectives: The Classification of Educational Goals: Handbook I. Cognitive Domain. New York: Longmans, 1956.
5. Hannafin MJ, Peck KL. The Design, Development, and Evaluation of Instructional Software. New York: Macmillan, 1988, p. 412.
6. Riding R, Grimley M. Cognitive style and learning from multimedia materials in 11-year children. Br J Educ Technol 1999;30:43–59.
7. Kolb DA. Experiential Learning. Englewood Cliffs, NJ: Prentice-Hall, 1984.
8. Kolb DA. Learning style inventory: Technical Manual. Boston: McBer, 1986.
9. Phillips DC, Soltis JF. Perspectives on Learning, Revised Edition. New York: Teachers College Press, 1998.
10. Knowles MS. Androgogy in Action. San Francisco: Jossey-Bass, 1984.
11. Wilson B. Constructivist Learning Environments. Englewood Cliffs, NJ: Educational Technology Publications, 1995.
12. Gardner H. Intelligence Reframed: Multiple Intelligences for the 21st Century. New York: Basic Books, 2000.
13. Najjar LJ. Multimedia information and learning. J Educ Multimed Hypermed 1996;5:129–50.
14. Nielsen J. Designing Web Usability: The Practice of Simplicity. Indianapolis, IN: New Riders, 2000.
15. Skinner H, Biscope S, Poland B. Quality of Internet access: barrier behind Internet use statistics. Soc Sci Med 2003;57:875–80.
16. Gray NJ, Klein JD, Cantrill JA, Noyce PR. Adolescent girls' use of the Internet for health information: issues beyond access. J Med Syst 2002;26:545–53.
17. Kalichman SC, Weinhardt L, Benotsch E, Cherry C. Closing the digital divide in HIV/AIDS care: development of a theory-based intervention to increase Internet access. AIDS Care 2002;14:523–37.
18. D'Alessandro DM, Dosa NP. Empowering children and families with information technology. Arch Pediatr Adolesc Med 2001;155:1131–6.
19. Mollica BM. The digital divide. Assist Technol 2000;12:93–5.
20. Brodie M, Flournoy RE, Altman DE, Blendon RJ, Benson JM, Rosenbaum MD. Health information, the Internet, and the digital divide. Health Affairs 2000; 19:255–65.

21. Winzelberg A, Eppstein D, Eldredge KI, et al. Effectiveness of an Internet-based program for reducing risk factors for eating disorders. J Consult Clin Psychol 2000;68:346–50.
22. Finkelstein J, O'Connor G, Friedmann RH. Development and implementation of the home asthma telemonitoring (HAT) system to facilitate asthma self-care. Medinform 2001;10 (Pt 1):810–4.
23. Arora NK, Johnson P, Gustafson DH, McTavish F, Hawkins RP, Pingree S. Barriers to information access, perceived health competence, and psychosocial health outcomes: test of a mediation model in a breast cancer sample. Patient Educ Couns 2002;47:37–46.
24. Gustafson DH, Hawkins RP, Boberg EW, et al. CHESS: 10 years of research and development in consumer health informatics for broad populations, including the underserved. Int J Med Inform 2002;65:169–77.
25. Nutbeam D. Theory in a Nutshell: A Guide to Health Promotion Theory. New York: McGraw-Hill, 1999.
26. Rudd R, Comings J. Learner developed materials: an empowering product. Health Educ Q 1994;21:313–27.
27. Rudd RE, Comings JP, Hyde JN. Leave no one behind: improving health and risk communication through attention to literacy. J Health Commun 2003;8(Suppl):104–15.
28. Kickbusch I. Health literacy: a search for new categories. Health Promot Int 2002;17:1–2.
29. Kickbusch IS. Health literacy: addressing the health and education divide. Health Promot Int 2001;16:289–97.
30. Kirsch I, Jungeblut A, Jenkins L, Kolstad A. Adult literacy in America: a first look at the results of the National Adult Literacy Survey. 1993, National Center for Educational Statistics, United States Department of Education: Washington, DC.
31. Baker DW, Gazmararian JA, Williams MV, et al. Functional health literacy and the risk of hospital admission among Medicare managed care enrollees. Am J Public Health 2002;92:1278–83.
32. Williams M, Parker RM, Baker DW, et al. Inadequate functional health literacy among patients at two public hospitals. JAMA 1995;274:1677–82.
33. Williams MV, Baker DW, Honig EG, Lee TM, Nowlan A. Inadequate literacy is a barrier to asthma knowledge and self-care. Chest 1998;114:1008–15.
34. Davis T, Meldrum N, Tippy P, Weiss B, Williams M. How poor literacy leads to poor health care. Patient Care 1996;30:94–127.
35. Weiss B, Hart G, McGee DL, D'Estelle S. Health status of illiterate adults: relation between literacy and health status among persons with low literacy skills. J Am Board Fam Pract 1992;5:257–64.
36. Williams MV, Baker DW, Honig EG, Lee TM, Nowlan A. Inadequate literacy is a barrier to asthma knowledge and self-care. Chest 1998;114:1008–15.
37. Williams MV, Baker DW, Parker RM, Nurss JR. Relationship of functional health literacy to patients' knowledge of their chronic disease. Arch Intern Med 1998;158:166–72.
38. Committee on Health Literacy. Health literacy: report of the Council on Scientific Affairs. JAMA 1999;281:552–7.
39. Baker DW, Williams MV, Parker RM, Gazmararian JA, Nurss J. Development of a brief test to measure functional health literacy. Patient Educ Couns 1999;38:33–42.
40. Golin C, DiMatteo MR, Duan N, Leake B, Gelberg L. Impoverished diabetic patients whose doctors facilitate their participation in medical decision making are more satisfied with their care. J Gen Intern Med 2002;17:866–75.
41. Davis TC, Williams MV, Marin E, Parker RM, Glass J. Health literacy and cancer communication.[see comment]. Ca Cancer J Clin 2002;52:134–49.
42. Doak C, Doak L, Root J. Teaching Patients with Low Literacy Skills. Philadelphia: J.B. Lippincott, 1995.
43. Forbis S, Aligne CA. Poor readability of written asthma management plans found in national guidelines. Pediatrics 2002;109:e52.
44. Gannon W, Hildebrant E. A winning combination: women, literacy, and participation in health care. Health Care Women Int 2002;23:754–60.
45. Foster D, Rhoney DH. Readability of printed patient information for epileptic patients. Ann Pharmacother 36:1856–61.

46. Hopper KD, TenHave TR, Tully DA, Hall TE. The readability of currently used surgical/ procedure consent forms in the United States. Surgery 1998;123:496–503.
47. Paasche-Orlow MK, Taylor HA, Brancati FL. Readability standards for informed-consent forms as compared with actual readability.[see comment]. N Engl J Med 2003;348:721–6.
48. Levie WH, Lentz R. Effects of text illustrations: a review of the research. Educ Commun Technol J 1982;30:195–232.
49. Pernotto D, Bairnsfather L, Sodeman W. Informed consent: interactive videodisc for patients having a colonoscopy, a polypectomy, and an endoscopy. MedInform 1995.
50. Liao L, Jollis JG, DeLong ER, Peterson ED, Morris KG, Mark DB. Impact of an interactive video on decision making of patients with ischemic heart disease. J Gen Intern Med 1996;11:373–6.
51. Graber M, D'Alessandro DM, Johnson-West J. Reading level or privacy policies on Internet health web sites. J Fam Pract 2002;51:642–5.

7
Qualitative Evaluation in Consumer Health Informatics

BONNIE KAPLAN

Approaches to qualitative evaluation for consumer health informatics are much like qualitative research for any purpose. Data collection and data analysis methods are similar for all projects. This chapter provides a general overview of these methods. But because qualitative research depends heavily on the research participants and contextual setting, each project is different. Examples throughout the chapter illustrate ways in which doing qualitative research to evaluate consumer health informatics projects is both similar and different from evaluating other kinds of projects.

Qualitative research involves data that, generally, are textual, but also may be visual or artifactual. There are ways to reduce this kind of data to numerical form, for example, by counting the occurrences of a particular phrase. Doing that often defeats the purpose of using a qualitative approach. Instead, qualitative data analysis employs procedures for producing an interpretation of the data. Qualitative research also involves conducting rigorous and detailed studies in natural settings. For example, a researcher might be investigating how people use health information Web sites and why they prefer some sites to others. Such a study might be done in a setting where people naturally use these Web sites, such as a library, their homes, or offices.

Many qualitative researchers attempt to understand something in the same way as the other participants involved in a study understand it. A research study on how people use Web sites and why people prefer some sites to others might investigate the way people think about a Web site's design, appearance, ease of navigation, trustworthiness, helpfulness, applicability to their own situation, overall tone of the content, and the like. Some of these dimensions can be made into variables and differences between them measured, for example, through a user satisfaction survey. That would not be considered qualitative research. If the survey also included open-ended questions such as "Please describe what you like about your favorite Web site," the data collected in answer to that question would be qualitative.

Other considerations are not investigated as easily. Even though people may rate a Web site as positive along whatever dimensions might appear on the survey, it might still give them a "bad" feeling, or there might be something far more important to them than anything the survey asks. Their sense that the information is trustworthy and reliable might make a difference, but what makes information seem trustworthy and reliable? Perhaps who else is around might make a difference, too, or what their friends think. It is difficult to anticipate what influences might be important. It also may be difficult to measure them. Qualitative methods are better than quantitative ones (such as a survey) in these circumstances. Further, although people may rate a site as trustworthy, it might be difficult to assess just why they do. Just what does "trustworthy" mean to different people? Perhaps people who use the Web site have different notions of what trustworthiness entails—different from each other, different from the site designers, and different from the researchers and evaluators. These kinds of questions, too, are better investigated through qualitative methods. Qualitative methods are particularly helpful when:

- You do no know what might be important to measure.
- You want to study something that cannot be measured easily.
- You want to determine why measured results are as they are.
- You want to know not only what happened, or what people are responding to, but also why.
- You want to understand how people think or feel about something and why they think that way, what their perspectives and situations are and how those influence what is happening.
- You want to investigate the influence of social, organizational, and cultural context on the area of study, and vice versa.
- You want to explore what a technology (such as a home health monitoring system) or practice (such as using a computer to access health information) means to people.
- You want to examine causal processes, and not simply what causal relationships exist. You are interested primarily in these processes as they develop and emerge, rather than in outcomes or impacts.
- You want the evaluation to parallel the development process for the application under study, for example, so that you can improve the application development as it progresses.

There are a variety of theoretical perspectives and practical approaches from which to approach these kinds of questions. The term "qualitative research," as used here, refers to all of them because this chapter is concerned primarily with what they have in common, what it is that defines them all as qualitative research. A variety of other terms describe these different perspectives and approaches: field research, naturalistic research, interpretive research, ethnographic research, postpositivistic research, phenomenological research, hermeneutic research, humanistic research, (some kinds of) case studies, and action research.

There are several common threads through all these. First, *the* primary research question is, "What is happening and why is it happening in this particular way?" This question will have numerous variants as it is asked in particular ways to address specific situations and research settings. Second, the focus is on what people think is happening and why they think that, as well as why they are responding as they are. Third, causality is multidirectional. There is no clear effect or impact of one factor on some specific outcome. Fourth, there are few predetermined analytic categories, explanatory theories, or even research questions. A variety of concerns is being addressed. The important questions, analytic categories, and theories develop over the course of research, rather than being imposed a priori. Fifth, data analysis is not clearly separated from data collection. A considerable element of continual interpretation and reinterpretation of data is required on the part of the researcher in making sense of things, as is collecting new data as well as revisiting data already gathered in order to check these interpretations. Lastly, qualitative research is particularistic, driven both by the research as it unfolds and by the context in which it is unfolding. Therefore, many aspects of the research itself may change as the research progresses.

Research Design

Qualitative research does not require the researcher to stick with a predetermined study design. Although a sound research plan is necessary, the exigencies of either the research itself or the researcher's developing sense of what and how to focus the research require flexibility. Five methodological guidelines can be useful when developing an evaluation plan [1]:

1. Focus on a variety of technical, economic, people, organizational, and social concerns.
2. Use multiple methods.
3. Be modifiable.
4. Be longitudinal.
5. Be formative as well as summative.

These guidelines allow the study to have the potential to track change over time, to be useful during the course of the project as well as afterwards, to change in focus or approach as the need arises, and to identify important concerns.

The guideline regarding multiple methods also is important for increasing validity. Multiple means of data collection can help ensure that interpretations of the data are comprehensive and, through triangulation, account for all important data. For example, in a study when a new clinical laboratory order entry and results reporting system was implemented, several sources of data were used [2–6]. I was a participant observer at laboratory management meetings. Colleagues and I also did observations in each laboratory. We surveyed laboratory technologists, and the survey included both Likert-scale and open-ended questions. Interviews with laboratory directors provided the key for interpreting data gathered from the Likert-scale survey questions. Similarly, interviews with patients using a health behavior counseling system suggested that there were important differences in reaction among people who used different versions of the system, and this was borne out by analyzing survey data [7]. In another case, when a new patient record system was tested, survey data and time–motion measurements did not agree. The researchers developed an explanation that encompassed these divergent data [8,9].

The Role of Theory

Because many qualitative researchers are interested primarily in understanding what is going on and what that means for the people involved, their studies may not involve testing theory. This does not make the research atheoretical. There are a variety of qualitative evaluation approaches that draw on different theories [10].

Theory is helpful in highlighting what is important each step of the way in a qualitative research study. Different theories have different emphases. Therefore, theories of knowledge and epistemologies underlying research approaches influence how the project is conceived, how the research is carried out, and how it is reported. Theory also can shape research questions and focus. Furthermore, theory can help in data analysis and interpretation. Lastly, theory may be generated from the study and across studies. What is important is that theory can serve as a guide, rather than as a framework into which findings are forced. On the whole, qualitative research is more data driven than theory driven, although it is widely recognized that data do not exist of and by themselves in the absence of theory.

Data Collection

Qualitative data are any data that are not to be analyzed solely numerically but are instead treated as text. Two main sources of data for qualitative research are interviews and observations, but any other sources, such as photographs and other images, company documents, e-mail messages, answers to open-ended survey questions, videotapes of meetings, and an observer's notes—anything—might be considered data. Often, more than one source of data is needed, as indicated earlier. I generally do both interviews and observations, at a minimum. One hallmark of qualitative research is that, at the outset, it is very difficult to know what might prove to be important, so nothing should be excluded as a possible data source at the beginning of a study. As the study progresses, it becomes clearer what to focus on, and the scope of data collection can narrow. Of course, you cannot collect *all* possible data. Instead, you decide beforehand what the important questions and issues are that you want to investigate, and you focus your efforts there. During the course of the study, you may need to change the focus in some ways perhaps because you find that something else is more important to investigate. It also may be difficult at the outset to know how much data to collect. Perhaps your approach is not producing results, in which case you try something different. Perhaps your approach was producing results, but you are no longer getting new material or insights. You should stop. Data collection is over when saturation is reached, that is, when nothing new is coming to light.

Interviewing

Qualitative interviewing also may be called ethnographic interviewing, elite interviewing, in-depth interviewing, unstructured interviewing, semistructured interviewing, or oral history interviewing. The main characteristic is that the interviewer does not, in general, constrain most of the interviewee's responses, as, for example, by asking the interviewee to rate something on a scale or say whether he or she agrees or disagrees with a statement.

Interviews can be conducted anywhere comfortable for the interviewee: the person's office or home, the cafeteria, while the interviewee is working, and so forth. Often, privacy is helpful, if only to make the interview more confidential and less likely to be interrupted. However, depending on the project, it can be helpful to choose a setting that also will provide information, as described later in the discussion of observation. For example, perhaps the number and nature of interruptions an interviewee experiences while working might be important. Interviewing often is done one-on-one, although I generally prefer to have another researcher present, for reasons explained below. Group interviews and focus groups are also possible.

When interviewing, I use a tape recorder if it will not interfere with the interviewee's comfort or willingness to talk. Whether or not I use a tape recorder, I take notes (again, unless it makes the interviewee uncomfortable), and try to write down as much as possible in the exact words used. Of course, there is no way I can write down everything as quickly as it is being said, let alone write it down while I am also trying to interview someone. There are several ways to help with this. When possible, I like to have another interviewer along with me. That way, we can both take notes and, if one of us is engrossed in writing, the other can keep the interview moving. Also, I may simply jot down a phrase or a few words to remind me what was said, and then I fill it in as soon after the interview as possible. My memory for reproducing what I heard has improved with practice.

Interviewees will have been contacted to give their permission for being interviewed before I meet them. Nevertheless, I start an interview first by explaining who I am, why

I am there, and what my relationship to the project is. I briefly explain the purpose of the project and what the rules for confidentiality will be. I always ask for permission to tape and take notes. Not everyone agrees to that. Regardless, I try to find some way to get comfortable talking to the person and have that person feel comfortable with me. For this, as for the rest of the interview, use your natural friendliness and conversational skills to develop rapport with the person you are interviewing. I simply use typical nonthreatening conversation starters. I may comment on a photograph of the family, or remark, based on a person's diplomas, that we used to live in the same city.

I come prepared with a list of a few broad questions I want to ask and a good sense of the general research questions firmly in mind. These questions are open-ended and are intended to create the opportunity to talk about the areas of research interest in that person's own words and own way. They should allow different people to give different kinds of answers. I may never ask all the questions I prepared, and I certainly will ask ones I had not prepared. Go with the flow. As the interviewee says something interesting or confusing, ask more about it. Probe and repeat what you are being told so that you get a good understanding of what the person is trying to say. You may not be able to ask directly what you think you want to know, but may need to go at it from one angle or another. You may need to let the conversation wander off in a seemingly irrelevant direction and come back to what you were interested in. Then again, you may find that what you thought was going to be irrelevant turned out to be very interesting and relevant after all.

Even though I may have the same set of broad questions, no two interviews are the same. Even what I say differs from interview to interview. I rarely can ask all questions in the same order. I use different wording, depending on the situation, our rapport, and the person I am interviewing. What I say influences the response, so I write down what I say as well as what the interviewee says. Also, as I conduct interviews, I learn that some questions do not work out well, and I stop asking those, or have to reword them, or find another way to get at what I am trying to find out. I learn that some questions I had not even thought of at the beginning are important questions to ask, and I ask those in later interviews.

In a study of a diet and exercise health advisory system [11], we wanted to see that system from the viewpoint of the people who used it. An interview partner and I used ethnographic in-depth interviewing to elicit how interviewees conceptualized, reacted to, and attributed meaning to their experience with the system. We started by asking interviewees to describe their use of the system and what a session with it was like. Then we asked questions to follow up on what they said. In the process, people spoke of changes in their dietary and exercise patterns and of their feelings about using the system. They talked about what they ate and what exercise they did. They talked about their family responsibilities and how those affected what they ate and what exercise they did, even though we had not specifically asked that. People talked about topics as varied as who did the cooking in their household, how they missed family when they left their country of origin, how they compared using this system to using an automatic teller machine, their divorces, their favorite recipes, their dogs, their favorite desserts, and what information they gave in response to queries from the system. Each interview was shaped by the personality of the interviewee and his or her personal circumstances, the relationship we developed with them, and the direction in which the conversation went, as well as by our steering it in directions of special interest to the research study. How to analyze such wide-ranging, disparate data is discussed in the paragraphs that follow.

When I started this study, I thought it might make a difference to ask people what their family members thought about the system, and whether they would recommend the system to their friends. Those turned out not to be fruitful questions. For me, one of the joys of qualitative research is the unanticipated things that can come up. This system involved hearing prerecorded messages on the telephone. I had not thought to ask interviewees what they thought of the voice, but that turned out to be a crucial question. In this case, familiarity with both the system and the people using it was important. My colleague had thought the sound of the voice would matter. Neither of us had anticipated, though, the depth or range of feeling people would have about it. As interviewees talked about their reactions, it became apparent, too, that their feelings about their interactions with the system over what they ate and what exercise they did or did not do also was a crucial issue.

Observation

Observation is similar to interviewing. Detailed notes are required. Videotaping may be helpful, if not too intrusive or costly, and has the advantage that you can observe repeatedly. Also, although you may have specific things you want to observe, there likely will turn out to be unanticipated things you observe that prove to be important, and things you wished you had noticed. You may be observing how someone uses a system, or how that person works and spends time. You may want to especially take note of where people sit at a meeting with the idea that that would tell you something about everyone's relative power and status. You may also observe who speaks during the meeting and when they speak, as well as note what they say.

You also may not be observing anything that specific or predetermined. In the project on the health behavior advisory system [12], I interviewed people in their homes. In one person's dining room, I noticed a border of shamrocks decorating the wall. As this interviewee was talking about having eaten food she knew was not healthy, I realized that she was feeling guilty about it, and that, for her, guilt involved confession. The shamrocks were the clue to me to consider guilt and confession as an important theme in this research. What she was saying, together with the shamrock decorations, made me realize that it was significant that this study was being done in an area with a large Irish Catholic population and that there were religious-based themes in the interviews. In another interview, another person told us about how he had changed his eating habits to consume more healthy food, in line with the guidelines provided by the system. Meanwhile, his wife was frying sausage for him. This apparent contradiction led us to check the system log to find out how often he had used the system. He had not used it. Observing what his wife was preparing raised the question of veracity, and we therefore checked system logs against what all other interviewees told us as well.

Another kind of observation is participant observation. Here, the researcher is not simply paying attention to the surroundings and people, but has deliberately joined the setting with the intent of both participating in it and paying attention to it. When I attended laboratory management meetings as a member of the department in which I was studying the clinical laboratory information system, I was a participant observer [2–6]. When I sat in the nursing station and watched as residents entered data into a psychiatric clinical decision support system [13], I was an observer, not a participant observer. In neither case was I solely an observer, though. I also interacted with the people, asked questions, and influenced what was happening simply by being there. I do not believe this influence could have been avoided, no matter what I did or did not do.

Both interviewing and observation are active. They could be very active indeed, as when I spent a week shadowing a physician for his entire work day in a hospital [14]. They can be rather limited, as when I interviewed two radiologists at a small hospital during one afternoon as part of a larger project involving several hospitals in more than one city. Both interviewing and observation require on-the-spot decisions about what to do next, what to record, what to say, and how to present yourself. For example, I unexpectedly interviewed two radiologists because the one with whom I had an appointment was not available. Instead, I found the other one and got his permission to talk with him. By then, the first radiologist had become available and I was able to interview him as well. What started out seeming problematic turned out to be fortuitous, because this way I was able to compare the responses of two radiologists instead of relying only on one.

Other Sources of Data

I have not discussed documents, images, and other data sources. Similar principles apply. You may be looking for specific things, and you certainly want to collect those. As you examine the materials, you may also find that new and interesting data are available that you will want to analyze as well.

Data Analysis

Although I am writing about data collection and data analysis separately, it should be clear from the discussion of data collection that it cannot be separated so neatly from data analysis. Deciding what to follow up, what question to ask an interviewee next, what observation to record and what to disregard, what document to keep—all these involve making decisions about the importance of the data, and that involves constant, ongoing analysis. This is one of the two main principles of qualitative data analysis: You cannot divorce the processes of data collection, data analysis, interpretation, and even research design from each other. They are intertwined and depend on each other. Data analysis proceeds iteratively, through a sequence of data collection, interpretation of that data as you are collecting it, checking that interpretation against the data you already collected and new data you are collecting with that interpretation in mind, more (or new, or changed) interpretation of the data, checking the interpretation against the data, and so forth. This so-called hermeneutic circle is the mainstay of qualitative data analysis, and especially distinguishes a qualitative study.

The second principle of qualitative data analysis is that the data are textual, or treated as a text, and are, therefore, both voluminous and not readily amenable to easy manipulation. That, at least, is the case if you are going to proceed as just described with the goal of creating a coherent account to answer the basic question, "What is going on here?" My previous description of an interview gives a sense of both the volume and range of data. Therefore, the main goal is to make sense of all this seemingly overwhelming morass of data. There are four standard methods of data reduction: coding, displays, contextual and narrative analysis, and analytic memos and writing. Although the process can be described, creativity and insight are involved as well, and that is not at all easy to describe. These four approaches may be used separately and in combination. They help in the process of identifying themes in the data, developing categories, and exploring similarities and differences in the data and relationships among them. Going through this process immerses you in the data, so you end up knowing it well and, in a way, living in it. That will help to stimulate the creativity and insight that can lead to an interesting and valid interpretation of the data.

Coding

Coding involves breaking up the data and rearranging them into categories. These categories are developed in interaction with, and tailored to, the particular data being analyzed. Some categories may be drawn from existing theory or prior knowledge of the setting and system. You develop others during the analysis. Still others are derived from the conceptual structure of the people studied, as evidenced in the data. Creating categories is a fluid process. You may develop categories you later decide were not useful, and you may need to add categories as you progress through the data. Also, categories are not mutually exclusive. They may overlap.

You may wish to organize the same data in different ways. In the study involving the clinical laboratory system [2–6], I organized data by laboratory as one part of the analysis. That way I could compare laboratories to see what was common among them and what was different. I also organized data by categories that cross-cut laboratories, such as categories for what laboratory technologists considered advantages of using the system.

As this example suggests, you may start with very large categories and then develop smaller ones. The "advantages of the system" category could be subdivided, for example, into different kinds of advantages, or by laboratory. In the health behavior advisory system study [12], "the voice" became a category. Anything anyone said about the voice was placed into this category. Some of that data also was placed into other categories, for example, the "guilt" category, which included anything anyone said about feeling guilty. When all data concerning the voice were put together into one place, it was easier to subdivide them into more categories and to develop a sense of the main ideas people were expressing about the voice.

Displays

Displays include formal tools such as matrices, flowcharts, and concept maps, and informal charts and diagrams. They are similar to memos in that they make ideas, data, and analysis visible and permanent. They also serve two other key functions: data reduction and the presentation of data or analysis in a form that allows it to be grasped as a whole. Creating displays, like categories, is a fluid process that may be done at different stages of data analysis. For example, sometimes I create displays as I work through the raw data. In my usability study of how medical residents tested a Web-based educational case [15], I first recorded all observations in sequence, noting the time, what was said, and what was done as the session progressed. Then, to analyze that data, I created a chart for each session. In one column I put the time. In another I put the part of the case that was being worked on. In another I put how the resident worked through the case. In another, I put whatever system difficulties or confusions were experienced. I had thought that I would be able to combine these displays into a master display showing how all residents worked their way through the case. That proved impossible. Part of the data analysis, and, consequently, part of the research itself, became figuring out how to make useful displays. Sometimes I create displays as a way of summarizing data into a table for publication. Note that displays may be very simple. I have made displays for myself in which I keep count of the frequency of various ideas that occur in the data.

Contextual and Narrative Analysis

In contextual and narrative analysis, instead of segmenting the data into discrete elements and re-sorting them into categories, you seek to identify and understand the relationships among these different elements and their meanings for the persons involved. Formal methods, such as discourse analysis, narrative analysis, profiles, or ethnographic microanalysis may be used. Less formally, the goal is to consider sections of the data as a whole. For example, rather than simply focusing on when interviewees mentioned "guilt," contextual or narrative analysis would also focus on the context in which they discussed feeling guilty, what they said that they related to feeling guilty, and so forth.

Analytic Memos and Writing

An analytic memo is anything you write in relationship to the research, other than direct field notes or transcription. It can range from a brief marginal comment on an interview transcript, or a theoretical idea incorporated into field notes, to a full-fledged analytic essay. Writing is key to data analysis. Writing gets your ideas down on paper so you can look at those ideas later. Writing facilitates reflection and analytic insight. You should begin writing as early as possible. Notes of your reactions, your ideas, your thoughts, your insights, and what puzzles you become part of the data. If you write these while collecting other data, you can include them in a well-defined area of your (interview or observation) notes so that it is easy to identify the data per se and your reactions to the data.

As with the other data analysis methods, writing involves experimentation and rewriting. For the clinical laboratory study [2–6], I wrote profiles of each laboratory and I wrote descriptions of the results in each category I created. For the heath advisory system study [12], I wrote summaries of each interview. I wrote profiles for each version of the system. I wrote descriptions of results of each category. I have done this sort of thing for each project. Eventually, some of this writing goes into a detailed report for the project sponsor. Developing a well-organized report is a step in developing a good interpretation of your data. Some of the text from a report gets further organized into a series of publishable research papers. Note, though, that all this writing comes after the other steps involved in data analysis. To write summaries, profiles, and reports requires a considerable degree of analysis. However, writing shorter bits as you go will help you do this, just as writing each of these provides a next level of analysis. The analysis is done when you have reached a level beyond which there is no further integration and interpretation of your data.

Validity

Although reliability and generalizability often come into question in qualitative studies, validity in qualitative studies often is stronger than in quantitative ones. Greater validity results from the researcher's flexibility, insight, and ability to use his or her tacit knowledge. Close attention to meaning, context, and process makes it less likely that the wrong research questions were asked or that important data were overlooked or excluded.

On the other hand, validity concerns in qualitative research also revolve around the special role of the researcher as an instrument of both data collection and data analysis. Therefore, your biases, interests, perceptions, observations, knowledge, and critical faculties all play a role in the study. They affect collecting and analyzing any data, but the subjective nature of qualitative research is very clear. The role of the researcher, therefore, needs to be explicit. I include in a research paper what my relationship is to the project, what experience I bring to it, what theoretical frames I am using that influenced either data collection or interpretation, and so forth so that others may consider their potential influence on study results.

It also is the responsibility of each of us to carefully consider previous beliefs and constantly question observations and interpretations so as to help avoid being blinded or misdirected by what we bring to the study. Moreover, we need to keep checking our analyses and interpretations. There are several ways to do this: rich data, triangulation, puzzles, and feedback and member checking. These approaches involve, as emphasized previously, testing ideas against existing data, against data collected specifically for this purpose, and others' interpretations. Qualitative studies are marked by rich data, that is, data that are as comprehensive and complete as possible. Data from multiple sources, or data collected by different methods (whether qualitative or not), also increase validity through triangulation. Some brief examples were mentioned earlier.

You also question the data, and yourself, by paying close attention to puzzles. One underlying assumption of qualitative methods is that things make sense to the people involved in the setting. It is your job to get to the point where they make sense to you as well. In particular, I find it very helpful to pay careful attention to surprises, puzzles, confusions, discrepant data, and negative cases. Figuring these out not only increases the validity of interpretation, but also, I have found, provides the most interesting insights. Also, get feedback. When I work with another researcher, we discuss the project as we go. We test ideas and interpretations against each other. Writing reports is another way to get feedback, in this case, from the project sponsor or other audience for the report. It also is very helpful to get feedback from participants in the study, if possible. This so-called member checking provides another opportunity for data collection and a way to see if your interpretation makes sense to the people whose ideas you are reporting.

Research Ethics

Much of what I have written relies on underlying ethical principles. General research ethics are addressed in another chapter. As in any research, it is necessary to gain the willing consent of the people involved in the study. However, because the methods involved in qualitative research can intrude into people's private lives, work spaces, and home, and probe their feelings and thoughts, personal issues may easily arise. Those who consent may not realize that, in the course of an interview, they may reveal aspects of their personal lives or personalities that they later wish they had not. This makes it all the more important for you to be sensitive to those issues and to conduct yourself and the project so as to not be unnecessarily voyeuristic, but to respect people's privacy and sensibilities. It also is incumbent on you to not promise more confidentiality than you can deliver, and to take significant steps to protect people's identities.

Other ethical issues arise specifically in the realm of consumer health informatics [16]. Part of an evaluator's role, I think, concerns helping to ensure that these applications, like any others, are designed and deployed in ways that actually help people. Yet, the potential users are a large population with diverse needs and attitudes. It is difficult to pay attention to such concerns as aspects of technology, values embedded into or projected onto applications, and not pushing applications on unwilling users, for a fairly homogenous and educated population, such as nurses, laboratory technologists, or physicians. It is especially difficult to do this with one application intended for populations that differ along many dimensions. Another important issue concerns the appeal of sus. If they are designed, as has been advocated, to be "seductive" or "persuasive" technologies, is that too manipulative [17,18]?

Sources on Methods

Coding

Glaser BG, Strauss AL. The Discovery of Grounded Theory: Strategies for Qualitative Research. New York: Aldine, 1967.

Strauss A, Corbin J. Basics of Qualitative Research: Grounded Theory Procedures and Techniques. Newbury Park, CA: Sage, 1990.

Displays

Miles MB, Huberman AM. Qualitative Data Analysis: A Sourcebook of New Methods. Beverly Hills: Sage, 1984.

Contextual and Narrative Analysis

Erickson F. Ethnographic microanalysis of interaction. In: LeCompte MD, Millroy WL, Preissle J, eds. The Handbook of Qualitative Research in Education. San Diego: Academic Press, 1992, pp. 201–25.

Gee JP, Michaels S, O'Connor MC. Discourse analysis. In: LeCompte MD, Millroy WL, Preissle J, eds. The Handbook of Qualitative Research in Education. San Diego: Academic Press, 1992, pp. 227–91.

Mishler E. Research Interviewing: Context and Narrative. Cambridge: Harvard University Press, 1986.

Seidman IE. Interviewing as Qualitative Research: A Guide for Researchers in Education and the Social Sciences. New York: Teachers College Press, 1991.

References

1. Kaplan B. A model comprehensive evaluation plan for complex information systems: clinical imaging systems as an example. In: Brown A, Remenyi D, eds. Proceedings of the Second European Conference on Information Technology Investment Evaluation. Henley on Thames, Birmingham, England: Operational Research Society; 1995, pp. 14–181.
2. Kaplan B. Impact of a clinical laboratory computer system: users' perceptions. In: Salamon R, Blum BI, Jørgensen JJ, eds. Medinfo 86: Fifth Congress on Medical Informatics. Amsterdam: North-Holland, 1986, pp. 1057–61.
3. Kaplan B. Initial impact of a clinical laboratory computer system: themes common to expectations and actualities. J Med Syst 1987;11:137–47.
4. Kaplan B, Duchon D. Combining qualitative and quantitative approaches in information systems research: a case study. Manag Inform Syst Q 1988;12:571–86.
5. Kaplan B, Duchon D. A job orientation model of impact on work seven months post implementation. In: Barber B, Cao D, Qin D, Wagner G, eds. Medinfo 89: Sixth Conference on Medical Informatics. Amsterdam: North-Holland, 1989, pp. 1051–5.
6. Kaplan B, Duchon D. Combining methods in evaluating information systems: case study of a clinical laboratory information system. In: Kingsland LC, III, ed. Proceedings of the Symposium on Computer Applications to Medical Care. Silver Spring, MD: IEEE Computer Society Press, 1989, pp. 709–13.

7. Glanz K, Shigaki D, Farzanfar R, Pinto B, Kaplan B, Friedman RH. Participant reactions to a computerized telephone system for nutrition and exercise counseling. Patient Educ Couns 2002;49:157–63.
8. Lundsgaarde HP, Fischer PJ, Steele DJ. Human Problems in Computerized Medicine. University of Kansas Publications in Anthropology, no. 13. Lawrence, KS: The University of Kansas, 1981.
9. Fischer P, Stratman W, Lundsgaarde H. User reactions to PROMIS: issues related to acceptability of medical innovations. In: Anderson JG, Jay SJ, eds. Use and Impact of Computers in Clinical Medicine. New York: Springer-Verlag, 1987, pp. 284–301.
10. Kaplan B, Shaw NT. People, organizational, and social issues: future directions in evaluation research. Methods Inform Med 2004;43:215–31.
11. Kaplan B, Farzanfar R, Friedman RH. Personal relationships with an intelligent interactive telephone health behavior advisor system: a multimethod study using surveys and ethnographic interviews. Int J Med Inform 2003;71:33–41.
12. Kaplan B. Addressing organizational issues into the evaluation of medical systems. J Am Med Inform Assoc 1997;4:94–101.
13. Kaplan B, Morelli R, Goethe J. Preliminary findings from an evaluation of the acceptability of an expert system in psychiatry. Extended Proc AMIA Symp (CD-ROM), 1997.
14. Kaplan B. Objectification and negotiation in interrupting clinical images: implications for computer-based patient records. Artif Intell Med 1995;7:439–54.
15. Kaplan B, Drickamer M, Marattoli RA. Deriving design recommendations through discount usability engineering: ethnographic observation and thinking-aloud protocol in usability testing for computer-based teaching cases. Proc AMIA Symp 2003, pp. 346–50.
16. Kaplan B, Brennan PF. Consumer informatics supporting patients as co-producers of quality. J Am Med Inform Assoc 2001;8:309–16.
17. King P, Tester J. The landscape of persuasive technologies. Comm ACM 1999;42:31–43.
18. Khaslavsky J, Shhedroff N. Understanding the seductive experience. Comm ACM 1999; 42:45–9.

8 Patient-to-Patient Communication: Support Groups and Virtual Communities

GUNTHER EYSENBACH

Virtual Communities

Virtual communities (or e-communities) have been defined as "social aggregations that emerge from the Net when enough people carry on . . . public discussions long enough, with sufficient human feeling, to form webs of personal relationships in cyberspace" [1]. Virtual communities can therefore be seen as social networks formed or facilitated through electronic media [2]. Although virtual communities already existed in the pre–World Wide Web era (e.g., in Bulletin Board systems), the primary medium for virtual communities is now the Internet. "Public discussions" leading to community building on the Internet take place in mailing lists, newsgroups/Usenet, or discussion forums with Web interface. Apart from these (asynchronous) venues, synchronous (real-time) community venues exist; for example, on Web sites such as *cancerpage.com* online support groups meet on designated days and at designated times in chat rooms.

In the health context, virtual communities often have the function and character of a self-support group and are then called electronic support groups (ESGs), where, for example, patients with a certain disease, consumers with a common health-related interest such as wanting to quit smoking or to lose weight, or informal (nonprofessional) caregivers exchange information and experiences. However, other communities primarily function as information exchange channels rather than serving as support groups (the latter of which involve providing and receiving emotional support). An example of an "information sharing" community is *remedyfind.com*, where consumers exchange personal experiences with medicines, diets, and treatments and rate the quality of these along the dimensions of effectiveness, lack of side effects, ease of use, effectiveness after long-term use, and cost-effectiveness. In addition, "wellness communities" exist, where healthy people exchange information and support on wellness and healthy lifestyles. Although most health-related virtual communities are unmoderated, some are facilitated by trained professionals.

As of August 2003, Yahoo!Groups listed 22.000 support groups in the Health & Wellness section. Among the most comprehensive online resource for electronic support groups is the Association of Cancer Online Resources (ACOR), founded by Gilles Frydman. After his wife was diagnosed with breast cancer, Frydman used a breast cancer mailing list that eventually led him to the conclusion that their physician was recommending far too radical a course of treatment, and he sought a second opinion. He was so impressed with the information he found on mailing lists that he tried to create a clearinghouse for mailing lists [3]. As of March 2003, the Web site (*http://www.acor.org*) hosts 235 cancer mailing lists, with 115,000 messages exchanged per day.

Virtual communities are an example of an entirely consumer-driven, consumer-developed health informatics application, rarely set up and run by health professionals. Community building features on hospital system, physician practice, or payer (HMOs, insurance) Web sites are the exception; most organizations fear negative discussions, libel, privacy violations, and potential liability arising from misinformation posted in these communities. Thus, setting up and managing communities (which is trivial from a technical standpoint, as it involves only a listserv software or a community-building website such as Yahoo!Groups) has been left largely to consumers. Still, as virtual communities are a low-cost intervention with potentially huge psychological benefits for participants, health researchers have increasingly become interested in understanding virtual peer-to-peer help processes and have set up and studied virtual communities.

Content Analysis of Messages

Content analysis is a method used primarily in the social and communication sciences to analyze text or transcripts. It has also been used to study e-mail exchanges [4] or for interactions in virtual communities (see later). To do a content analysis, researchers typically develop a coding framework (either starting from an a priori existing coding system such as from a prior publication, more often an iteratively developed framework as they go along) and code the themes of the messages. It is important to remember that in qualitative research the "what" is more important than the "how often". The text should ideally be coded independently by two researchers and the intercoder reliability should be reported. In addition to such manual analyses, a variety of software tools exist that can help to process and semiquantitatively analyze large amounts of texts. In the future, content analysis modules may be built into more sophisticated community platforms. While present community software suites typically provide message boards, chats, and polls, such advanced tools could provide the community manager with a content analysis tool just as standard statistical tools measure page views, members, and so forth.

According to a content analysis study of an electronic cancer support group, 80% of messages contained information giving/seeking, personal opinions, encouragement/support, and personal experiences, while the remaining 20% contained thanks, humor, and prayer [5]. An emphasis on the two pillars "information" and "support" was also found in other content analysis studies [6,7], mirroring findings from the literature on face-to-face self-help support groups [8]. Klemm notes interesting gender differences in the content of the messages, with women engaging in supportive messages more frequently than men, who used the electronic community primarily for information exchange [9], which again is similar to findings from face-to-face groups [8].

It has been suggested that virtual communities present an excellent opportunity for researchers to learn about preferences and experiences of patients—provided that the material it is obtained in an ethical manner [10]. Content analysis of messages exchanged on mailing lists or other virtual community venues can be a rich source for researchers interested in understanding experiences and views of people and patients, and is an opportunity not only to understand helping processes, but also to analyze where and why gaps exist between evidence-based medicine and consumer behavior and expectations, to identify priorities for patient education, and to identify outcomes that are important for patients. Such research may elicit a wealth of valuable data that may inform priorities for research, health communication, and education [10].

Ethical Issues of Content Analysis

Unfortunately, many studies have been published without appropriate ethical considerations or Institutional Review Board (IRB) approval. Many IRBs are also ignorant concerning the issues.

Three different groups of Internet-based research methods can be distinguished, and ethical considerations have to take into account different levels of "intrusion" of the researcher [11]. The least intrusive method is passive analysis, such as studies of information patterns on Web sites, or interactions on discussion groups, without the researchers actually involving themselves, for example, to study helping mechanisms and content of online self-help groups for colorectal cancer [5], breast cancer [6], Alzheimer's disease [12], and eating disorders [13]. Another kind of online research—slightly more intrusive—is through active analysis, in which researchers participate in the communications process incognito and post messages to analyze reactions, for example, to determine the accuracy of Usenet responses to a health question [14]. This method has an element of deception, as the researcher may pretend to be a consumer. The third group consists of methods in which researchers identify themselves as such and gather information in the form of online semistructured interviews or from online focus groups and Internet-based surveys, or use the Internet to recruit participants for "traditional" research.

In all of these cases, informed consent, a basic ethical tenet of scientific research on human populations [15–17], and the question whether it can be waived is an issue.

Although it is clear that in the third kind of research informed consent is a must, the "matter is less clear in the first and second kind of research. To determine whether "informed consent is required, one has first to decide whether postings on an Internet community are 'private' or 'public' communications. This distinction is important, as informed consent is required when behavior of research participants occurs in a private context where an individual can reasonably expect that no observation or reporting is taking place" [18]. On the other hand, "researchers may conduct research in public places or use publicly available information about individuals (e.g., naturalistic observations in public places, analysis of public records, or archival research) without obtaining consent" [18] and "research involving observation of participants in, for example, political rallies, demonstrations or public meetings should not require Research Ethics Board review since it can be expected that the participants are seeking public visibility" [19].

Although publication on the Internet may have parallels to publishing a letter in a newspaper, or saying something in a public meeting, there are important psychological differences, and individuals participating in an online discussion group cannot be assumed to be "seeking public visibility." In fact, on the Internet the dichotomy of "private" and "public" sometimes may not be appropriate; rather, communities may lie in a continuum between both. Several yardsticks can be considered to estimate the perceived level of privacy:

First, if a subscription, or some form of registration, is required to gain access to the discussion group, then the great majority of the subscribers are likely to regard the group as a "private place" in cyberspace [20].

Second, the number of (real or assumed) users of a community determines how "public" the space is perceived; a posting to a mailing list with 10 subscribers is different from a posting to a mailing list with 100 or 1000 subscribers. However, as sometimes messages sent to mailing lists are also stored in Web-accessible archives, the actual number of people accessing the messages may be greater than assumed and may in fact be impossible to determine.

Third, and perhaps most importantly, the perception of privacy depends on the individual group norms and codes, target audience, and aim of the particular mailing list, often laid down in the "frequently asked questions" or information files of Internet communities. For example, SickKids is a discussion list for children who are ill. The information file about the mailing list states that "adults will NOT be permitted to participate on this list as its purpose is to provide kids with their own personal place to share." It seems clear that those children who send messages to this list are very unlikely to be "seeking public visibility." Similarly, a virtual self-support group of sexual abuse survivors was reported to have a group policy explicitly discouraging interested professionals who were not sexual abuse survivors from joining the group [21], yet postings were analyzed without prior or retrospective consent having been obtained from the group members [22].

If it is felt that the community may be perceived "private," the next question is whether informed consent for passively analyzing the postings is needed or whether this requirement can be waived. In the medical area, nonintrusive medical research such as retrospective use of existing medical records may be ethically conducted without the express consent of the individual subjects if anonymity of the content is ensured at the earliest possible stage, if there is no inconvenience or hazard to the subjects, and if the IRB has reviewed and agreed on the research protocol [23]. Similar considerations may be applied to passive analysis of messages on mailing lists. When considering potential hazards to group participants or the community as a whole, privacy issues are especially important, and it should be considered whether publication of the results (especially when the group name is mentioned) may negatively affect group members or harm the community as a whole. Much will depend on which data will be collected and how they will be reported, how vulnerable the community or sensitive the topic is, and also on the degree to which the researcher interacts with group individuals.

Once it has been decided that informed consent should be obtained, there are basically two possibilities: The first is to send an e-mail to everyone on the mailing list, describing the research prospectively and giving participants the opportunity to withdraw from the list. The second is to ask retrospectively each individual whose postings have been or would be used, giving him or her an opportunity to withdraw from the analysis. Obtaining permission from the "listowner" (the individual responsible for maintenance of the mailing list) or moderator (if any) is rarely an adequate way for a researcher to obtain "community consent," as neither of them can properly claim to speak for all of the participants in a mailing list. Both approaches have disadvantages [10], but given that the first approach is very intrusive, the second approach is preferable. The third and perhaps best option is to build a community anew that is specifically created for the purpose of research, with appropriate consent obtained from each participant at the outset.

Proposed considerations for researchers and Institutional Review Boards before doing research on Internet communities. Researchers should explicitly address these issues in their research protocol [10].

1. **Intrusiveness:** Discuss to which degree the research conducted is intrusive ("passive" analysis of Internet postings versus active involvement in the community by participating in the communications).
2. **Perceived privacy:** Discuss—preferably with consultation with individual members of the community—the level of perceived privacy of the community (consider: closed group requiring registration? number of group members? group norms?).
3. **Vulnerability:** Discuss how vulnerable the community is. For example, a mailing list for sexual abuse victims or AIDS patients will be very vulnerable community.
4. **Potential harm:** As a result of considerations 1–3, discuss whether the intrusion of the researcher or mere publication of results have the potential to harm individuals or the community as a whole.
5. **Informed consent:** Discuss whether informed consent required or can be waived. If required, how will it be obtained?
6. **Confidentiality:** How can the anonymity of participants be protected? (If verbatim quotes are used, originators can be identified using search engines; thus informed consent is always required.)
7. **Intellectual property rights:** In some cases, participants may not seek anonymity, but publicity, so that use of postings without attribution may not be appropriate.

Advantages and Disadvantages of ESGs over Face-to-Face Groups

Advantages of virtual communities for patients over face-to-face self-support groups include absence of geographic and transport barriers, anonymity for stigmatizing, embarrassing or sensitive issues, increasing self-disclosure, and encouraging honesty and intimacy, and that even patients with rare diseases can find peers online. Electronic support groups seem to attract more men than traditional face-to-face support groups, where women participants outnumber men four to one [8]. The anonymity (or more accurately pseudonymity, as people often use pseudonyms) of virtual communities may facilitate participation of men, who may be culturally and socially conditioned not to ask for help and support in person.

Disadvantages of virtual communities include a large volume of mail with a considerable amount of "noise," negative emotions ("flaming," harassment of participants who do not agree with the majority opinion, encouraged by the veil of pseudonymity), and lack of physical contact and proximity [24]. As with content on the Web, there have been concerns over inaccurate or "non–evidence-based" information exchanged in virtual communities (see later) [12,25]. A recent topic analysis of messages from a mailing list for brain tumor patients found that alternative treatments were the most frequently discussed topics (15%), followed by debates about therapeutic strategy and about symptoms [26].

Quality Issues

As other Internet venues, electronic communities have been scrutinized by health researchers under the aspect of "quality." In one early study, investigators analyzed a drug information newsgroup, and concluded that about one half of the drug information was found to be correct in this newsgroup. Although 68% of the drug information was found to result in no harm, 19.4% was classified as harmful [27].

Even if the proportion of "harmful" messages is in fact lower in other communities, many communities are in fact flooded with messages offering dubious commercial products. Contrary to the popular believe that big pharmaceutical companies regularly infiltrate these communities pitching their products, the majority of advertising is in fact "peer-to-peer"—by consumers to consumers. The motivation of consumers to advertise even the most dubious health product (from shark cartilage to slimming soap) is often a financial incentive: an abundance of "affiliate" programs exist on the Web, paying referrers a commission (kickback). The more abstruse the product—from breast enlargement pills (*http://www.ultra-enhance.com/*) to penis enlargement pads (*http://www.enlargepatch.com*)—the higher seems to be the commission, and the more likely one of these "affiliates" abuses health communities for pitching these products.

The only possibility to avoid this is to "moderate" the community. Different levels of moderation exist; in some instances the moderator has to approve every message before it is posted and in other instances the moderator only screens the content and either reacts to or deletes messages deemed inappropriate.

Impact of Virtual Communities on Well-Being and Health Outcomes

While little rigorous evidence exists on the effectiveness of virtual communities [28], in the opinion of the author virtual communities may well be the one Internet application area with the biggest impact on health outcomes. Figure 8.1 illustrates the conceptual framework of how Internet use may affect health outcomes, illustrating the central role of communities (apart from the other two domains of the Internet, communication and content) to improve psychological, social, and health outcomes through facilitation of social networks, decreasing loneliness and depression [29]. Further, virtual communities not only have an (emotional) support function, but are also crucial in information exchange and help consumers to assess content found on other venues such as Web sites. (Questions such as, "I read *x* on *y*; can I believe this information?" are common, and the resulting discussions may help consumers to appraise information before asking a health professional.) Anecdotal reports from patients support the notion that they can benefit enormously from these interactions [3,30].

Virtual communities can also help individuals to seek professional care for problems not previously recognized as medical issues. (However, the opposite may sometimes also be true—people may delay professional help while relying on peer support.) In a cross-sectional analysis of participants in a depression community on various national partnersites of a major European health portal (Netdoktor), it was found that most of the respondents actually suffered from major depression (varying by country from 40% to 64%). However, almost half (49%) of users meeting criteria for major depression were not receiving treatment, and 35% had no consultation with health services in the previous year. On the other hand, 36% of repeat community users who had consulted

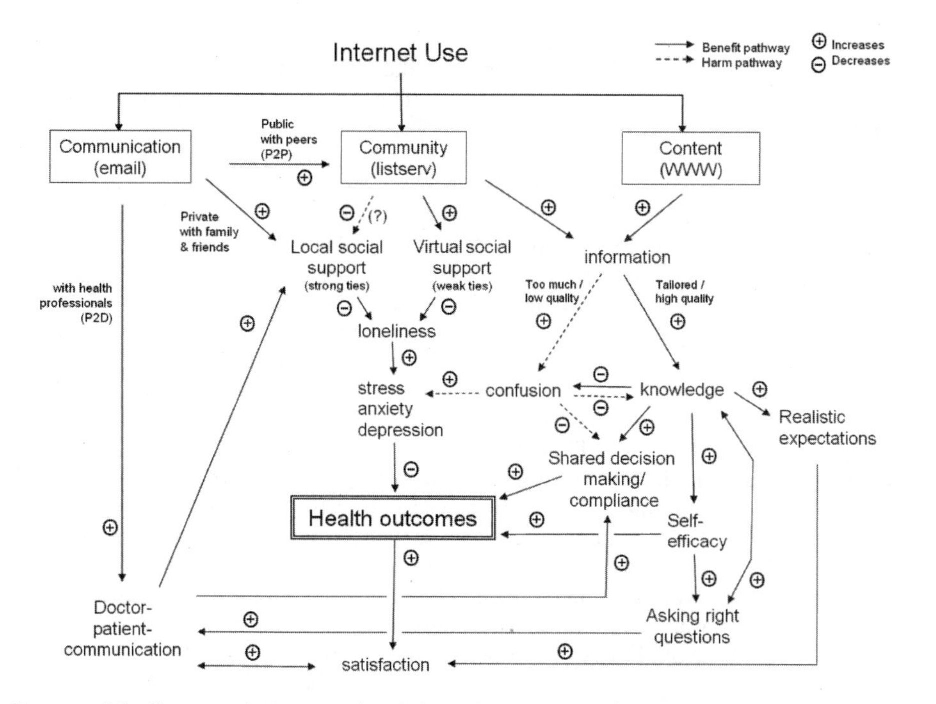

FIGURE 8.1. Conceptual framework of how Internet use (communication—community—content) may affect health outcomes, illustrating the central role of virtual communities. (Adapted from Eysenbach [30].)

a health professional in the previous year felt that the Internet community had been an important factor in decisions to seek professional help [31].

There is an ongoing debate on whether electronic communities in fact lead to social isolation and reduced well-being rather than strengthening social support. These concerns are based mainly on the controversial "Internet paradox" publication reporting results from a longitudinal study of the impact of the HomeNet project at Carnegie Mellon University, in which a sample of 169 persons were provided free computers and Internet and followed over a period of 1 to 2 years. The study provided alarming evidence of the possible harmful effects of Internet use [32]. The paradox was that a "social technology" (e-mail, newsgroups, and chat rooms) used primarily for interpersonal interaction apparently increased social isolation and decreased mental health and psychological well-being among its users. Heavy Internet use was associated with increases in loneliness and depression and tended to increase stress. To explain the paradox, the researchers reasoned that superficial relationships (weak ties) formed online displaced meaningful (strong tie) relationships in the real world.

It should be pointed out that the HomeNet study was conducted with healthy participants and not with patients. However, in a cross-sectional study looking at cancer patients in ESGs and face-to-face groups, Klemm and Hardie have recently noted a significant higher proportion of depressed cancer patients in ESGs (92%) compared to 0% depressed participants in face-to-face cancer support groups [33]. Does this mean that ESG participation causes depression? Or that face-to-face groups reduce depression, whereas ESGs do not? Or only that depressed individuals are primarily turning to electronic groups while staying away from face-to-face groups? Obviously, an association does not tell us anything about the causation sequence, and the latter explanation—or selection bias of the study participants—might be the most plausible explanation for this finding. Longitudinal studies or randomized trials are needed to investigate this question further.

On the other hand, there are numerous patient narratives [3,30] and studies reporting benefits for cancer patients that are incompatible with the notion that Internet use leads to depression. Fogel reports that Internet use in breast cancer patients is associated with increased perceived social support and decreased loneliness [34,35]. The most impressive study to date, a randomized controlled trial with participants of a breast cancer mailing list, suggests that a Web-based support group can be useful in reducing depression and cancer-related trauma, as well as perceived stress [36].

In summary, the overall "net benefits" of virtual communities—in particular in the health context—are unclear, and there is a lack of high-quality controlled trials addressing these questions [8,28]. It is likely that the majority of patients benefit from virtual communities, while a minority may prefer local face-to-face support and might not feel comfortable using computers to build up social relationships. In fact, when the authors of the original Internet paradox publication recently revisited their HomeNet study population after 3 years, which is now more experienced with Internet and computers, higher Internet use was associated with lower depression, and no significant association with loneliness was observed. The authors speculate that the negative findings from the early study phase might have been only a result of the novelty of the Internet and the fact that in the early years of the Web the nature of the Internet was different. The authors have also expanded their analysis and now argue that Internet use has positive effects on well-being for extroverted, highly sociable individuals, who have existing social support in "real life," while the opposite is true for introverted individuals, where the Web might interfere with real-life relationships [37]. Cancer patients participate more in online communities when they perceive that support received from a face-to-face partner was low [38]. In this situation it is unlikely that time spent to build up a virtual support network compromises local support, in particular as some ESGs actually lead to face-to-face meetings and "virtual" interactions can turn into strong and long-lasting social and emotional support relationships.

References

1. Rheingold H. The Virtual Community. New York: Harperperennial Library, 1993.
2. Wellman B. An electronic group is virtually a social network. In: Kiesler S, ed. Cultures of the Internet. Mahwah, NJ: Lawrence Erlbaum, 1997, pp. 179–205.
3. Landro L. Alone together. Cancer patients and survivors find treatment—and support—online. It can make all the difference. Oncologist 1999;4:59–63.
4. Eysenbach G, Diepgen TL. Patients looking for information on the Internet and seeking teleadvice: motivation, expectations, and misconceptions as expressed in e-mails sent to physicians. Arch Dermatol 1999;135:151–6.
5. Klemm P, Reppert K, Visich L. A nontraditional cancer support group. The Internet. Comput Nurs 1998;16:31–6.
6. Sharf BF. Communicating breast cancer on-line: support and empowerment on the Internet. Women Health 1997;26:65–84.
7. Weinberg N, Schmale J, Uken J, Wessel K. Online help: cancer patients participate in a computer-mediated support group. Health Soc Work 1996;21:24–9.
8. Klemm P, Bunnell D, Cullen M, Soneji R, Gibbons P, Holecek A. Online cancer support groups: a review of the research literature. Comput Inform Nurs 2003;21:136–42.

9. Klemm P, Hurst M, Dearholt SL, Trone SR. Gender differences on Internet cancer support groups. Comput Nurs 1999;17:65–72.
10. Eysenbach G, Till JE. Ethical issues in qualitative research on Internet communities. Br Med J 2001;323:1103–5.
11. Eysenbach G, Wyatt JC. Facilitating research via the Internet. In: McKenzie B, ed. Internet and Medicine. Oxford: Oxford University Press, 2002.
12. White MH, Dorman SM. Online support for caregivers. Analysis of an Internet Alzheimer mailgroup. Comput Nurs 2000;18:168–76.
13. Winzelberg AJ. The analysis of an electronic support group for individuals with eating disorders. Comput Human Behav 1997;13:393–407.
14. Seaboldt JA, Kuiper R. Comparison of information obtained from a Usenet newsgroup and from drug information centers. Am J Health Syst Pharm 1997;54:1732–5.
15. World Medical Association. Declaration of Helsinki: Ethical Principles for Medical Research Involving Human Subjects (last amended Oct 2000). *http://www.wma.net/e/policy/17-c_e.html* (accesses January 20, 2001).
16. Jones RA. The ethics of research in cyberspace. Internet Res 1994;4:30–5.
17. Frankel MS, Siang S. Ethical and Legal Issues of Human Subjects Research on the Internet—Report of an AAAS Workshop. Washington, DC, 1999.
18. American Sociological Association. American Sociological Association's Code of Ethics. *http://www.asanet.org/members/ecoderev.html.* 1997 (accesses January 12, 2001).
19. Tri-Council Policy Statement: Ethical Conduct for Research Involving Humans. *http://www.sshrc.ca/english/programinfo/policies/Index.htm.* 2000.
20. Mayer M, Till JE. The Internet: a modern Pandora's box? Qual Life Res 1996;5:568–71.
21. King SA. Researching Internet communities: proposed ethical guidelines for the reporting of results. Inform Soc 1996;12:119–28.
22. Finn J. An exploration of helping processes in an online self-help group focusing on issues of disability. Health Soc Work 1999;24:220–31.
23. Royal College of Physicians Committee on Ethical Issues in Medicine. Research based on archived information and samples. Recommendations from the Royal College of Physicians Committee on Ethical Issues in Medicine. J R Coll Phys Lond 1999;33:264–6.
24. Han HR, Belcher AE. Computer-mediated support group use among parents of children with cancer—an exploratory study. Comput Nurs 2001;19:27–33.
25. Culver JD, Gerr F, Frumkin H. Medical information on the Internet: a study of an electronic bulletin board. J Gen Intern Med 1997;12:466–70.
26. Mursch K, Behnke-Mursch J. Internet-based interaction among brain tumour patients. Analysis of a medical mailing list. Zentralbl Neurochir 2003;64:71–5.
27. Desai NS, Dole EJ, Yeatman ST, Troutman WG. Evaluation of drug information in an Internet newsgroup. J Am Pharm Assoc (Wash) 1997;NS37:391–4.
28. Eysenbach G, Powell J, Englesakis M, Rizo C, Stern A. Health related virtual communities and electronic support groups: systemic review of the effects of online peer to peer interactions. BMJ 2004;328:1166.
29. Eysenbach G. The impact of the Internet on cancer outcomes. CA Cancer J Clin 2003; 53:356–71.
30. Penson RT, Benson RC, Parles K, Chabner BA, Lynch TJ, Jr. Virtual connections: Internet health care. Oncologist 2002;7:555–68.
31. Powell J, McCarthy N, Eysenbach G. Cross-sectional survey of users of Internet depression communities. BMC Psychiatr 2003;3:19.
32. Kraut R, Lundmark V, Patterson M, Kiesler S, Mukopadhyay T, Scherlis W. Internet paradox: a social technology that reduces social involvement and psychological well-being? Am Psychol 1998;53:1017–31.
33. Klemm P, Hardie T. Depression in Internet and face-to-face cancer support groups: a pilot study. Oncol Nurs Forum 2002;29:E45–E51.
34. Fogel J, Albert SM, Schnabel F, Ditkoff BA, Neugut AI. Internet use and social support in women with breast cancer. Health Psychol 2002;21:398–404.

35. Fogel J, Albert SM, Schnabel F, Ditkoff BA, Neugut AI. Racial/ethnic differences and potential psychological benefits in use of the Internet by women with breast cancer. Psychooncology 2003;12:107–17.
36. Winzelberg AJ, Classen C, Alpers GW, et al. Evaluation of an Internet support group for women with primary breast cancer. Cancer 2003;97:1164–73.
37. Kraut R, Kiesler S, Boneva B, Cummings J, Helgeson V, Crawford A. Internet paradox revisited. J Soc Issues 2002;58:49–74.
38. Turner JW, Grube JA, Meyers J. Developing an optimal match within online communities: an exploration of CMC support communities and traditional communities. J Commun 2001; 51:231–51.

9 Electronic Patient-Centered Communication: E-Mail and Other E-Ways to Communicate Clinically

Daniel Z. Sands

From a 47-year-old attorney:

I love this Dr/e-mail thing. I enjoy bragging to my colleagues, family, and friends about communicating with my doctor via e-mail. Every one asks how it works and all seem enthusiastic about finally being able to communicate without traveling or catching the doctor by using the phone. It's really the best thing to happen to my personal health concerns. I now can enjoy house (or office) calls directly with the doctor and all without an appointment. Beat that!

Electronic mail and other forms of asynchronous electronic communication provide a channel complementary to other forms of communication through which patients and clinicians can communicate. Such electronic patient-centered communication (ePCC) can be useful in treating nonurgent medical issues, following up ongoing conditions, monitoring the impact of therapy, managing chronic conditions, and handling administrative tasks. Although nonsecured e-mail can be used, it is prudent when possible to use encrypted e-mail or a secure messaging gateway. The majority of online patients would like to communicate with their physicians electronically; physicians, on the other hand, have been reluctant to adopt this technology, citing reasons such as lack of remuneration, additional workload, and issues of liability. For physicians who have used this technology, however, these concerns have not generally been realized. Published guidelines are available to help physicians and organizations who are considering the use of electronic patient-centered communication. Electronic patient-centered communication will be increasingly adopted as physicians experience its benefits and become more comfortable with computer technology.

Background: E-Mail in Society

E-mail is the most popular activity among those who use the Internet, with well over 100 million e-mail users in the United States alone [1]. E-mail enables people to communicate asynchronously, or without regard for time. Using e-mail, parties can send and receive messages when it is most convenient for them, while allowing participants to stay in close touch. E-mail has enhanced communication among social networks and within extended families and has motivated people of all ages to acquire computer skills.

E-mail was first developed in the 1970s for use on the ARPANET (the predecessor to the Internet) and was initially used among academic and government researchers. E-mail systems were used early on in some medical facilities [2] and companies, and e-mail was rapidly adopted throughout the corporate world. It is hard to imagine not being able to use e-mail to communicate with friends, family, colleagues, and even customer service at companies with which we do business.

E-mail is as commonly used within health-related payer organizations as in the rest of the corporate world. According Vincent D. Plourde, Vice President, Provider Service Division, Blue Cross/Blue Shield of Massachusetts, "In today's fast-paced, highly competitive marketplace, the lack of immediate access to real-time information is a competitive disadvantage. Simple e-mail capabilities have transformed the way that business is conducted forever. I can't imagine how we operated without it" [3]. It is used between health care administrators and many provide it to their employees and affiliated physicians, who find it useful for administrative and interclinician communication.

E-Mail in Patient Care

In one major Boston teaching hospital, a large proportion of e-mail used by clinicians centered on patient care [4]. Despite the widespread use of e-mail among clinicians, recent surveys of physicians show that fewer than one quarter have used e-mail with patients [5], and well under 10% do so regularly. Between 45% and 90% of patients who use the Internet would like to e-mail their physicians [6,7], yet only about 5% are able to do so [6]. Lest we think that only healthy patients wish to use e-mail with their physicians, a survey of patients with chronic illness suggested that they too found e-mail communication with their physicians particularly useful [8]. In fact, for the disabled, who may find it difficult to go to see their physician or communicate once there, e-mail can be more useful than an office visit or a phone call. Furthermore, in another survey, 44% of patients who were not using e-mail with their physicians said that they would be willing to change physicians to find one who used e-mail [9].

E-Mail Characteristics

E-mail has properties that make it useful in clinical practice. Most important among these is asynchrony. This means simply that when communicating, parties do not need to be available at the same time. E-mail fulfills an important need in health care because the most commonly used channels of communication—telephone calls and office visits—are synchronous, requiring parties to exchange information simultaneously. Because both physicians and their patients are busy and highly mobile, this leads to frustration from "telephone tag" and unnecessary office visits. (Of course, another form of asynchronous electronic communication, the fax machine, is ubiquitous in medical offices, although meaningful communication outside of paperwork rarely takes place via fax. One notable exception to this is an offering from a company called MDHub, which permits patients to send messages to physicians via fax [10].)

Because it is asynchronous, e-mail permits communication at the convenience of both the patient and the clinician. This is important for physicians because it allows them to "time shift" and manage their time better. In addition, patients may prefer to send messages to their physicians at night, after they return from work and have put their children to bed. Whereas it would be inappropriate to call about a nonurgent issue at night, it is perfectly acceptable to send e-mail. Physicians also benefit from being able to give careful consideration to the responses they give to patients. This is in contrast to a telephone conversation or appointment, during which answers may be either incomplete or incorrect owing to time constraints beyond the physician's control.

A concern about time shifting is that patients or their physicians might inappropriately use e-mail to communicate about an urgent or time-sensitive issue. For example, a patient who has crushing substernal chest pain, which might represent a heart attack, should not use e-mail to communicate. Likewise, a physician should not use e-mail to contact a patient with a dangerously abnormal blood test result. If both parties remember that this is not real-time communication, problems should not occur. It is also possible that a patient would use e-mail to communicate about a constellation of symptoms that, unbeknownst to him or her, represents a medical emergency. However, the same problem occurs with telephone messages left on voice mail or with non-medically trained secretaries or medical assistants. Yet like e-mail, these forms of communication remain so useful that the risk is outweighed by the overall benefits.

E-mail is also comfortable. Many people have been using it long enough that sending messages becomes as casual and comfortable as placing a telephone call, which makes e-mail a democratizing medium that breaks down barriers to communication. But despite the comfort that a clinician might feel when composing an e-mail message to a patient, he or she should make certain that the message will not be misunderstood and will maintain an appearance of professionalism.

Despite its informality, e-mail is permanent. Copies of electronic messages can be recovered from both the sender's and recipient's computers, even when the users have deleted them. Copies can also be retrieved from mail servers used to send or receive e-mail. Because e-mail is digital, it is easily replicable and can be transmitted to others who may store copies that can be recovered. E-mail can also be printed and stored as hardcopy.

The permanence of e-mail may be of concern to physicians, who may recall recent legal trials in which accused politicians and high-level executives were incriminated by e-mail messages that were uncovered during investigation. E-mail, like any written information, is legally discoverable. But the advantages of permanence are many. For example, physicians who typically document only a minority of telephone messages with their patients could have difficulties when defending themselves against malpractice suits. In contrast, e-mail is self documenting: it provides a transcript of the dialog and can be readily printed and stored in the paper record or in a computer-based record system.

Patients also benefit from the permanence of e-mail; it allows them to review and reflect on messages from their physicians. Typically, patients recall less than half of what their physicians tell them in the office or on the telephone. Despite this, physicians almost never encourage patients to video- or even audiotape encounters. E-mail permits leisurely review of the physician's words in the comfort of home and with the input of loved ones.

The accessibility of electronic communication is also one of its weaknesses; the security of e-mail is less than optimal for health-related communication. First, it is easy to "spoof" identity with e-mail, so that a message might appear to be from a physician or a patient when in fact it originated from someone else. Second, e-mail can be intercepted, although with the great volume of e-mail messages being sent this is not likely to occur unless a particular clinician or patient is targeted. If intercepted, nonencrypted e-mail can be easily read. (Employers are legally permitted to intercept and read e-mail messages sent on their computer systems.) Third, e-mail can be misaddressed. If the incorrect e-mail address is not a legitimate e-mail account, the message will be returned to the sender; however if the address corresponds to an existing recipient, inappropriate disclosure of health information will result. Finally, it is difficult to ensure that the intended recipient received and read the message. An e-mail message intended for a patient might be read by a family member with a shared computer or e-mail account. Technological solutions to these shortcomings are available in the form of encrypted e-mail and secure messaging portals, which are discussed in the paragraphs that follow. In the absence of some form of secure communication, it would be prudent to adopt a policy that prohibits the use of unencrypted e-mail for sensitive issues, such as those involving psychiatric disease, substance abuse, sexually transmitted disease, HIV, and domestic violence.

Electronic messaging is also different from face-to-face communication in that it does not permit the use of visual or aural cues, which can be important for conveying warmth, bad news, and humor. In addition, it is less than useful when messages are long or require negotiation. Despite these limitations, e-mail messages are a powerful transmitter of information when used appropriately.

Appropriate Use of E-Mail

For electronic messaging to be effective in patient care, it must be used in appropriate situations:

- Prescription renewals
- Appointment requests
- Referrals to specialists
- Name, address, phone number, or insurance information changes
- Non-urgent medical issues
- Monitoring chronic conditions (e.g., diabetes, asthma, headaches)
- Monitoring effects of therapy
- Follow-up on behavioral interventions (e.g., smoking cessation, dietary changes)

Because of the properties of electronic communication, it becomes apparent that there are situations in which electronic communication should not be used, which include:

- Medical emergencies or time-sensitive issues because of its asynchronous nature
- Issues requiring lengthy messages
- Issues requiring negotiation through long volleys of messages that become cumbersome
- Communicating bad news, which is best done in person
- Sensitive issues at risk of disclosure due to potentially weak security mechanisms
- When confronted with an electronic message from a patient that does not lend itself to electronic response, it is important that clinicians using electronic communication with patients be unafraid to explain to the patient (via telephone, if necessary) that an appointment or phone call may be necessary.

Alternatives to E-Mail

Electronic mail is a readily available, comfortable, asynchronous communication technology, making it useful in nonurgent clinical communications. However, there are several caveats when e-mail is used for electronic patient-centered communication.

First, plain text e-mail does not readily support forms, templates, or questionnaires that can help patients to more effectively structure their messages. With branched-logic questionnaires, Patients can answer questions relevant to their specific health problems, and avoid the need for multiple back and forth messaging volleys. Responses to questionnaires can then present information concisely to the clinician to help with efficiency [11]. Forms can be used to acquire structured information for prescriptions renewals, specialty referrals, and other requests. On the clinicians' side, tools such as templates can allow them to provide patients with reusable or structured health information more efficiently.

Second, as mentioned earlier, e-mail is not secure. Although for the most part e-mail can be used safely without difficulties, there is substantial risk of inappropriate disclosure. The Health Insurance Portability and Accountability Act (HIPAA) mandates the encryption of electronically transmitted patient information. Although HIPAA suggests that e-mail transmission between patients and clinician be encrypted, the legislation does not prohibit patient–clinician use of e-mail. In fact, the administrative simplification act of HIPAA was actually intended to *encourage* electronic communication in health care, with the proviso that appropriate attention be given to issues or privacy and security [12]. If encrypted communication is not to be used, a policy must be in place to explicitly state the rationale for its omission and any safeguards that are in place in its stead. As discussed, many of the security threats are user rather than technology based, so encryption solves only part of the problem.

Most popular e-mail applications allow the use of digital certificates, which permit the use of encryption with a public–private key technique. Unfortunately, this method requires a trusted certificate authority and necessitates an awkward process of obtaining and then installing the certificates, something that is cumbersome in practice and is not supportable in an open system in which not all parties are under the jurisdiction of a single enterprise. Technological solutions to this problem have been implemented, often using "plug-ins" or modules that work with popular e-mail systems. Those not registered within the enterprise mail system can send and receive messages using an ordinary Web browser. An advantage of this method is that each person can use his or her own e-mail program. Although this resolves the security issues of e-mail, it is still text-based communication and not easily capable of using questionnaires, forms, and templates. In addition, this solution is most powerful when used within an organization or with trusted outside partners. Examples of this technology are available through Zix Corporation [13], Sigaba [14], and Kryptiq [15].

A simpler solution is to establish a secure Web server that allows authorized users to communicate using browsers at both ends of the interaction, a solution referred to as a "secure messaging portal" or "secure messaging gateway." When a message is sent on a secure messaging portal, the recipient is generally notified via regular e-mail that there is a message waiting to be retrieved from the server. The recipients then click on the link in their e-mail message, their browser opens to the login page of the portal, and they log in with their username and password. The encryption technology is the same used to provide secure interactions with financial institutions. Secure messaging portals have a number of advantages over e-mail: they can effectively and securely deliver interactivity, questionnaires, and multimedia information; they can easily acquire structured data; they can display data from multiple sources; they do not require special programs or plug-ins to be installed on users' computers; they can support the workflow of the practice including the automatic routing of messages within the system; and they use commonly available technology. Examples of companies offering secure communication portals are MyDocOnline [16], RelayHealth [17], and Medem [18]. While these portals resolve the problems of unecrypted e-mail, they introduce the conundrum that the messaging application is different from the e-mail application that is used comfortably and conveniently for all other communications. However, these systems can be very useful as secure, structured communication tools.

Because secure messaging portals can display data from multiple sources, they lend themselves to integration with electronic health records, permitting patients to see their health records, including test results. One example is *PatientSite*, which was developed at Beth Israel Deaconess Medical Center and CareGroup Healthcare System and has been in use since April 2000 [19,20]. As of this writing, *PatientSite* is being used by more than 20,000 patients and 200 clinicians in almost 50 practices. Although very few health provider organizations are attempting to build systems like this on their own, a number of the major electronic health record (EHR) vendors—including Epic, GE Medical Systems, and Cerner—now have modules that are designed to provide this functionality to patients and their clinicians who use their EHR systems. The clinician or provider organization should determines which of the communication options they wish to implement, based on their functional needs and budget, and the population with whom they will be communicating [21]. For example, a small practice of modest means might choose to use unencrypted e-mail (with a policy on file explaining why encryption is not being used) or better, an encrypted e-mail application. More complex practices or healthcare provider organizations would be better served utilizing a secure messaging portal. A good fit between the system chosen and the needs of the organization will facilitate the implementation process. A comparison of the features of various types of patient-provider communication is shown in Table 9.1 [22].

Implementation

Three sets of stakeholders that need to be involved with implementation of an electronic communication system: the patients, the clinicians, and the practice staff. Each of these constituencies has its special needs that must be addressed, and representatives of each group should be involved with all aspects of the implementation.

Regardless of the technology, everyone in the practice should have access to the system so that they can send and receive messages. In that way, even if ordinary e-mail is used, messages can be forwarded to support staff who can manage tasks such as prescription renewals and appointment requests.

Organizations must decide who should be the first contact for various types of messages coming into the practice. This depends on which technology the practice is using. With e-mail, all messages can be directed to the physician, who can then forward them as appropriate. Alternatively, an alias can be set up for all incoming messages (e.g., *info@drjohnsmith.com*). Messages can then be reviewed by a triage nurse or secretary and routed to the appropriate staff. If the message volume is manageable, all messages can be directed to the physician, who can then route them as appropriate. Having the doctor as the focal point may be acceptable, though physicians who are reluctant to use e-mail may be hesitant to do this for fear of being overrun by messages. Multiple aliases can also be established, such as *appointments@drjohnsmith.com* or *rx@drjohnsmith.com*, with the disadvantage that this requires that patients remember these various e-mail addresses and use them appropriately.

Secure messaging portals can generally route different types of messages automatically to the groups of personnel within the practice who can best handle the messages. Still, a decision must be made about who should handle clinical messages, that is, which ones can be managed by physicians or clinical support staff, such as triage nurses or

Table 9.1. Attributes of various types of patient-clinician communication (from NEJM).

Current Attributes			Future Evolution
Telephone	Conventional E-Mail	Secure Messaging	
Synchronous	Asynchronous	Asynchronous	Secure synchronous and asynchronous, sometimes substituting for personal encounters
Almost universally accessible	Increasingly accessible	Not yet widely available	
Highlights vocal expression and nuance; lacks visual and written content	Encourages informal, written expression; lacks aural and visual content	Encourages informal, written expression; lacks aural and visual content	Integrated with patient-controlled personal health record Video conferencing and messaging
Good for urgent communication	Not good for urgent communication	Not good for urgent communication	Instant voice transcription into written record
Not automatically documented in records	Self-documenting	Self-documenting; readily linked to electronic records	Full patient access to notes and reports
Messages may be heard by others; call triage can be automated through menus	Susceptible to interception; messages manually routed to others	Secure; automated forwarding to professionals and support staff	Automated access to medical glossaries Translation into different languages
Rarely reimbursed	Reimbursed by some payers	Reimbursed by some payers	Connectivity to multiple data sources
		Platform for reminders, questionnaires, medication refills, appointments, test results, educational material	Incorporation of multimedia educational material Data from home-based diagnostic technology sent to clinicians

physicians' assistants. In larger organizations, one must decide if these will be handled at the practice level or in a central call center.

Once the practice has determined how incoming messages will be routed and handled, clinicians must decide if they will offer electronic messaging to all patients immediately or if they will limit the number of patients at first, until they feel more comfortable with using the system. This latter approach is likely to be more acceptable to those physicians who are reluctant to try this new technology. On the other hand, this deprives the excluded patients of the benefits of electronic communication until it is can be offered more widely in the practices.

The process of enrolling patients in the communication system requires several steps. If e-mail is being used, there is no registration involved; one only needs to provide an e-mail address and record the patient's e-mail address. The patient's e-mail address should be verified frequently, since e-mail addresses change even more often than home addresses or telephone numbers. If a secure messaging portal is being used, there will be a defined process for patient registration. In some cases, patient demographic information will be imported from a practice management system or EHR, but in other cases this will need to be reentered (introducing the possibility of errors). Once this is done, the patient can be given a username and temporary password, either in person, through the telephone, or via postal mail. Once patients log in for the first time, they are requested to change to a password of their choice.

When registering patients, the identity of the patient must be firmly established, especially when portals are used that permit patients to see parts of their medical record.

dsands@caregroup.harvard.edu

Please Follow These Rules to Improve Communication

1. Use alternative forms of communication for:
   - emergencies and other time-sensitive issues
   - sensitive information (do not assume e-mail is confidential)
   - situations in which my response is delayed (I may be away)
2. Be concise
3. Put your name and BI number in the subject line
4. Keep copies of e-mail you receive from me
5. I may save e-mail I send and receive in your record
6. I may share your messages with my office staff or with consultants (if necessary)

FIGURE 9.1. Back of business card with e-mail guidelines.

The people most likely to want to have inappropriate access to this information are those close to the patient, who know enough about the patient to enable them to masquerade in his or her place. Because of this, every attempt must be made to verify patient identity through personal contact or telephone communication prior to giving account information.

There are legitimate reasons that family or other caregivers may need to communicate on behalf of a patient. This *proxy access* is important for parents of children or those responsible for elderly or disabled patients or for those unable to use a computer. A properly established proxy access would indicate on each e-mail message that the message was sent from the proxy on behalf of the patient. These messages should then be stored in to the patient's record, not the record of the proxy.

A critical component of the implementation process is agreement between the patient and the clinician about the guidelines for the use of this technology, including an understanding of the potential risks. Guidelines for the use of e-mail in patient care have been available since 1998 [23–26]. A discussion about electronic communication policy can be conducted either by the clinician or by office staff, but the discussion should be documented in the medical record much like any informed consent agreement. Some practices may choose to have the patient sign a standard agreement that can be filed in the office and a copy given to the patient. If a secure messaging portal is in use, the process of explaining appropriate use can take place online through the Web site, and the system can record patient assent to the guidelines automatically. In my practice, since 1998 I have been providing a summary of the guidelines on the back of my business card (see Fig. 9.1).

Other Practice Issues

Other issues arise in the use of e-mail in health care. As previously discussed, copies of e-mail conversations must be stored in the patient's medical record. This is important for reasons of medico–legal risk management but also for communication with colleagues who may be caring for patients. Patients must be informed that their messages will be stored in their medical records.

Clinicians and their practices need to determine service guarantees for response time, with reasonable policies being anything from one to three business days. Patients should be made aware of these time delay policies. Because not all of a patient's concerns require the same alacrity of response, one might institute a policy that allows the patient to dictate his or her expectations: if patients do not receive their responses soon enough, they should be advised to escalate communication to a telephone call or visit. When clinicians are unable to check messages for more than a day, there should be a function (often built into e-mail programs and secure messaging portals) that allows them to let senders know about their absence and to direct messages to clinicians who are covering for them.

Electronic messaging is useful for sharing messages among members of a healthcare team, but patients need to understand that their messages may be shared. When using unencrypted e-mail, certain additional issues arise that must be addressed by policy. For example, clinicians must take great care that messages are not misaddressed. A safeguard against this is for physicians to reply to messages sent by patients but never initiate messages themselves, thereby avoiding such misdirection. Messages must not be sent to more than one patient; otherwise, patients' identities will be revealed to other patients. (The blind copy [BCC] function of e-mail prevents recipients' e-mail addresses from appearing on any message other than the one intended for them.)

Physician Concerns: Real and Imagined

Physicians remain reluctant to use electronic communication with their patients: as mentioned, only about a quarter have communicated electronically with patients and few regularly do so [5] for reasons that include concerns about time, money, legal liability, and security [27]. In addition, physicians are concerned about the time needed to learn to use this "new" technology in their practices.

The most valuable commodity to most physicians is time. Because of this, physicians fear that introducing electronic communication into their practices will increase the time they will be working. There are a few misconceptions about this. First, it is more efficient to respond to an e-mail message than to handle a telephone call. Typically, an e-mail message will take 1 to 5 minutes to handle, whereas a telephone call, if the patient and physician can connect, will rarely be less than 5 minutes in duration and often longer. Next, *when* that time is spent is almost as important as how much time is spent. Electronic communication permits users to *time-shift*, handling communication when it's most convenient for them. In some cases, this might be early in the morning or late at night, times when one should not call patients on the telephone. Furthermore, experience has shown that patients do not for the most part overload their physicians with messages. In our institution we have found that for every 100 patients able to send a clinical message, a physician will receive less than one message per day on average [28]. Moreover, these messages are concise, in contrast with telephone conversations, because it is more difficult to ramble in written communication. Structured communication and customized online interviews that can be offered through a secure messaging portal make this type of communication even more efficient.

Having stated that, many physicians believe they should be reimbursed for the care they deliver electronically: 66% of physicians would adopt this technology if reimbursed [5]. Arguably, physicians should be reimbursed for all nonvisit care, whether delivered by telephone, fax, e-mail, or videoconference [29]. We have had billing codes to bill for telephone care for quite some time, but very few payers will reimburse for this activity. Arguably, it is more compelling to bill for electronic communication since there is a better "paper" trail of the care that was delivered. In 2004, the American Medical Association issued a code for reimbursements for online consultations [30]. It remains to be seen whether insurers, including the federal government, will reimburse for the care that is delivered this way.

In the meantime, some payers are studying the impact of reimbursement for structured electronic communication, generally with a portion (copay) paid by the patient, much like what takes place in an office visit [31,32]. Early results show satisfaction among both clinicians and patients and a cost savings to the healthcare system.

Outside of these well-defined pilot projects, some physicians are charging their patients for electronic communication. While some do this by message or incident of care, others are opting for a monthly or annual subscription fee that may cover other services in addition to e-mail as a communication option. One step up from this, of course, is concierge medicine, in which patients pay a subscription fee to get care from a practice that offers deluxe services, among which is electronic access to their physicians.

Another concern of physicians is their legal liability through the use of this new technology. While there is no tort case yet involving electronic communication [33], certainly there will be. Already, e-mail messages are routinely subpoenaed during malpractice cases, but more often these are communications between clinicians and not between patient and clinician. The use of electronic communication does not actually increase liability exposure; it just provides better documentation of interactions between patient and physician, making the details of these interactions more apparent. This is actually an advantage for reducing liability: although improving documentation does not eliminate all liability, better documentation reduces malpractice exposure. Furthermore, improving communication between patients and their clinicians by whatever means reduces the risk of a malpractice suit [34,35]. Spielberg has written extensively about legal issues in physician patient communication using electronic mail [36,37].

Physicians are also concerned about the security of this new technology; "hacker attacks" and security leaks are fodder for the evening news. As discussed earlier, the low-tech risks to security are actually more common and more likely to occur than malicious security breaches. Nevertheless, prudence would dictate that physicians use encrypted e-mail or secure messaging portals unless there is a compelling reason not to do so.

The last issue for consideration is physicians' reluctance to incorporate a new technology into their practices. Using electronic communication with patients takes practice, and physicians aren't comfortable fumbling with a new technology, particularly when others (patients, support staff) may see their mistakes. Furthermore, using electronic communication requires a change in workflow. Physicians are creatures of habit and often slow to change. This conservatism can serve patients well, since physicians are often reluctant to try new drugs or order new tests until they've become convinced of their safety and efficacy, but even then they can be slow to adopt [38]. They will try things sooner if they see benefit to themselves. In the case of e-mail with their patients, not enough has been done to prove to physicians the benefits of this technology, although research is ongoing.

Evaluation of Benefits

There are as yet few studies of the benefits of electronic patient-centered communication, and they are hampered by selection bias, because only those who already like this technology are using it. Although surveys of physicians who do not use this technology have elicited concerns, studies thus far suggest that there are benefits to patients, to clinicians, and even to payers.

Physicians who use ePCC regularly feel that it is a good way to communicate with patients [39,40]. For example, Houston et al. interviewed/surveyed physicians who were already regularly using e-mail with their patients and found that three fourths were satisfied with it, particularly when they believed that e-mail saved time or improved care delivery. Satisfied physicians were more likely to adhere to published guidelines. Dissatisfaction was associated with physician use of electronic communication when the only reason for their use was that their patients requested it.

A qualitative analysis of physician interviews by Patt et al. concluded that e-mail can be useful with select groups of patients. Further work was suggested to determine which clinical issues lend themselves to asynchronous management, how to best integrate messaging into workflow, and reimbursement for electronic messaging. Whether e-mail volume offsets telephone message volume or visit volume is controversial. In my experience, electronic messaging does offset telephone messages among patients who can use electronic messaging, but since many patients cannot yet use this communication channel, the reduction in telephone messages overall is negligible. Katz et al. [41] found in their study of a triage-based e-mail system that e-mail volume did not offset telephone volume or visits. Users of the system were satisfied, however.

RelayHealth and a number of payers commissioned a case-control study of online care for more than 5000 patients for one year. They found that patients reported reduced absenteeism, reduced telephone calls, and reduced numbers of physician visits. Most impressive was the finding that total healthcare spending was reduced by over $3 per patient per month. Both physicians and patients were satisfied. A smaller but peer-reviewed study of the same secure messaging portal by Liederman and Morefield showed that physicians and patients were satisfied and that physicians did not find the message volume problematic. Satisfaction among patients was correlated with speed of response. The system did not adversely affect physician productivity.

More work remains to be done to study the impact of ePCC on relationships, workflow, productivity, physician reimbursement, and patient preferences [42]. However, preliminary results are promising.

In a Patient's Own Words

Patient comments are often quite instructive. One patient, a 61-year-old retired minister with advanced diabetes, chronic pain syndrome, gait disturbance, and osteoarthritis, spent quite a bit of time reflecting on what the use of e-mail (in this case through *PatientSite*) meant to him:

Case Study

1. With e-mail you don't have to stress over calling your doctor, and bothering him or her, or feeling that simple questions that you need an answer to seem to be requiring you to push a panic button.
2. I feel in touch with my doctor, simple questions used to take cumbersome phone calls, visits, or long lists of questions at visits. Now with short and simple notes in e-mail to my doctor my follow-up visits take much less time and are more productive.
3. With e-mail, I can take the time at home to think out my questions, achieving the detail I feel needed to be specific, short, and direct. Using my time, and not my

doctor's. That takes a lot of pressure off of me, because I am always tongue tied at my doctor's office.

4. With e-mail, I can get my questions and symptoms all together in a simplified manner, and e-mail my notes to my doctor just before our visit.

a. In this, I get the chance to tell my doctor what I need to express, [. . .] and I feel comfortable that I have told my doctor everything I needed to say.

b. Because of simple e-mail communication with my doctor, I never leave a visit anymore feeling that I forgot to mention important thoughts or symptoms. I feel relieved that my doctor is in better control, because my communication was in better control. This is worth a million dollars!

5. Making a list for my doctor's visit, or dealing with less urgent matters through e-mail just before my visit, makes for much shorter and less complicated visits. That makes me feel as if I've helped my doctor by saving time. That's a good feeling; it really is.

6. As a patient, I often let physical problems go until they get very complicated, for fear of disturbing my doctor with phone calls. Sometimes the time and confusion it will take to try and get a call through causes me to put things off.

Now I send a few simple e-mails, but I have far less problems. I can e-mail my doctor at any time, day or night. If it's late at night, I can send an e-mail off to my doctor, knowing that he or she will get it at some point. With e-mail communication I get my message out, and I feel better doing it when I was feeling bad—that helps a great deal! I know my doctor will answer when [he or she gets] the chance next day. That is a very big comfort!!! Emergencies are a different matter!

7. The horror of phone tag! There is nothing worse for a patient than having to call your doctor for medication questions, simple medical issues, or something that is important to you! Your doctor is busy, and you know that.

You may wait all day for the doctor's call. You don't dare leave your phone; you can't get anything done because you're waiting for that doctor's call. You don't dare to use your phone; you quickly cast your friends' calls off so as not to tie up the phone. You ask your family not to use the phone.

With a quick and simple e-mail, you and your doctor can be about your business. No pressure for the patient or doctor; when the doctor has a chance he or she will e-mail you; you won't miss that e-mail, and you know that.

This method of communication with your doctor offers great relief for the patient and allows you to take calls and get things done. This is an important factor!

8. E-mail with my doctor has allowed me to feel more secure and in touch with my doctor and my whole medical team. A whole medical system is a very large thing to a patient. Direct e-mail communication with my doctor, brings it all together, because your doctor brings it together. You feel welcome, not [like] an intruder.

9. E-mail communication with my doctor and medical team has given me control over my medication refills, which allows me to request my prescriptions be sent to the necessary person. That keeps my pharmacist happy, and saves him or her time, and it saves my doctor time. For me, it's so much easier, less complicated, and prevents a much larger number of errors. That helps everyone, and avoids the need for repeated trips to your drug store because things weren't ready.

10. E-mail through *PatientSite* helps me keep track of my appointments by listing them and by reminding me when they are coming up. For a person with memory problems, that is a great help!

11. E-mail through *PatientSite*, allows me to graph my diabetic control, weight control, fluid control, and other issues. That helps me a great deal and provides a record for my doctor to check out at our visits.

12. [T]hrough *PatientSite* [I have] been able to check labs and test results, which helps me to ask intelligent questions.

13. Through [. . .] *PatientSite* it is very helpful for me to be able to check drug interactions, and look up many of the things my doctor explains to me. I get greater detail, become more informed, and that helps me a great deal.

E-mail, and doctor–patient communications through it, has made my life less complicated, given me greater hope, and has helped me to see just how much help there is behind me and my doctor.

I have a lot of medical issues, and this e-mail system has left me feeling comfortable, and in good hands! Otherwise, I would feel as cold, depleted, and alone, at the lifeless tree in my front yard, in the deepest of winter!

For me, this e-mail system is a warm hearth in the storm. Never underestimate its importance to your patients!

Future Directions

Within the next few years, Internet use will become increasingly ubiquitous among our patients. These connected patients will demand that their physicians communicate with them and provide services electronically, just as they expect all companies and professionals with whom they interact to offer online services. At the same time, healthcare clinicians will discover that computers are as indispensable to medical practice as a stethoscope and that the Internet is as useful as the telephone and fax machine. These parallel tracks of adoption will foretell the widespread use of electronic patient-centered communication.

Physicians will adopt electronic communication as they discover that it allows them to be more efficient and that it supports the provision of better care for their patients. Rather than being controlled by technologies that require synchronous communication, physicians will be able to deliver care to patients whenever and wherever they and their patients happen to be.

Electronic patient centered communication will come to include attached images, documents, sounds, waveforms, videos and other objects, enabling patients and physicians to share important health-related information. Secure messaging portals will make it easy for patients to upload almost any type of information from their personal health record or home monitoring equipment, which would then be easily shared with their physicians. When necessary, synchronous communication modalities, such as telephone conversations, instant messaging, and videoconferencing will be utilized to enhance information transfer. And all of this will be as commonplace as our use of a fax machine and telephone today.

Physicians will also gravitate to online consultations because of financial incentives. These will be the result of payment for individual online "visits," subscriptions for unlimited online consultation, concierge practice arrangements, reduced malpractice premiums, or reimbursement for managing panels of patients rather than payment for visits. Furthermore, physicians who use these technologies will be at a competitive advantage over their technology-averse colleagues.

Patients who do come into the office will be there because that the office visit is the best way to manage their problems. In some cases, the choice of channel through which to communicate may be a function of patient or physician preference for face-to-face interaction. Since physicians will be reimbursed regardless of the channel of their care delivery, they will have little incentive to overfill their schedule and their waiting rooms with patients who could be better managed online. In the end, there may be fewer office-based encounters, but those that do occur will be of higher quality or intensity.

Electronic patient-centered communication is a technology whose time has come and physicians must learn how to integrate it into their practices.

Acknowledgments. The author wishes to acknowledge Kayla Cytryn, RN, PhD, and Warner Slack, MD, for their invaluable assistance with the manuscript for this chapter.

General References

In addition to the cited references below, the following are good general references on this topic:

Sands DZ. Electronic patient centered communication resource center. At *http://www.e-pcc.org*, (accessed March 24, 2004).

MacDonald K, Case J, Metzger J. E-Encounters. California HealthCare Foundation. At *http://www.chcf.org/topics/view.cfm?itemID=12863* (accessed March 22, 2004).

References

1. Pew Internet & American Life Project Tracking surveys (March 2000–present). At *http://www.pewinternet.org/reports/chart.asp?img=Internet_Activities_3.22.04.htm* (accessed April 18, 2004).
2. Bleich HL, Beckley RF, Horowitz G, et al. Clinical computing in a teaching hospital. N Engl J Med 1985;312:756–64.
3. Plourde, Vincent, Vice President, Provider Service Division, Blue Cross Blue Shield of Massachusetts. Personal communication, January 5, 2004.
4. Sands DZ, Safran C, Slack WV, Bleich HL. Electronic mail use in a teaching hospital. In: Proceedings of the Symposium on Computer Applications in Medical Care, 1993, pp. 306–10.
5. Manhattan Research, LLC. Taking the Pulse 3.0: Physicians and Emerging Information Technologies. New York, 2003.
6. Manhattan Research, LLC. CyberCitizen Health v3.0: Targeting Today's eHealth Consumers, Understanding Tomorrows Impact. New York, 2003.
7. Harris Interactive. Patient/physician online communication: Many patients want it, would pay for it, and it would influence their choice of doctors and health plans. Harris Interactive Health Care News 2002;2:8.
8. Patt MR, Houston TK, Jenckes MW, Sands DZ, Ford DE. Doctors who are using email with their patients: a qualitative exploration. J Med Internet Res 2003;5:e9.
9. Manhattan Research, LLC. Cybercitizen® Health v2.0: The Integration of Information Technology and Consumer Healthcare. New York, 2002.
10. MDHub at *http:///www.mdhub.com* (accessed November 17, 2004).
11. Slack WV. Cybermedicine: How Computing Empowers Doctors and Patients for Better Health Care (revised and updated edition). San Francisco: Jossey-Bass, 2001.
12. Goldman J. Doctor/Patient E-mail: The Right Prescription With Privacy Safeguards. iHealthBeat Jan. 6, 2004. At *http://ihealthbeat.org/index.cfm?action=lookupID&id=26300* (accessed Nov. 17, 2004).
13. *http://www.zixcorp.com*
14. *http://www.sigaba.com*
15. *http://www.kryptiq.com*
16. *http://www.mydoconline.com*
17. *http://www.relayhealth.com*
18. *http://www.medem.com*
19. Sands DZ, Halamka JD, Pellaton D. *PatientSite*: a Web-based clinical communication and health education tool. Health Information Management Systems Society 2001 Annual Conference; HIMSS, Chicago, IL, 2001.

20. Sands DZ, Halamka JD. *PatientSite*: patient centered communication, services, and access to information. In: Nelson R, Ball MJ. Consumer Informatics: Applications and Strategies in Cyber Health Care. New York: Springer-Verlag, 2002.
21. First Consulting Group. Online patient–provider communication tools: an overview. California HealthCare Foundation. At *http://www.chcf.org/topics/view.cfm?itemID=12863* (accessed March 22, 2004).
22. Delbanco TL, Sands DZ. Electrons in Flight—e-mail between doctors and patients. N Engl J Med 2004;350:1705–7.
23. Kane B, Sands DZ for the AMIA Internet Working Group, Task Force on Guidelines for the Use of Clinic-Patient Electronic Mail. Guidelines for the clinical use of electronic mail with patients. J Am Med Inform Assoc 1998;5:104–11.
24. Sands DZ. Guidelines for the use of patient-centered electronic mail. In: Leading the Way to Information Exchange in the Electronic World; Massachusetts Health Data Consortium, April 1999, pp. 28–40.
25. eRisk Working Group for Healthcare. Guidelines for online communication. At *http://www.medem.com/phy/phy_eriskguidelines.cfm* (accessed March 22, 2004).
26. American Medical Association. Guidelines for physican–patient electronic communications. At *http://www.ama-assn.org/ama/pub/category/2386.html* (accessed March 22, 2004).
27. Sands DZ. Electronic patient-centered communication: managing risks, managing opportunities, managing care. Am J Manag Care 1999;5(12):1569–71.
28. Sands DZ, Halamka JD. *PatientSite*: patient centered communication, services, and access to information. In: Nelson R, Ball MJ. Consumer Informatics: Applications and Strategies in Cyber Health Care. New York: Springer-Verlag, 2002.
29. American College of Physicians. The changing face of ambulatory medicine—reimbursing physicians for computer-based care: ACP analysis and recommendations to assure fair reimbursement for physician care rendered online. Philadelphia: American College of Physicians Policy Paper, March 2003.
30. Anonymous. New CPT code covers online consults. Health data management 1/5/2004. At *http://www.healthdatamanagement.com/html/news/NewsStory.cfm?DID=11126* (accessed April 1, 2004).
31. RelayHealth, Inc. The RelayHealth webvisit study: final report. 2003. At *http://www.relayhealth.com/rh/specific/physicians/studyResults.aspx*. (Accessed March 29, 2004).
32. Liederman EM, Morefield CS. Web messaging: a new tool for patient–physician communication. J Am Med Inform Assoc 2003;10:260–70.
33. Luria SV. Legal concerns surrounding e-mail use in a medical practice. JONAS Healthc Law Ethics Regul 2003;5:53–7.
34. Hickson GB, Clayton EW, Entman SS, et al. Obstetricians' prior malpractice experience and patients' satisfaction with care. JAMA 1994;272:1583–7.
35. Beckman HB, Markakis KM, Suchman AL, Frankel RM. The doctor–patient relationship and malpractice: lessons from plaintiff depositions. Arch Intern Med 1994;154:1365–70.
36. Spielberg AR. On call and online: sociohistorical, legal, and ethical implications of e-mail for the patient–physician relationship. JAMA 1998;280:1353–9.
37. Spielberg AR. Online without a net: physician-patient communication by electronic mail. Am J Law Med 1999;25:267–95.
38. Balas EA, Boren SA. Managing Clinical Knowledge for Health Care Improvement. Yearbook of Medical Informatics. Stuttgart: Schattauer, 2000, pp. 65–70.
39. Houston TK, Sands DZ, Nash B, Ford D. Experiences of physicians who frequently use E-mail with patients. Health Commun 2003;15:515–25.
40. Moyer CA, Stern DT, Dobias KS, Cox DT, Katz SJ. Bridging the electronic divide: patient and provider perspectives on e-mail communication in primary care. Am J Manag Care 2002;8:427–33.
41. Katz SJ, Moyer CA, Cox DT, Stern DT. Effect of a triage-based e-mail system on clinic resource use and patient and physician satisfaction in primary care. A randomized controlled trial. J Gen Intern Med 2003;18:736–44.
42. Mandl KD, Kohane IS, Brandt AM. Electronic patient–physician communication: problem and promise. Ann Intern Med 1998;129:495–500.

10
Consumer Health Vocabulary

Catherine Arnott Smith and P. Zoë Stavri

Patrick et al. [1] have called the "consumer vocabulary problem" a fundamental issue in health information provision. This is the problem of mismatch between terms used by healthcare professionals and those used by the consumers who receive their services. Compatibility, between consumer and clinical terminology, or the lack of it, has been investigated in domains including Web site usability [2–4], information prescriptions [5], and HMO report cards [6]. The issue is seen as so important that one packaged consumer vocabulary was advertised as the "Rosetta Stone for the consumerization of healthcare" [7].

In fact, the consumer vocabulary problem is a very old one. Mazur [8] notes that "basic communication . . . has perplexed medical science, doctors and patients since at least the late 1700s" and Andrews spoke of the old dichotomy between scientific and "lay" terminology in his classic *History of Scientific English*:

> The background of medical English . . . is utterly at variance with the usual ancestry of a language . . . Ordinary speech is controlled from below; the masses make and remake it in defiance of scholars who reluctantly have to accept the speech of the populace as their own. With the scientist, however, the written word rules the spoken word, and regular regeneration of older changing words is a steady process. [9]

The first consumer health vocabulary may in fact have been English. Words that had "escaped" from scientific books with the advent of the printing press soon became part of popular speech; so, for example, in the fifth act of Shakespeare's *Henry IV*, Part II, the clown Mistress Quickly addresses the First Beadle: "Thou atomy, thou!" using lay slang for *anatomy* or *cadaver*, while her colleague Doll Tearsheet cries synonymously "Goodman bones" [10]! Greenberg [11] looked at the effect of Gutenberg's printing press on public health information dissemination in 17th-century London: health information for the first time *expressly intended for the public*, printed in English and not solely for the Latin-speaking physicians of the day.

Historically, the terminology for consumer terminology in health has been *lay language*. Mazur ascribes the origins of this term to the judicial system and defines it as "scientific description for nonscientists . . . the nontechnical language of consumers, patients and others" [12].

Language, meaning, relationships between terms, and disease models all contribute to the comprehensibility of health information being transmitted. We understand new information by applying the new knowledge to preexisting cognitive models. If the disease model is not congruent with the prevailing one, it may not be understood. One complication, however, is that the perspective of the objective scientific researcher may inadvertently bias his or her understanding of the patient's model. Tedlock [13] investigated the presence of the "hot–cold" categorization of Galenic humoral medicine in Latin American traditional healing practice, a model being blamed for purported interference with orthodox Western healthcare. He found that contrary to anecdote, highland Guatemalan traditional healers "did not include hot–cold categories in their explanatory models of illness etiology," but that anthropologists who asked questions of *patients* that incorporated these dichotomous categories were likely to receive appropriately hot and cold answers. Ironically, for the purposes of this chapter, the confusion of practitioner language with lay language was part of the research problem.

With that caveat in mind: Is there such a thing as a consumer health vocabulary? Are there in fact unique concepts that are not already represented by professional, clinical vocabularies? These questions are addressed in the following section, through discussion and review of relevant research.

Research Themes

We can structure our discussion of vocabulary issues in consumer health in three main areas:

1. Patient–physician communication: information flow from physician to patient, for example, in the context of obtaining informed consent
2. Patient interpretation of print and media: the information itself observed in transit
3. Consumer health vocabulary: information flow from consumer to information retrieval system and back again, for example, in the context of information seeking online

Central to each of these themes is patient interpretation—with affective overtones—of medical concepts.

We understand concepts or retain vocabulary differently based on our state of mind. If we are under stress, we might need someone with us when we talk to the doctor, and a written summary of what we are being told so that we can refer to it later. Even when we are not under stress, we may not understand the now increasingly more readily accessible medical information we come across when attempting to self-diagnose. Do current vocabularies, such as those represented in the Unified Medical Language System (UMLS), already incorporate concepts that a consumer might use? The affirmative posits that although there might be some "consumer terms" unavailable through the UMLS, as the concepts are already represented, it is simply a question of adding synonyms. The opposing argument suggests that it is likely additional concepts need to be constructed, arising from the different cultural models of health, disease, treatment, and mortality found in the United States population.

What is under discussion in this chapter is consumer vocabulary in service of communication, understanding, and information seeking. This chapter does not provide an exhaustive review of these topics, but rather approaches a synthesis of the critical issues that must be addressed.

Patient–Physician Communication

Patient participation in the decision making process is vital in today's healthcare system. The key to participatory health care is communication, and the key to communication is informed participation in the dialogue. Informed participation is bidirectional: the patient must understand what the physician and the literature say, and the physician must understand what the patient says.

Mazur [12] proposes that patient–physician communication must begin with "the patient's understanding of the information disclosed, *in lay language*" (italics added). This is an ancient concern: language that was intended for physicians was considered actively harmful when applied to nonphysicians. Connor in 1963 voiced the typical attitude of medical librarians when he wrote: "The average patient normally does himself more harm than good when he tries to determine even in a scientifically sound tome his own diagnosis and therapy. The avenues of approach are so many and the language so highly technical that even the intensely trained physician frequently must work hard to comprehend and make the appropriate choice among many alternatives" [14] and even today, Williams et al. [5] cite "terminology" as one reason for providing librarian-mediated translations in Vanderbilt's PICS (Patient Informatics Consult Service). However, this is not simply a matter of vocabulary; in other words, use of a common language at a level of comprehension appropriate to the person may not be enough. The education of patients may not be successful if, for example, written material is not comprehensible to the patients' own belief system: If a patient and her physician have different conceptual models of illness and health, then any ensuing dialogue will only be as effective as the fit between the patient's cultural model and the physician's. Language barriers were one of the four factors cited by Buchanan et al. as "stand[ing] in the way of effective doctor–patient communication" [15]. Not only have the linguistic forms of medical language been implicated in the creation of distance during treatment [16] but the very name of the illness has historically been known to have an effect on the patient [17,18]. Chapple et al. [19] addressed the emotional ramifications of clinical terminology in the "anxiety and confusion" among families in genetic counseling situations. Their work goes beyond identification and definitional experiments, taking into account the anxiety accompanying the patient's search for understanding of a disease or condition; and how the words chosen in trying to present information can go a long way to diminish that anxiety. In an online environment, we might consider replacing the term *abnormality* (worst possible scenario unfolding) with the term *chromosome variation* (understood as "something different"). Do we know whether this replacement will not only diminish anxiety, but also enhance understanding? We have nonverbal cues to go by in a face-to-face encounter, to which we can quickly adjust; but we do not have that advantage with printed text shared at a distance, nor do we know how consumers really interpret the content of Web sites such as *ClinicalTrials.gov*.

Communication and Vocabulary

Even if clinical terminology does exist to represent a particular consumer-oriented concept, its placement or context in a controlled vocabulary determines, to a certain extent, its meaning. *Tobacco* illustrates how contextual placement in a thesaurus represents the conventional meaning of the term. Hypothetically, both an allopathic view of medicine and a more traditional (for example, Native American) perspective would place *tobacco* in an agricultural, or crop, context. The allopathic view would also place it in a context representing an ingredient in cigarettes, a recreational or carcinogenic substance, something marketed and sold to people who may become addicted to the carcinogenic substances that are byproducts of the smoke. In traditional Native

American culture, however, tobacco has religious significance used ceremoniously; its primary function is not as a recreational substance.

The use of clinical terminology itself can be a signal of context: AHCRQ (the Agency for Healthcare Research and Quality) and the Kanter Foundation, in their publication "Now You Have a Diagnosis: What's Next?" note that patients must beware of documents relying on "the use of medical-ese – impressive technical terms to help make treatment decisions" [20]. Contrast this, however, with the interesting finding of Ogden et al. [21], who presented 740 patients in 3 English counties with 2 prepared scenarios of clinical diagnoses, randomly expressed in lay terminology, medical terminology, or a combination of the two (for example, *stomach upset* as opposed to *gastroenteritis*). These authors found considerable differences between lay and medical labels for the same diagnoses; patients consistently rated the medical labels as beneficial for the validation of their "sick role" and improving their confidence in their doctor. Lay labels, on the other hand, were associated with assumption of responsibility and taking of blame.

Patient Interpretation of Print and Media

In a landmark study published in 1970, Boyle [22] published a study that is relevant today to the way in which patients may interpret the written word. Two hundred and thirty-four outpatients and 35 doctors completed multiple-choice questionnaires aimed at evaluating differences in interpretation of commonly used medical terms. Part of the instrument asked patients and doctors to select which of four figures portrayed the correct anatomical placement of certain organs. One finding of the study was that patients had trouble locating various body parts, suggesting, for example, that in the absence of active communication, a patient might misconstrue the site of an unexplained pain. To add to the confusion about terminology presented in print, not all physicians in this study were able to correctly identify the heart! Similarly, not all physicians agreed on the definitions for either *constipation* or *diarrhea*. In fact, doctors and patients disagreed on most definitions except what is meant by *a good appetite*. Hadlow and Pitts [23], working in England, found similar results from 120 patients and 100 doctors and support staff asked to define common medical and psychological terms; these authors found significant differences in levels of understanding strongly associated with the level of medical education.

A person in a state of grieving brings an emotional overlay to any information-seeking task. The affective component of the terminology needs to be sensitive to such potentially emotional states. "Misconceptions cannot be easily addressed using a static, printed handout" [24].

Consumer Health Vocabulary and Information Seeking

Sievert et al. [25] start to address consumer health information seeking from the information retrieval perspective. They have brought the common term *conundrum* to the query formulation stage and demonstrate that search results can be confounded by the way most search engines deal with lexical variants, particularly as they have become more sophisticated and often err on the side of recall over precision.

Finding Out What Consumers Say

One guiding assumption in this research domain is that consumers have their own "language" susceptible to analysis. Any study of consumer "language" will beg the question of what terms consumers actually use.

Therefore, two significant challenges to consumer terminologists are the definition and the capture of terms that accurately reflect consumer reality. One straightforward strategy used by a number of researchers in different disciplines has been to ask the consumers themselves. Both Barrett and Wellings and Fischer et al., for example, surveyed the relationship between intentional achieving of pregnancy and the terms the pregnant women used to describe those pregnancies, finding them "highly correlated to social and cultural influences" [25,26]. Two British studies have used this same approach and discovered that consumers don't particularly want to be called consumers. In England, Batra and Lilford [27] asked 100 pregnant women what they would like to be called and found *mother-to-be* and *pregnant woman* more popular than *client*, *consumer*, or *maternant*. Four years later in Wales, Byrne et al. [28] also found *patient* the most popular term for "women attending antenatal clinics," with *consumer* being the least favored of all.

Similarly, several studies have investigated the cultural dimensions of consumer language. Schorling and Saunders [29] asked 1031 rural African Americans if they had "sugar" or "diabetes." Of those who responded affirmatively to "sugar," 31% answered "No" when asked subsequently if they had diabetes. Interestingly, those subjects who used the term *sugar* also believed their condition to be less serious. Blumhagen [30] posited the existence of a physical illness called "hyper-tension," "characterized by excessive nervousness caused by untoward social stress" and used by some people in his study to explain and justify particular social behaviors. Thirteen years later, Heurtin-Roberts [31] delineated a chronic folk illness among elderly African-American women in New Orleans that they called "high-pertension" and believed to involve "blood and nerves."

Another strategy to enhance usability of information targeted at consumers is to involve patients themselves in the development of their own educational material, for example, clinical practice guideline composition [32]. Content analysis of query log files and e-mail messages can also provide a new perspective on consumer vocabulary. For example, McCray et al. [3] examined 3 months' worth of queries submitted to the National Library of Medicine's home page. These authors were able to identify common terminological problems in query formulation, ranging from translation errors ("psicology") to transcribed verbal slips ("prostrate cancer"). Patrick. Sievert et al. [1] looked at e-mail messages and extracted words and phrases from print publications explicitly authored by consumers, raiding the *Dictionary of American Regional English* for their folk equivalents. Smith et al. [33] examined e-mail messages submitted to a Web-based cancer information service marketed to the general public at the University of Pittsburgh Medical Center. Messages in which writers self-identified as healthcare providers (doctors, nurses, medical students) were eliminated from analysis. In this study of 139 e-mail messages, the terms these e-mail writers used to express their health information needs overlapped in 96% of the cases with terms from the 92 healthcare terminologies comprising the 2001 UMLS.

Is the Consumer Different?

Many researchers contend, conversely, that there is no "consumer vocabulary." The results of Smith et al. [33] showed almost universal consonance between lay terminology and that of healthcare professionals. In fact, two unique e-mail writers used the same word to describe their cancer diagnosis—*cribriform type*—a phrase not found in any UMLS source vocabulary, but a perfectly correct clinical term meaning *sieve-like* (for the appearance of the cancer cell). Far from demonstrating a preference for slang, in this case two consumers excelled the UMLS in granularity of expression.

Zeng et al. [34], however, found poor matches between the UMLS and terms that patients used to search a hospital Web site. These authors' recommendations included the development of vocabulary tools to assist in the search process. Patrick et al. [1] studied controlled vocabulary resources to evaluate their potential to accommodate the consumer terminology used to describe *diabetes*. This study emphasized differences between consumer and physician terminology and how the latter helps to focus retrieval on the World Wide Web. This work also suggested that the addition of "vernacular terms" would enhance searching on the Internet.

Conclusion

"Lay conceptions of disease," as Chapple et al. call them [19], may be based on many factors beyond sound—or shared—medical facts. Shared decision making is subverted when doctors and patients understand the meaning of certain terms in different ways. Computer-based programs designed to facilitate decision making need to take this divergence into account. However, to facilitate the process of context provision, the transmitter of the information must understand the model that will be infiltrated; then the words used will be related to each other in strings and sentences in a meaningful way. The problem of understanding a concept but not remembering the correct word for it is one that can be addressed during the communication process. If the consumer can communicate a given concept to a healthcare provider, then translation into clinical terminology is still possible.

References

1. Patrick TB, Monga HK, Sievert ME, Houston Hall J, Longo DR. Evaluation of controlled vocabulary resources for development of a consumer entry vocabulary for diabetes. J Med Internet Res 2001;3:E24.
2. Miller N, Lacroix EM, Backus JE. MEDLINEPlus: building and maintaining the National Library of Medicine's consumer health web service. Bull Med Libr Assoc 2000;88:11–7.
3. McCray AT, Loane RF, Browne AC, Bangalore AK. Terminology issues in user access to Web-based information. Proc AMIA Symp 1999:107–11.
4. McCray AT, Dorfman E, Ripple A, et al. Usability issues in developing a Web-based consumer health site. Proc AMIA Symp 2000:556–60.
5. Williams MD, Gish KW, Giuse NB, Sathe NA, Carrell DL. The Patient Informatics Consult Service: an approach for a patient-centered service. Bull Med Libr Assoc 2001;89:185–93.
6. Hochhauser M. Can consumers understand managed care report cards? Manag Care Interface 1998;11:91–5.
7. Health Language, Inc. Health Language, Inc. licenses consumer healthcare terms for use in Cyber+LE language engine technology. Press release, November 20, 2000. Available online: *http://www.healthlanguage.com/press/PR_-_PRIMETIME.PDF.*

8. Mazur DJ. The New Medical Conversation: Media, Patients, Doctors, and the Ethics of Scientific Communication. Lanham, MD: Rowman & Littlefield, 2003, p. xii.
9. Andrews E. A History of Scientific English: The Story of Its Evolution Based on a Study of Biomedical Terminology. New York: Richard E. Smith, 1947.
10. Shakespeare W. *King Henry IV* (Part II, Act V, Scene IV).
11. Greenberg SJ. The "dreadful visitation": public health and public awareness in seventeenth-century London. Bull Med Libr Assoc 1997;85:391–401.
12. Mazur DJ. Op. cit.: 129.
13. Tedlock B. An interpretive solution to the problem of humoral medicine in Latin America. Soc Sci Med 1987;24:1069–83.
14. Connor J. The medical society library. Questionable medical literature and the library: a symposium. Bull Med Libr Assoc 1963;51:467–71.
15. Buchanan J. Doctor–patient communication. N Z Med J 1991;104:62–4.
16. Mintz D. What's in a word: the distancing function of language in medicine. J Med Hum 1992;13:223–33.
17. De Crespigny L. Words matter: nomenclature and communication in perinatal medicine. Clin Perinatol 2003;30:17–25.
18. Wood M. Naming the illness: The power of words. Fam Med 1991;23:534–8.
19. Chapple A, May C, Campion P. Lay understanding of genetic disease: a British study of families attending a genetic counseling service. J Genet Couns 1995;4:281–300.
20. Agency for Healthcare Quality and Research and The Kanter Foundation. Now you have a diagnosis: What's next? Using health care information to help make treatment decisions. Rockville, MD: Author, 2000.
21. Ogden J, Branson R, Bryett A, et al. What's in a name? An experimental study of patients' views of the impact and function of a diagnosis. Fam Pract 2003;20:248–53.
22. Boyle CM. Difference between patients' and doctors' interpretation of some common medical terms. Br Med J 1970;1:286–9.
23. Hadlow J, Pitts M. The understanding of common health terms by doctors, nurses and patients. Soc Sci Med 1992;34:339.
24. Sievert ME, Patrick TB, Reid JC. Need a bloody nose be a nosebleed? Or, lexical variants cause surprising results. Bull Med Libr Assoc 2001;89:68–71.
25. Barrett G, Wellings K. What is a 'planned' pregnancy? Empirical data from a British study. Soc Sci Med 2002;55:545–57.
26. Fisher RC, Stanford JB, Jameson P, DeWitt MJ. Exploring the concepts of intended, planned, and wanted pregnancy. J Fam Pract 1999;48:117–22.
27. Batra N, Lilford RJ. Not clients, not consumers and definitely not maternants. Eur J Gyn Reprod Biol 1996;64:197–9.
28. Byrne DL, Asmussen T, Freeman JM. Descriptive terms for women attending antenatal clinics: mother knows best? Br J Obstet Gynecol 2000;107:1233–6.
29. Schorling JB, Saunders JT. Is "sugar" the same as diabetes? A community-based study among rural African-Americans. Diab Care 2000;23:330–4.
30. Blumhagen D. Hyper-tension: a folk illness with a medical name. Cult Med Psychiatr 1980;4:197–224.
31. Heurtin-Roberts S. "High-pertension": the uses of a chronic folk illness for personal adaptation. Soc Sci Med 1993;37:285–94.
32. Van Wersch A, Eccles M. Involvement of consumers in the development of evidence based guidelines: practical experiences from the North of England evidence based guideline development programme. Qual Health Care 2001;10:10–16.
33. Smith CA, Stavri PZ, Chapman WW. In their own words? A terminological analysis of e-mail to a cancer information service. Proc AMIA Symp 2003;697–701.
34. Zeng Q, Kogan S, Ash N, Greenes RA, Boxwala AA. Characteristics of consumer terminology for health information retrieval. Methods Inform Med 2002;41:289–98.

11
Disability Informatics

RICHARD APPLEYARD

So what is disability informatics? Disability informatics is a yet undefined/emerging field and one that this chapter will begin to describe. The purpose of this chapter is to present not a comprehensive review of the research and developments in the areas associated with disability informatics, but more of an overview of the areas contained in this new field and an introduction to some of its potential applications with a focus in the area of medical and consumer health informatics.

Disability informatics can be thought of as another subspecialty of informatics, or the science of information, which has been defined elsewhere (refer to Chapter 1 for a definition of consumer health informatics). A more practical way of looking at the field of informatics is to consider it the study of how people use, manage, and process information to "get things done." Individuals might talk to other people, refer to a book, make a phone call, use a computing device, or go online. Disability informatics is then simply a case of studying this for people with disabilities. Disability informatics also interfaces with other traditional disability fields such as rehabilitation services and assistive technology (as shown in Fig. 11.1).

As a general goal, disability informatics seeks to understand better how individuals with disabilities can use information technology and information systems to address any functional issues they encounter, improve their self-efficacy, and empower them to be as independent as any other persons. But disability informatics broadly defined can be any application that collects, manages, and distributes information related to disability to persons with disabilities, as well as to care providers and family and to healthcare and rehabilitation professionals.

In many instances, accessible information systems will be equally applicable to the nondisabled population. In fact, one of the major reasons for considering universal design principles and accessibility in design is that everyone is subject to different types of functional limitations in various environments; for example, design requirements for noisy environments are very similar to those for people with hearing impairments, and for environments in which it is not safe to look at a device (such as driving a car) are very similar to those for people with visual impairments [1]. But whereas these systems provide a convenience or make something easier for the abled population, they are essential for the disabled population to function independently. A major area of disability informatics involves identifying and addressing the particular needs and requirements of the disabled population to utilize general information systems. The main resolution is then educating and raising awareness of these issues to information technology professionals and the information technology (IT) industry.

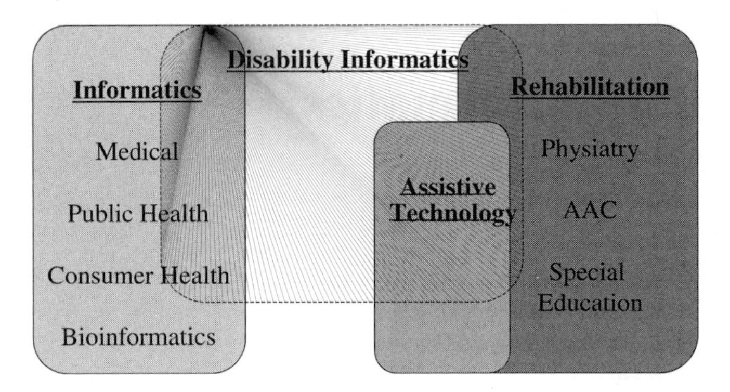

FIGURE 11.1. Relationship of disability Informatics to other fields of expertise.

Defining Disability

There are as many definitions of disability as there are organizations involved with people with disabilities [2]. Disability status can be "determined by medical category, by functional limitation, or by use of assistive technology. It can be based on self-report or require a diagnosis by a healthcare professional. In the United States, being disabled can be determined by eligibility for Medicaid and can vary from state to state. A person may be regarded as disabled under the ADA legislation but not under Social Security work disability criteria" [3]. There is no gold standard that defines disability. Statistics on prevalence and types of disability are gathered by federal and private organizations that use different criteria for self-reporting disability.

People with disabilities can be broadly defined as those with limitations in human actions or activities resulting from physical or mental impairments [4]. The most commonly cited definition is the 1976 definition of the World Health Organization [5]. This, along with other definitions of disability, are listed below.

An **impairment** is any loss or abnormality of psychological, physiological or anatomical structure or function; a **disability** is any restriction or lack (resulting from an impairment) of ability to perform an activity in the manner or within the range considered normal for a human being; a **handicap** is a disadvantage for a given individual, resulting from an **impairment** or a **disability**, that prevents the fulfillment of a role that is considered normal (depending on age, sex and social and cultural factors) for that individual. World Health Organization [5]

A physical or mental impairment that substantially limits one or more of the major life activities. American with Disabilities Act of 1990 (ADA) [6]

A health problem or disability which prevents [you] from working or which limits the amount of work that [you] can do. Census Bureau, Bureau of Labor Statistics [7]

Any disability, handicap, or chronic disease that keeps you from participating fully in work, school, housework or other activities. Pew Internet and American Life Project [8]

It is significant that by one estimate there are now 50 million people in the United States (age 5 and older according to Census 2000) self-reporting some form of disability (as defined by the US Census Bureau) [7]. As currently 14 million of the 50 million people with disabilities are 65 years of age and older (equivalent to 42% of this age group), and this number is expected to increase as the baby-boom generation continues to enter retirement, there is a potential for the disabled population to grow at a significant rate. Although these are significant numbers of the general population, there are many types of disability that express very different levels and types of function. This presents a challenge when trying to accommodate people with disabilities, as the needs and types cover such a wide spectrum and therefore seems to be an impossible undertaking.

Medical Classification of Disability

Predominant definitions of and attitudes toward disability are from a medical perspective. This is often referred to as the "medicalization of disability" and stems from a strong hope for cures and rehabilitation from the tremendous advances in the field of medicine, which became institutionalized by the implementation of the social assistance programs that were set up to provide support within this perspective. The medical classification is certainly appropriate for researching the etiology of, and development of treatments for, disabilities; however, it is not well suited to other efforts such as self-determination or health promotion, which are in reality independent of the specifics of disability.

Functional Classification of Disability

In contrast, a more recent attitude is the functional classification of disability that focuses on the function rather than that which affects the disability, for example, disease, trauma, and so forth [9–11]. For example, research on mobility limitations might include people whose mobility was impaired as a result of spinal cord injury, spina bifida, cerebral palsy, and so forth. The relative level of functioning is the focus of this classification where the model of the disabling process moves from pathophysiology, through impairment, to functional limitation and finally to disability. A functional conceptualization of disability served as the framework for the Institute of Medicine's (IOM's) landmark report "Disability in America" [11] and is the underpinning of the current National Institute on Disability and Development Research (NIDDR) long-range plan [12].

The functional types of disability can be divided into three categories: mobility, sensory, and cognitive. These are by no means exclusive, and disabilities are generally represented on a continuum of level of function. A brief overview is provided here. More detail on the different disabilities can be found elsewhere [13,14].

Mobility—Physical Motor and Speech Communication

Mobility problems faced by people with physical motor disabilities can be the consequences of traumatic injury, for example, spinal cord or loss of limb, or of disease or birth defect, for example, cerebral palsy, muscular dystrophy, multiple sclerosis, spina bifida, amyotrophic lateral sclerosis, Parkinson's disease, or epilepsy. Problems faced from these disabilities stem from impaired muscle control and can range from simple weakness and fatigue to difficulty in walking, sensing, grasping, and speaking/communication. The more severe disabilities may prevent direct operation of devices and require assistive technologies such as wheelchairs, manipulation aids, communications aids (voice synthesis), and computer interface aids, for example, sip-puff switch or eye/head-motion tracking.

Sensory—Visual and Aural

Sensory impairments are divided further into visual (sight) and aural (hearing). Visual disabilities can range from correctable (with the use of eyeglasses, contact lenses) to not correctable (very poor vision) impairments, to perceiving light but not shapes, to perceiving no light at all ("totally blind"). Two categories are commonly used: "low vision" and "legally blind." "Low vision" includes extreme near- or far-sightedness, dimness of vision, haziness (e.g., cataract), tunnel vision (e.g., glaucoma), and spots before the eyes (e.g., diabetic retinopathy). The "legally blind" category includes those whose visual acuity is worse than 20/200 after correction, or whose field of vision is less than 20 degrees. Many of the diseases causing visual impairment are common in the aging population, which makes this disability more significant among baby boomers.

Braille has been the traditional remedial strategy for information access for those who are blind. However, less than 10% of the blind population now uses Braille (printed or refreshable Braille devices) [15,16], and its drawbacks include cost (of printers and refreshable Braille devices) and speed. With advances in computer technology, Braille is being largely replaced by voice synthesis and screen readers. Another drawback to Braille is that it is a remedy only for those with language skills and relatively good cognitive skills.

A third less severe visual disability that is often overlooked is "color blindness." This doesn't pose much of a problem except where information is color coded with poor relative intensities.

Aural disabilities can range from mild hearing loss (less than 30 decibels), moderate (less than 50 decibels), severe (less than 80 decibels), to profound (less than 95 decibels). Someone who is considered deaf falls in the severe to profound hearing loss range. Mild and moderate hearing loss is considered "hard of hearing." The type of hearing impairment can be conductive (the moving parts or bones of the inner ear) or neural (cochlea, auditory nerve, or brain) damage. The cause of deafness can be congenital genetic (hereditary) or a result of traumatic injury or middle ear infections (otitis media) and other diseases. It is also a common part of the aging process, and again significant for the baby-boomers.

Cognitive—Intellectual and Language Communication

The concept of cognitive disabilities is extremely broad and not always well defined. At a general level, a person with a cognitive impairment has greater difficulty with one or more types of mental tasks that an average individual. These can range from severe retardation to a simple inability to remember, and may involve the loss of any number of cognitive functions. Cognitive functions include memory, language, perception, problem-solving, hand–eye coordination, conceptualizing, attention, and executive function. Cognitive disabilities are broadly categorized as follows:

1. Learning and developmental disabilities (also referred to as mental retardation, intellectual disabilities); language problems such as reading, writing (e.g., dysgraphia), and spelling (e.g., dyslexia); hand–eye coordination problems (e.g., dyspraxia); attention deficit hyperactivity disorder (ADHD); autism; Down's syndrome
2. Brain injury, traumatic brain injury (TBI), stroke, and disease (meningitis, tumors)
3. Age-related brain diseases: Alzheimer's (progressive intellectual decline) and dementia (progressive loss of mental functions beginning with memory, learning, attention, and judgment)

Multiple Impairments

It is common for a cause of a single impairment to cause others as well. This is particularly true in the case of severe brain trauma and age-related brain diseases and developmental disabilities.

Deaf–blindness is the condition of being both aurally and visually disabled. Most individuals who are labeled "deaf–blind" are neither totally blind nor totally deaf: the designation implies that the usual strategies for deafness or blindness alone do not work because they usually involve compensating for one impaired sense by relying heavily on the other. Tactile modes are often the most appropriate methods of delivering information to individuals who are deaf–blind. Many individuals labeled "deaf–blind" also appear to have cognitive limitations. People with severe developmental disabilities may experience impairments of motor, sensory, and cognitive skills, as in CHARGE association syndrome.

Sociological Classification of Disability

There is a third, emerging sociological classification of disability. The field of "Disability Studies" was born out of a need to counterpoint the medicalization of disability with a more social construction view of disability. But in addition to the corrective nature of this field, it is also the "socio-political-cultural model of disability incarnate" with a firm basis in the liberal arts [17].

Related Fields of Expertise

Medical Informatics

Whereas medical informatics tends to focus on the management and use of information in health and biomedicine by the healthcare provider, disability informatics focuses on the management and use of information by people with disabilities. Disability is often viewed within the medical model, and therefore disability informatics could be thought of as a pure subfield of medical informatics. However, disability issues are not restricted to medical or health issues, and therefore informatics can be applied to other problems faced by the disability community, for example, technologies that assist with the navigation of their physical environment.

A major secondary effect of disability is poor health status and increased personal healthcare needs. This provides an overlap of disability informatics with other subfields of medical informatics, public health informatics, and consumer health informatics. Consumer health informatics is an area of growing significance for people with disabilities. The increased communication and patient education possible in the online world afford greater impact and benefit to these individuals, who are often isolated and ostracized from the usual community support systems. Finally, because many disabilities are rooted in genetic heredity and diseases, bioinformatics has large long-term implications in the education and ethics around genetic screening and gene therapy treatments.

Rehabilitation

To address the issues individuals with disabilities face, a number of rehabilitation fields have developed. Assistive technology (AT) and information technology (IT) can be applied in each of these rehabilitation areas and some of the different technologies available have been mentioned in the Functional Classification section.

Physical medicine and rehabilitation (PM&R), also called physiatry, is the medical specialty that deals with the evaluation and treatment of patients with a neurologic, musculoskeletal, or cardiopulmonary disease, disorder, or injury that impairs normal, functional capacity. Using a multidisciplinary team, physiatry covers everything from cardiac rehabilitation to pain management in recovery from a stroke to restoring cognitive function lost with Alzheimer's disease. Team members can include a physiatrist, audiologist, clinical social worker, occupational therapist, physical therapist, recreational therapist, and/or speech/language pathologist.

Augmentative and alternate communication (AAC) is an area of rehabilitation that specifically addresses the loss of the ability to speak and communicate. This can be due to a loss of a physical motor ability required to generate speech or to a loss of the cognitive ability to generate and process speech, or a combination of both. In fact, there is often some debate as to when physical communication ends and cognitive communication begins. AT can involve dedicated communication devices that can be programmed with different limited sets of functions and operated through a touch pad or communication board to computers that can perform text to speech synthesis.

Assistive Technology (Computer Accessibility)

any item, piece of equipment, or product system, whether acquired commercially, modified, or customized, that is used to increase, maintain, or improve functional capabilities of individuals with disabilities. AT Act of 1998 (Section 508) [18]

AT is focused on the individual and seeks to address the loss of a particular human function. In terms of computers and information technology use, AT addresses the disconnect in the human–computer interface that is present as a result of the disability. As such, AT addresses mobility and sensory impairments and provides augmentative and alternate communication (AAC) and adaptive access for computers (with alternative human–computer interfaces). AT is too large a field to be covered in any detail here, and a number of good resources are available for those who wish to learn more [19].

The human–computer interface issues can be thought of from two perspectives: input and output.

Input

Standard computer input centers around the WIMP (windows, icons, mouse, pointers) "desktop" metaphor provided by most modern computer operating systems, and the main input devices are a keyboard and a mouse. Where the loss of function impairs or prevents use of these devices, alternatives have been developed: alternative and adaptive keyboards, on screen keyboards, touch screens, tablets, joystick (pointer), switch access, and speech recognition.

Output

Standard computer output again centers on using a computer screen to display images. In the case of visual impairments, screen magnification, printed and refreshable Braille, and speech synthesis can be used. In this case it is not just a matter of a technology or device, but that the content and information being imparted is divorced from the presentation so that the AT can communicate it in a nonvisual format.

AT is an integral part of disability informatics and often a prerequisite to the use of information systems by people with disabilities. The overlap therefore centers on computer accessibility or the AT required to make the computer usable by a person with disabilities. In most informatics applications, one will generally assume that an individual has the necessary interface devices for him or her to interact with the computer, electronic device, or information technology being employed. Of course, this will not always be the case, as the implementation of new IT can always introduce new environmental interface issues that were not present or have not been encountered before. So it will always be necessary to have an assistive technologist or engineer on hand to advice and develop new ideas and solutions.

AT will become more sophisticated as technology continues to shrink in size and increase in complexity and power. There is a tremendous amount of potential for integration of different technologies to allow for much more sophisticated AT systems. Handheld computing power and the ubiquity of wireless telecommunications is reaching a point where information can be delivered "just-in-time" to and obtained "on demand" by the user. Add to this intelligent, location-aware capabilities, and you have the ability to provide "guardian angel"-like support for people with disabilities.

Universal Design (Computer Usability)

The main issue around the use of computers by people with disabilities has been around simple accessibility, the ability to access or own a computer that is equipped with the necessary AT to allow use with an individual's particular impairments. The next step is the improvement and refinement of technology to ensure maximum utility and ease of use. The preoccupation with computer accessibility for people with disabilities has tended to leave out or distract attention away from the usability issues. In fact, it is only relatively recently that an increased focus on usability and human–computer interface issues has occurred across the general population.

There has been a heavy focus on visual impairments and the use of screen readers in Web accessibility, in large part because the Web is so visual in nature. However, the increasing amount of multimedia and video that is becoming available on the Web, and the desire in the design community to make the Web more like the television in presentation (with animation platforms such as Flash and SMIL), is introducing more inaccessible content to those with aural impairments. In fact, in contrast to the broadcast and cable distribution, most of the video on the Web is not subtitled. There are also still many other types of impairments, for example, cognitive impairments and intellectual disabilities, that are not as well studied, nor as well known to the Web development community at large.

One of the other challenges has been incorporating universally accessible design requirements into the general design process rather than as an afterthought prompted by actual or threatened litigation under the ADA [6]. A number of cases have shown that dealing with accessibility issues retroactively is vastly more expensive than incorporating accessibility principles into the initial requirements gathering phase of a project plan.

It is impossible to attain 100% accessibility. Generally the amount of effort versus the percentage of accessibility curve is a classic asymptote (tending to infinity). Designers therefore tend to attempt to identify and target the specific users of the system. However, an understanding of the prevalence of people with disabilities within the general population and the design issues is often not present and easily passed over for other design requirements. Unfortunately, this is like playing Russian roulette. You might be able to get away with inaccessible design 9 times out of 10, but that 10th time could be a very stressful and expensive wake-up call.

Areas of Disability Informatics

In contrast to AT, disability informatics and IT for people with disabilities are more "group focused." It is certainly possible to have a "group of one," but this is just one end of a spectrum of the number of users possible. And there is certainly a symbiosis between and mutual dependence of AT and IT; AT is needed to access IT, and IT provides capabilities and services beyond what individual AT devices can do.

It is instructive to categorize the IT applications and issues in disability informatics into four broad areas of environment: virtual, personal, physical, and social/intellectual. The virtual environment covers primarily the online, digital telecommunications world of the Internet and the World Wide Web. The personal environment covers support systems aimed at the individual such as time and task management. Finally, the physical environment covers support systems aimed at helping the individual move around his or her physical environment (both in the home and within the community).

Virtual Environment

The digital revolution has had, and will continue to have, a profound impact on the self-efficacy and empowerment of people with disabilities. Although we are certainly not without access issues in the new digital realm, the digitization of information in order to allow computers to manage and manipulate it also means that people with disabilities can have equal access much more easily and with less dependence on others. AT can simply and easily allow the information to be represented in an accessible form; for example, a computer can read the text to a person with a visual impairment. No special accommodation is required, such as the production of specialized, alternate media, for example, Braille.

Of course, the reality is that presumptive design decisions in electronic media are to a certain extent re-creating comparable barriers that exist in the physical world. Therefore a major effort in online accessibility and usability is building awareness and providing education around best practices and basic universal design principles. In addition, the cost of assistive technology and the lower incomes of people with disabilities are continuing to create a "digital divide." This is of particular concern because people with disabilities have the most to gain from access to these new technologies through mitigation of the impairment and in some cases making it obsolete.

World Wide Web (Network) Accessibility

The WWW or Web has had a strong accessibility advocacy from early on in its evolution, probably as a result of the vision of the father of the Web:

> The power of the Web is in its universality. Access by everyone regardless of disability is an essential aspect.
>
> —Tim Berners-Lee, W3C Director and inventor of the World Wide Web [20]

The Web has had a profound impact in how information is published and transmitted all over the world and continues to have an increased role in all aspects of our daily lives. The Web has open standards for data request and response, and for the markup language used to define the page layout, there are no standards or restrictions on who can access or post to the Internet. Webmasters were very creative in how they used the initially very limited set of tools, and the HyperText Markup Language (HTML) has rapidly expanded in complexity to meet the demands of developers. However, it soon became obvious that guidelines were needed to ensure that people with disabilities were not excluded from accessing the Web. The World Wide Web Consortium (W3C) responded by launching the Web Accessibility Initiative (WAI) [20] and forming a working group to draft the first Web Content Accessibility Guidelines. WCAG version 1.0 became a W3C recommendation on May 5, 1999 and has had an important influence over the subsequent Web accessibility laws and policies. It was heavily used in the Web Accessibility Standards for the US Federal Government in Section 508 of the Reauthorized Rehabilitation Act [21].

A very useful "cheat sheet" for the Web Content Accessibility Guidelines, version 1.0, is the WAI Quicktips Reference Card [W3C, 2003, no. 153] with the 10 top to-dos listed here:

- Images and animations: Use the alt attribute to describe the function of each visual.
- Image maps: Use the client-side map and text for hotspots.
- Multimedia: Provide captioning and transcripts of audio and descriptions of video.
- Hypertext links: Use text that makes sense when read out of context. For example, avoid "click here."
- Page organization: Use headings, lists, and consistent structure. Use CSS for layout and style where possible.
- Graphs and charts: Summarize or use the longdesc attribute.
- Scripts, applets, and plug-ins: Provide alternative content in case active features are inaccessible or unsupported.
- Frames: Use the no frames element and meaningful titles.
- Tables: Make line-by-line reading sensible. Summarize.
- Check your work: Validate. Use tools, checklist, and guidelines at *http://www.w3.org/TR/WCAG*

WCAG version 1 contained guidelines and requirements that were very specific to HTML. Although this was appropriate at the time, there has since been a growth of other media markups and standards on the Web, for example, Adobe PDF, Macromedia Flash, Scalable Vector Graphic (SVG) format, and Java. The WAI working group is currently working on a draft of version 2 of the guidelines [22] that will have a broader scope and be media format independent so as to be more adaptive and robust to future technological developments.

A number of accessibility checking tools are available on the Internet. The best known is Bobby [23], which was developed at the Center for Applied Special Technology (CAST) and recently purchased by Watchfire. This online tool allows you to enter a URL and have an accessibility report generated based on the compliance of the Web page with the WCAG 1.0 and Section 508. There are other tools [24] including WAVE [25], Cynthia Says [26], and Lift [27] that provide accessibility extensions for common HTML editors.

An alternate approach is to improve the accessibility and usability of the Web browser or client software. Standard Web browsers are not very accessible to people with cognitive disabilities that rely on skills beyond the abilities of these individuals, such as reading, spelling, or complex multistep tasks. Davies et al. [28] at AbleLink Technologies have developed a Web browser called WebTrek [29] that has been customized to the needs and requirements of people with cognitive disabilities. Initial studies [28] determined that the Webtrek browser provided better access to the Internet for individuals with mental retardation than did Internet Explorer.

Socioeconomic Accessibility (Digital Divide)

The personal use of the Internet has continued to increase over recent years, even more so than the use of computers, and now broadband (high-speed) connections are beginning to gain in market share.

A growing digital divide has been documented in the United States [8,30,31]. According to the latest report from the National Telecommunications and Information Administration, although computer and Internet use continues to grow across the United States, there are still significant subpopulations (the elderly, persons of certain race and ethnicity or with low income and education) for whom the digital divide continues to be a major problem. And in particular "people with a disability are only half as likely to have access to the Internet as those without a disability: 21.6% compared to 42.1%. And while just under 25% of people without a disability have never used a personal computer, close to 60% of people with a disability fall into that category" [32] (see Fig. 11.2).

In fact, the digital divide is compounded for people with disabilities because they are also likely to be of lower economic status and less well educated as a result of their disability. But even taking this into account, disability status has as much impact on digital access as age, race, and ethnicity. Another factor is the additional expense associated with AT for a particular disability. Given the lower average income for people with disabilities, this can make access to the digital realm prohibitively expensive.

Personal Environment

Personal Management

Personal management covers the realm of procedures (how to perform a task), task management (when and where to perform tasks), and decision support (different

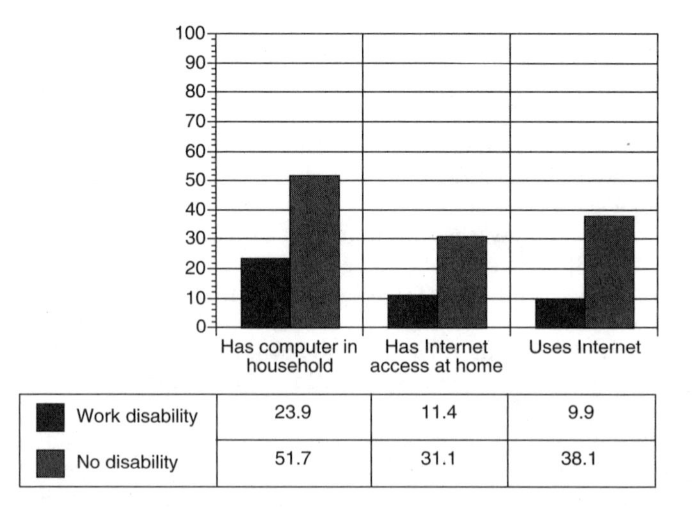

	Has computer in household	Has Internet access at home	Uses Internet
Work disability	23.9	11.4	9.9
No disability	51.7	31.1	38.1

FIGURE 11.2. Computer and Internet access overall. (From Current Population Survey, 1998 Computer and Internet Use Supplement & 1999 Annual Demographic Supplement.)

options to choose from in a task). Decision support is an important field in medical informatics, where the volume of medical information is such that it is impossible for an individual doctor to be familiar with all aspects of knowledge. In disability informatics, decision support is also important in assisting individuals with cognitive impairments in their ability to make every day decisions that the average person takes for granted. This would include tasks such a taking medication or brushing one's teeth.

The MAPS (Memory Aid Prompting System) project [33] provides a simple prompting system for the user and an interface for caregivers designed to effect high rates of integration into daily life.

Health and Disability Information and Education

Quality Online Information

Depending on people's perspective, the Web has become either a treasure trove of useful resources or a veritable dumping ground of questionable and dubious information. This issue is covered in more detail elsewhere, and is certainly applicable to people with disabilities.

Bioinformatics

One technology area that will have a large impact on health and disability education is bioinformatics. With the completion of the Human Genome Project, an increasing number of congenital disabilities are having their genetic markers and profiles identified, and it is highly likely that in the future this will lead to treatments being developed. This will lead to a concurrent demand for understanding and education around this knowledge in order for the general public to make "informed decisions." With the increasing move to put all information online, there will need to be additional research around the most effective way to provide this information. This will need to involve clinical providers, health educators, and genetic counselors.

Health Monitoring

One area where biomedical engineering is being applied is in "gerontechnology" in a high tech nursing home [34,35]. Oatfield Estates is located outside of Portland, Oregon and is home to around three dozen residents. It was opened in September 2000 and was the first wired rest home in the United States. Touchscreen PCs are installed in all the living spaces that not only allow access to the Internet but also provide internal information services (directory of names and faces) and controls (lights, ceiling fans). Other data can also be monitored, such as an individual's vital signs and a constant fix on their location within the facility.

One of the major efforts was to make the technology as unobtrusive as possible, and at first glance, Oatfield appears no different than other higher-end assisted living facilities. The main goal of the technology is to assist in the monitoring and management of both the caregivers and the residents. At Oatfield everyone wears an infrared/radiofrequency tracking badge that constantly transmits their location to the local-area network. But it would be preferable to remove the inconvenience of having to remember to wear an item. Biomedical engineering can be used to develop monitoring technologies that are nonintrusive by hiding or embedding them in the environment [36], for example, items of clothing that are worn, or within furniture such as sensors in the bed.

All these attempts to monitor individuals would at first inspection seem to be an invasion of privacy. But it turns out that they provide the Oatfield residents with unprecedented freedom to move about and perform more risky tasks than in a traditional nursing home. Residents can use the tracking badge to call for help, but also the system intelligently monitors the individual and alerts care providers in the event of an unwanted behavior, such as leaving the grounds without prior arrangements, or wandering into a kitchen area for someone known to be at risk of self-injury.

Physical Environment

Major opportunities exist in using technology to overcome the physical or cognitive barriers that exist, through enabling the individual to get to a service (technology helps them to get around) or through using technology to bring the service to him or her (technology helps others to get to him or her).

Community Navigation

The ADA has gone a long way to improving physical accessibility. However, getting around the physical environment is still fraught with many problems and barriers, for example, long inclines with areas to rest and lack of curb cuts. Several efforts are underway to address this problem using assistive information technology. MAGUS is a project that uses a geographical information system (GIS) to inform users about wheelchair access in urban areas [37]. It in effect provides the same type of functionality to the car-based GPS wayfinding systems, only it finds the best route for a wheelchair. The project both surveyed a large number of wheelchair users to identify the barriers in urban environments and also conducted field observations of wheelchair users navigating through town centers. These data, along with other measurements such as rolling resistance on difference surface types, were used to build and program a GIS database, and then finally a user-friendly interface was designed. An interesting side effect of the project was that the highlighting the accessibility black spots on the urban landscape gave urban planners a novel diagnostic tool.

Most, if not all, public transportation systems are now wheelchair accessible. However, for a number of other individuals, physical access is not so much the problem. Persons with cognitive disabilities have many different barriers to accessing public transit [38]; for example, it is necessary to comprehend and process maps, schedules, bus labels and signs, and clocks as well as adapt to errors and changing circumstances such as a bus being late or breaking down. Again assistive information technology can be used to mitigate these barriers. Global positioning satellite (GPS) technology is getting to the point that handheld units are feasible. Many public transit systems now also manage their operations using GPS-equipped buses. Finally, wireless telecommunications are ubiquitous in urban areas and now allow data transmission in addition to voice.

Telehealth/Telerehabilitation

With the increased ability to do unobtrusive health monitoring (see earlier section on Personal Health Monitoring), it becomes more easier to do remote care Telehealth and/or Telerehabilitation. In the past, the level of sophistication and training required to operate even the automated blood pressure cuff was a barrier to use. Telehealth technologies, such as patient monitoring, medical vital sign monitoring, sensors, e-mail communication with healthcare providers, as well as increasingly common video teleconferencing, are empowering the individual to take an active role as the patient.

Also if developed properly, Telehealth methods have the potential to take the hassle out of the health encounter for people who have difficulty with transportation, availability of personal assistants, and so forth. It is also possible to increase efficiencies by making support services more effective by centralizing them and providing services remotely via telecommunication.

References

1. Vanderheiden GC. Anywhere, anytime (+ anyone) access to the next-generation WWW. Comput Network ISDN Syst 1997;29:1439–46.
2. Pfeiffer D. The problem of disability definition, again. Disabil Rehabil 1999;21:392–5.
3. Krahn G. Oregon Health & Science University. Available at *http://www.healthwellness.org/training/sciconf_presentations/gkkeynote/text/page1.htm*(accessed on September 12, 2003).
4. LaPlante MP. How Many Americans have a disability? Washington, DC: U.S. Department of Education, National Institute on Disability and Rehabilitation Research (NIDRR), 1992, p. 4.
5. WHO. Document A29/INFDOCI/1. Geneva, Switzerland: World Health Organization, 1976.
6. ADA. US Department of Justice. Available at *http://www.usdoj.gov/crt/ada/adahom1.htm* (accessed on September 12, 2003).
7. US Census Bureau. Available at *http://www.census.gov/main/www/cen2000.html* (accessed on September 12, 2003).
8. Lenhart A, Horrigan J, Rainie L, et al. The ever-shifting Internet population: a new look at Internet access and the digital divide. Washington, DC: The Pew Internet & American Life Project, 2003, p. 46.
9. Nagi S. An epidemiology of disability among adults in the United States. Milbank Mem Fund Q 1976;6:493–508.
10. Nagi SZ. Disability concepts revisited: implications for prevention. In: Pope AM, Tarlov AR, eds. Institute of Medicine: Disability in America. Washington, DC: National Academy Press, 1991, pp. 309–27.
11. Pope AM, Tarlov AR. A model for disability and disability prevention. Institute of Medicine: Disability in America. Washington, DC: National Academy Press, 1991, pp. 76–108.
12. NIDRR. National Institute on Disability and Rehabilitation Research. Available at *http://www.ncddr.org/new/announcements/nidrr_lrp/* (accessed on September 12, 2003).
13. Vanderheiden GC, Vanderheiden KR. Trace R&D Center, University of Wisconsin-Madison. Available at *http://www.tracecenter.org/docs/consumer_product_guidelines/consumer.htm* (accessed on September 12, 2003).
14. WebAIM. Web accessibility in mind. Available at *http://www.webaim.org/techniques/.* (accessed on September 12, 2003).
15. Foulke E. Is it too late to rescue Braille literacy? The Braille Monitor 1996;39:Article no. 5.
16. APH. Distribution of federal quota based on registration of eligible students. Louisville, KY: American Printing House for the Blind, 1963–1998.
17. Linton S. Claiming Disability: Knowledge and Identity. New York University Press, 1998, p. 203.
18. Section 508. Available at *http://www.section508.gov/docs/AT1998.html* (accessed on September 12, 2003).
19. AbleData. AbleData. Available at *http://www.abledata.com/* (accessed on September 12, 2003).
20. W3C. World Wide Web Consortium. Available at *http://www.w3c.org/WAI/* (accessed on September 12, 2003).
21. ATBCB. Architectural and transportation barriers compliance board. Available at *http://www.section508.gov/* (accessed on February 17, 2003).
22. W3C. World Wide Web Consortium. Available at *http://www.w3.org/TR/2003/WD-WCAG20–2003062/* (accessed on September 12, 2003).

23. Watchfire. Watchfire. Available at *bobby.watchfire.com/bobby/* (accessed on September 12, 2003).
24. W3C. World Wide Web Consortium. Available at *http://www.w3.org/WAI/ER/existingtools.html* (accessed on September 12, 2003).
25. WebAIM. Web accessibility in mind. Available at *wave.webaim.org/* (accessed on September 12, 2003).
26. HiSoftware. The International Center for Disability Resources on the Internet (ICDRI), Internet Society Disability and Special Needs Chapter and HiSoftware Company. Available at *http://www.cynthiasays.com/* (accessed on September 12, 2003).
27. UsableNet. UsableNet. Available at *http://www.usablenet.com/* (accessed on September 12, 2003).
28. Davies DK, Stock SE, Wehmeyer ML. Enhancing independent Internet access for individuals with mental retardation through use of a specialized Web browser: a pilot study. Educ Train Ment Retard Dev Disabil 2001;36:107–13.
29. AbleLink. AbleLink Technologies, Colorado Springs, Colorado. Available at *http://www.ablelinktech.com/ProductPage.asp?SelectedProduct=WebTrek.* (accessed on December 8, 2003).
30. Kaye HS. Computer and Internet use among people with disabilities. Washington, DC: US Department of Education, National Institute on Disability and Rehabilitation Research, 2000:13.
31. NTIA. A nation online: how Americans are expanding their use of the Internet. In: Cooper KB, Victory NJ, eds. Washington, DC: US Department of Commerce, Economics and Statistics Administration, National Telecommunications and Information Administration, 2002, p. 92.
32. NTIA. Falling through the Net: toward digital inclusion. Washington, DC: US Department of Commerce, National Telecommunications and Information Administration, 2000, p. 122.
33. Carmien S. MAPS: PDA scaffolding for independence for persons with cognitive impairments. Paper presented at 2002 Human Computer Interaction Consortium (Pervasive communication access: availability and its consequences), Winter Park, CO, 2002.
34. Shellenbarger S. Available at *http://www.careerjournal.com/columnists/workfamily/20020719-workfamily.html.* (accessed on September 12, 2003).
35. Fox C. Technogenarians: The pioneers of pervasive computing aren't getting any younger. Wired 2001 November. Available at *http:www.wired.com/wired/archive/9.11/aging-pr.html.*
36. Winters JM, Wang Y, Winters JM. Wearable sensors and telerehabilitation. Engng Med Biol Mag IEEE 2003;22:56–65.
37. Matthews H, Beale L, Picton P, Briggs D. Modelling Access with GIS in Urban Systems (MAGUS): capturing the experiences of wheelchair users. AREA 2003; 35:34–45.
38. Fischer G, Sullivan J. Human-centered public transportation systems for persons with cognitive disabilities: challenges and insights for participatory design. In: Binder T, Gregory J, Wagner I, eds. Proceedings of the Participatory Design Conference (PDC'02). Malmö University, Sweden: CPSR, P.O. Box 717, Palo Alto, CA 94302, 2002:194–8.

12
Ethical Issues in Consumer Health Informatics

Holly B. Jimison

Principles of Ethics as a Framework for Consumer Health Informatics

Medical ethics are used to guide conduct and action. Many stakeholders come into play when considering how consumers obtain their health information. In addition to the consumer, we must consider the spectrum of clinicians (physicians, nurse educators, physical therapists, dieticians, etc.), as well as those people and organizations who create information materials for consumers (e.g., pharmaceutical companies, publishers, government groups, Web companies). With the growth in use of the Web for health information, it becomes critical to consider the ethical roles and responsibilities of the various stakeholders. Five guiding ethical principles form the basis for evaluating moral conduct in health care: autonomy, veracity, beneficence, nonmaleficence, and justice [1–3,22,23].

- **Autonomy**: self-determination, right to privacy, individual freedom, fundamental to informed consent
- **Veracity**: telling the truth, keeping promises, open patient–physician relationship
- **Beneficence**: doing good, promoting the well-being of others, professional obligation to help those in need
- **Nonmaleficence**: avoiding harm to others; protecting patients from danger, pain, and suffering (Hippocratic oath)
- **Justice**: fairness, respect for equality of all humans, equitable allocation of scarce resources, consideration of social policy.

Autonomy is relevant because it is the patient who is making choices about his or her own health care based on good quality information. Inasmuch as the physician and patient decision aids provide information about available treatment options, the principle of veracity is also important. The respect for autonomy and duty to inform truthfully are intimately related and concordant in patient decision aids and Web sites. As agents for the benefit of the patient, in the course of treatment both information tools and physicians must be beneficent and nonmaleficent. The moral obligations of fairness, respect, equality, and equity all play a role in the recommendation of treatments in the context of shared decision making and within computer tools for consumers.

Relating Ethical Principles to Consumer Health Informatics

In this chapter we discuss ethical issues relating to how consumers use Internet technology for health information, obtaining medicine or therapy and social support. Several topics at the forefront of consumer health informatics have important ethical implications. For example, the privacy and security of a consumer's medical information is a clear concern to the vast majority of consumers. Privacy and security of information are explicit goals of the ethical principle of autonomy. The quality and reliability of the information found on the Web is highly variable and difficult for consumers to judge. Conflict of interest on health Web sites is a rampant problem. Oftentimes it is difficult to distinguish sites that are selling or promoting a medical product from those attempting to provide unbiased material and recommendations. Health Web site developers have an ethical responsibility to convey accurate and current information. Interestingly, even for organizations without a product or advertising, creating and maintaining Web sites takes significant funding and effort to do well. Beyond fundamental honesty, some interesting questions would be to determine how good is "good enough" or how current is "current enough." Similarly, from the programmer's point of view, there is a question as to how much testing to ensure accurate performance is required to be "good enough." Oftentimes, ethical goals are confronted by practical business goals, and it is important to create clear policy to promote ethical principles. This type of policy can be set as voluntary guidelines or as regulations enforced by a governmental organization.

Ethical issues are particularly challenging in the environment of consumer health applications for several reasons: health is important and the stakes are high, consumers are not the experts in the domain of knowledge required to judge value and to protect themselves, Web sites can be created quickly and inexpensively by nearly anyone, both regulation and verification by experts are difficult because of an extremely large number of sites and the dynamic nature of material on the Web; and finally the technologies are constantly changing, creating new capabilities with further ethical implications.

Ethics and Quality Assurance on Consumer Health Sites

Judging the quality of information we receive in our daily lives is always difficult. Our information comes from a variety of sources (TV, newspapers, magazines, professional journals, books, and the Internet). However, judging the quality of health materials on the Web is particularly challenging for consumers. There are minimal monetary and skill barriers to creating Web sites, and it is fairly easy to make a site look quite professional and indistinguishable from those of larger, well-established organizations. Not all sites are "peer reviewed," published, or created by professionals with expertise in the topic covered. Because the quality of health information is so critical for consumers, several organizations have created guidelines for judging the quality of information on the Web for consumers [4–6,24]. Some of the criteria included in all of these guidelines are topical relevance, currency of the information, accuracy, and authoritativeness or objectivity.

The accuracy of health information on a Web site, insofar as it can be ascertained, is a basic concept relating to quality. Some professional health sites (both for-profit and nonprofit) have professional writers with domain expertise and also a board of reviewers to ensure accuracy of their material. Oftentimes, consumers are advised to judge sites with .gov or .edu extensions as having more accurate and unbiased information, as compared with .com sites. Naturally, although this heuristic may be useful as a first pass, it is oversimplified. Unless a health Web site has funding for both quality development and maintenance of content, it is very easy for information to go through a careful quality assurance process and still become outdated [21]. For the consumer of information, trying to find proxies for quality can be difficult. The following are some criteria that have been suggested:

- Credentials of information provider (Is there an advisory board?)
- Qualifications of advice providers (Are they licensed health care professionals?)
- Credibility of content (no wild promises)
- Full disclosure of sponsor of Web site (purpose of the Web site)
- Attribution clearly noted, including copyright.

From the consumer's point of view, topical relevance is certainly important when assessing the usefulness and quality of a Web site. The relevance of a site is context specific and depends on the particular question an individual consumer has in mind. To find appropriate materials, sites must be clearly organized and/or have intelligent search functions. In addition, the relevance of material on a Web site depends on the degree to which it is tailored to the individual and appropriate to his or her specific needs. Most health material on the Web is generic and not interactively tailored to individuals. This basically replicates what could be found in a textbook or brochure. The final aspect of relevance to an individual has to do with whether the material is action oriented and helps the consumer either make a healthcare decision that may lead to an action or a health behavior change.

Currency or the timeliness of information on a Web site itself is an important consideration. It is often difficult to have a generalized policy on how often health materials need to be updated. However, most professional sites ensure at least quarterly review of all materials. Consumers may judge the currency of Web site information by looking for date stamps or a notice of date of creation and/or update. On the ethical front, it is important to note that some Web sites use algorithms to update their time stamp automatically even if the material has not been changed or even reviewed, giving the impression that the information is current.

Thus, from the developer's point of view there are substantial ethical issues in creating health information sites for consumers. In addition to navigating conflict of interest, fraud, and inaccuracies, there are also the more murky decisions on the time and resources to put into Web site development and testing. Providing health information and interventions over the Internet is becoming an increasingly important component of health care. Ensuring that the materials are unbiased, accurate, relevant, and timely is fundamental to providing quality health care.

Ethics and Shared Decision Making

Shared decision making is now acknowledged by many as a viable alternative to what used to be a typical doctor-centered "paternalistic" model of care [7–11]. Shared decision making involves a two-way flow of information: from doctor to patient regarding treatment options, positive and negative effects, and the likelihood of such effects; and from patient to doctor regarding such factors as personal preferences, values, and constraints. Shared decision making also includes a shared deliberation or negotiation about the preferred treatment and a choice. Thus, shared decision making relates to the self-determination aspects of the ethical principle of autonomy.

The drive toward a paradigm of sharing treatment decision making has come about because of the realization that in many clinical situations (most often involving chronic diseases) there is no one best treatment option for all patients. Outcomes for many treatments are inherently uncertain at the individual patient level, and individual patients have differing risk tolerances, which affect their treatment preferences [8]. In circumstances in which multiple treatment options exist, making a decision often involves making tradeoffs between various attributes and outcomes. This process is value laden and based on patient preferences. In addition, it is now recognized that many patients wish to actively participate more fully in decision making and become more explicitly informed about their illness and options for treatment [12]. Nevertheless, the fact that not all patients prefer to play an active role in the decision making process or in making the final choice must not be neglected in the context of shared decision making.

The guiding ethical principles that serve as the foundations of shared decision making and patient decision aids are sometimes challenged and present dilemmas that must be addressed when they are incorporated in the patient–doctor decision making process. A useful approach to guiding ethical decision making in medicine was developed by three clinical ethicists (a philosopher—Jonsen, a physician—Siegler, and a lawyer—Winslade) [13]. The process can be thought of as the "ethics workup," similar to the "History and Physical" skills that all medical students come to use when learning how to "work up" a patient's primary complaints. Although this method has deep philosophical roots, the approach closely reflects how clinicians actually think through difficult cases. It is also appropriate for structuring knowledge content development for computer tools for patients.

The approach is to consider the following four topics as a way to organize the facts of the particular case at hand.

- *Medical indications*: a review of diagnosis and treatment options
- *Patient preferences*: how a patient values the potential health outcomes
- *Quality of life*: the objective of all clinical encounters is to improve, or at least address, quality of life for the patient
- *Contextual features*: the wider context beyond physician and patient which includes the family, law, hospital policy, insurance companies, and so forth.

These four topics are present in every clinical problem domain. In the design of computer tools for consumer use, it is important to incorporate the ethical concepts related to shared decision making in an explicit manner. These guidelines argue for interactivity, tailoring, and assessing patient preferences for potential health outcomes.

Privacy and Security of Patient Data

A recent survey on the attitudes of consumers on healthcare Web sites administered by the California Healthcare Foundation found that 88% of consumers do not want their health information shared without their consent [14]. In addition, the California Healthcare Foundation found that the privacy policies and practices of many prominent healthcare Web sites lacked proper protective measures for consumers' health information.

The Federal Trade Commission (FTC) is the governmental organization that regulates privacy practices. In its recent review of prominent Web sites, it found that several of the organizations were sharing information about their users with third parties (such as advertisers) without the permission of the users of their site. In fact, three of these sites were health Web sites [15]. The California Healthcare Foundation has also found that many Web sites, including those of pharmaceutical companies, have not ensured adequate privacy protection for consumers. The main findings of their report include [14]:

- Visitors are not anonymous, even if they think they are.
- Privacy policies fall short of truly safeguarding consumers.
- An inconsistency between policies and practices exists.
- Security is not adequate to protect health information.
- Few sites disclaiming liability for third parties can guarantee those entities are protecting visitors' health information.

The ethical principle of autonomy includes the notion of a patient's right to privacy, but clearly this principle is often violated in consumer health applications. In response to these reports and ongoing press coverage, many sites have begun to adhere to ethical codes and guidelines, signified by a posted code on their Web page. Examples of self-regulatory initiatives include [6,16–19]:

- Hi-Ethics: emphasizes privacy, security, credibility and reliability
- American Medical Association's Principles Governing Web Sites
- Health On the Net Code of Conduct: emphasizes reliability and credibility
- Internet Healthcare Coalition's eHealth Code of Ethics
- Verified Internet Pharmacy Practice Sites Program: for pharmaceutical companies

The Web sites that have adopted these voluntary guidelines and regulations have been proactive in responding to the public's concern about the privacy and security of information. The primary piece of legislation and regulation in this area is the Health Insurance Portability and Accountability Act of 1996 (HIPAA). This act creates very strict requirements for ensuring the security and privacy of patient information. Although it is not clear how HIPAA may apply to the full spectrum of health Web sites, most organizations with Web sites for patients are taking care to be in full compliance proactively.

Ethics and Etiquette of Online Virtual Communities

Online virtual communities are growing in importance in health care. Many of these communities are focused on specific diseases or conditions, where social support and problem solving are important components of care. These include both electronic bulletin boards for posting messages or real-time online chat rooms. Some of the communities are facilitated or moderated by healthcare professionals. In other cases, there may be an experienced patient who serves as a coach or facilitator. Social support and online problem solving by patients contributes significantly to improving health outcomes. However, several ethical concerns merit clarification as new participants join a group. Some sample issues are covered in the World Wide Web's Virtual Library site [20] covering the Ethics and Etiquette of Internet Resources. These include guidelines for social interactions (netiquette), copyright information, as well as advice on how to protect privacy while participating in online virtual communities. Although there may be no formal regulations for a health Web site, the guidelines around respect and privacy are similar to those for face-to-face group support meetings. Many organizations that provide forums for virtual communities employ moderators for these groups to ensure that ethical principles are followed.

Conclusion

The guiding ethical principles discussed in this chapter are considered essential as the moral underpinnings of guidelines and regulations that serve as codes of ethical conduct for all parties involved in the delivery of health information and health interventions via the Internet. We have examined the ethical issues from the perspective of patients, clinicians, Web site developers, and Web site sponsors. The dynamic nature of the Web environment, and of technology development in general, offers continual new challenges for ethicists and stakeholders in this area. It is encouraging to see the grassroots efforts of the consumer health informatics community to self-regulate and help ensure that patients have an opportunity to access unbiased, secure, and high-quality health information and interventions. The ethical challenges we face are not always clear cut, but the five guiding ethical principles have served as a useful framework for facilitating a powerful new component of health care—consumer health informatics.

References

1. Beauchamp TL, Childress JF. Principles of Biomedical Ethics, Fourth Edition. New York: Oxford University Press, 1994.
2. Reich W, ed. Encyclopedia of Bioethics, Second Edition. 5 vols. New York: Simon & Schuster/Macmillan, 1995.
3. Veatch RM, ed. Medical Ethics, Second Edition. New York: Bartlett and Jones, 1994.
4. Discern Online. Discern quality criteria for consumer health information. *http://www.discern.org.uk/* (accessed November 2004).
5. Health Summit Working Group. Criteria for assessing the quality of health information on the Internet *http://www.bmlweb.org/internet_medical_critere.pdf* (accessed November 2004).
6. Health on the Net Foundation, Hon (Health on the Net) Code, *http://www.hon.ch/HONcode/* (accessed November 2004).
7. Charles C, Gafni A, Whelan T. Shared decision-making in the medical encounter: what does it mean? Soc Sci Med 1997;44:681–92.
8. Charles C, Whelan T, Gafni A. What do we mean by partnership in making decisions about treatment? Br Med J 1999;319:780–2.
9. Charles C, Gafni A, Whelan T. Decision-making in the physician–patient encounter: revisiting the shared treatment decision-making model. Soc Sci Med 1999;49:651–61.
10. Coulter A. Partnerships with patients: the pros and cons of shared clinical decision-making. J Health Serv Res Policy 1997;2:112–21.
11. Coulter A. Paternalism or partnership? Patients have grown up-and there's no going back. Br Med J 1999;319:719–20.
12. Sculpher M, Gafni A, Watt I. Shared treatment decision making in a collectively funded health care system: possible conflicts and some potential solutions. Soc Sci Med 2002;54:1369–77.
13. Jonsen AR, Siegler M, Winslade WJ. Clinical Ethics: A Practical Approach to Ethical Decisions in Clinical Medicine, Fourth Edition. New York: McGraw-Hill, 1998.
14. California HealthCare Foundation. Ethics Survey of Consumer Attitudes about Health Web Sites. Conducted by Cyber Dialogue and the Institute for the Future. January 2000. Available at *http://www.chcf.org/documents/consumer/surveyreport.pdf* (accessed November 2004).
15. PriceWaterhouseCoopers. Protecting online privacy. *http://www.pwcglobal.com/extweb/manissue.nsf/DocID/16F59A741FF1198C85256A64004B9D36* (accessed November 2004).
16. American Medical Association. Guidelines for health information sites on the Internet. *http://www.ama-assn.org/ama/pub/category/1905.html* (accessed November 2004).
17. Hi-Ethics. About Hi-Ethics. *http://www.hiethics.com/About.asp* (accessed November 2004).
18. Internet Healthcare Coalition . eHealth Code of Ethics. *http://www.ihealthcoalition.org/ethics/ethics.html* (accessed November 2004).

19. National Association Boards of Pharmacy. VIPPS. *http://www.nabp.net/vipps/intro.asp* (accessed November 2004).
20. World Wide Web Virtual Library. Ethics and etiquette of Internet resources. *http://www.ciolek.com/WWWVLPages/QltyPages/QltyEtiq.html* (accessed November 2004).
21. Eysenbach G, Köhler C. Does the internet harm health? Database of adverse events related to the internet has been set up. Br Med J 2002;324:239.
22. Eysenbach G. Towards ethical guidelines for e-health. J Med Internet Res 2000; 2:e7.
23. Goodman KW, Miller RA. Ethics and health informatics: users, standards, and outcomes. In: Shortliffe EH, Perreault LE, eds. Medical Informatics: Computer Applications in Health Care and Biomedicine. New York: Springer-Verlag, 2000.
24. Internet Healthcare Coalition. Tips for health consumers: finding quality health information on the Internet. *http://www.ihealthcoalition.org/content/tips.html* (accessed January 20, 2004).
25. Kliever LD, ed. Dax's Case. Essays in Medical Ethics and Human Meaning. Dallas: Southern Methodist University Press, 1989.

13 Social Informatics and Consumer Health

STEVE SAWYER

The dominant contemporary conceptualization of consumers is as individual seekers of health information for their personal use. This individualistic view informs the development and deployment of technically sophisticated systems and is flawed in two ways. First, an individualistic view overlooks the socially embedded nature of consumer health engagements. Second, such a view reifies the rather problematic expert-centric view of health care. In this chapter I focus on how social informatics helps to both illuminate these issues and redress them through alternative conceptualizations.

Working groups focused on Consumer Health Informatics with the American Medical Informatics Association and the International Medical Informatics Association advocate for a range of needs relative to consumer's health information needs [1,2]. However, they focus on helping individuals make decisions about personal health issues (e.g., [3]). Conversely, the Pew Internet and American Life Project's reports note that women and well-educated people are seeking health resources information, primarily to help inform others [4]. Further, the Pew's empirical findings make clear that people use the Internet as a forum for emotional support and for practical, daily help in coping. Finally, the findings of the Pew researchers are that these searches are done via search engines, with little fact checking, and convenience and anonymity are valued above breadth and validity.[1]

This contrasting view on consumer health behavior is problematic. Evidence supporting a view of consumers as embedded in a web of social relationships, set in physical and temporal contexts, and often seeking information on behalf of others is difficult to reconcile to the current discourse on consumer health-information–seeking behavior. To help address this gap, in this chapter I introduce you to the concepts and findings of social informatics. I do so to help reframe your understanding of, and issues with, consumer's information seeking regarding health and medical information and their use of information technologies and information systems to support this information-seeking behavior. To these ends, in this chapter I:

---

[1] The Pew findings reflect more the missions of the American Medical Informatics Association: People and Organizational Issues working group (see *http://www.amia.org/working/poi/main.html*) and the International Medical Informatics Association's Organizational and Social Issues working group (see *www.imia.org/search.lasso?-database=organizations.fp5&-response=WG_profile.html&-layout=CGI&-sortField=workgroup_SIG&-sortOrder=ascending&-op=bw&type=WGSIG&-maxRecords=1&-skipRecords=13&-search_*. These groups' Web sites note that there is a long tradition of research into, and a cumulative body of evidence on, the larger social and organizational dynamics surrounding individuals who seek health information and interact with health-information-providing systems.

1. Define and explain the concepts and findings of social informatics.
2. Examine consumer health opportunities and unexplored issues from a social informatics perspective.

Thus, this chapter serves as an introduction to social informatics, and in doing so provides a lens for consumer health informatics scholars, systems developers, and policy makers to reflect on the current approaches to engaging issues in (and with) consumer health.[2] My premise is simple: social informatics can assist consumer health informatics scholars, systems developers, and policy makers in developing more robust and useful theories, applications, and policies.

Social informatics is the body of rigorous empirical research that focuses on the relationships among information and communications technologies (ICT) and the larger social context in which these ICT exist. By using ICT I include formal information systems such as medical records systems through to the informal and often highly personalized collection of devices such as phones, cellular phones, personal digital assistants, and so forth, that people use to find and share information. Thus, ICT is a plural and fluid placeholder that I use to evoke the concept of a web of computing [5]. Focusing on context highlights that ICT exist within a larger social milieu through which the uses of that ICT can be understood. In saying this I explicitly connect social with technical: in the rest of this chapter I refer to this intimate interdependency as a sociotechnical relationship.

Social informatics research shares a common perspective and often common findings, as others and I have noted. Social informatics work, however, is found in a range of disciplinary literatures. In this way, social informatics is transdisciplinary. Acknowledging this helps to give voice to common findings found in dispersed bodies of related research literatures. For example, I summarize three studies, each from relevant literatures, focused on different social settings and using different ICT to showcase the commonalities of social informatics research.

Kaplan et al. [6] report on a study of patients interacting with a telemedicine system (the trial being done in the New England region of the Unites States). The system was designed to provide an automated and interactive response to patients dealing with changes in their physical activity and eating (in response to medical procedures). The interactive system was driven by an expert system that had both diagnostic and response questions about health and physical activity. Kaplan found that this clinical system was much more than a fact-dispensing interaction with its clientele. Participants reported developing an attachment to the automated voice, looking forward to the social interactions with the system, and even developing personal feelings toward the voice, often asking questions far beyond the range of responses anticipated by the designed (leading to odd interpretations of what was reported by the automated clinician). Many of the participants were lonely and isolated, and this clinical system served as much more than the clinical expert its designers anticipated. The automated system became a friend and confidant—valued more because it "listened" than for its medical advice.

Patterson et al. [7] report on a study of automated (barcoding) systems used by nurses in a US veteran's hospital. The system, hosted on a personal digital assistant, was used to help automate the work flow of nurses, better monitor patient interactions

[2] As I will discuss, social informatics is not a theory, a method, or a domain. Social informatics research spans disciplines and research domains. My particular interest in the relationships between uses ICT and organizational effects shapes the literatures I cite and examples I present.

and medications, and reduce human errors in the practice of medicine. Patterson and her colleagues found that the design of the system and its hosting device did not fit the nurse's work. The device masked details of the medical record and the limited interface made it difficult to search, read, and record information. The predesigned workflow system did not accommodate moves (such as demanding medicine to be administered to patients when the patient was in another part of the hospital for test. This would be recorded as a nurses' error). This led to nurses using work-arounds and often increasing the number of possible mistakes (not reducing them). Simply, the information system did not account for the complex coordination needs, importance of worker-to-worker social interactions, and the structural demands of the organizational settings.

Etzioni and Etzioni [8] focus on computer-mediated-communication (CMC) and report that the creation of sustainable (stable) communities of participants (stakeholders) is critical to the CMC system. They explore the role of community and extend observations of behavior in face-to-face communities to what they mean in a computer-mediated world. Their analysis maps aspects of community with features of ICT that support computer-supported communities. In doing this they raise both ICT design and ICT use issues, reflect on the ways that the social context formed by these communities shapes CMC use, and suggest several hybridized CMC designs that would better meet the needs of virtual communities.

The Kaplan, Patterson et al., and Etzioni and Etzioni articles focus on different types of problems, look at different types of ICTs, draw on different literatures, use different theories, and are set in different contexts. However, these studies highlight similar conceptual issues and their findings have much in common. For example, these studies suggest that ICT uses leads to multiple and sometimes paradoxical effects. All three studies describe how ICT use shapes thought and action in ways that benefit some groups more than others and these differential effects. Third, all three studies depict a reciprocal relationship between ICT and their context. We return to these points later.

What Is Social Informatics?

Six elements help to both define and bound what is meant by social informatics.

The Problem-Oriented Nature of Social Informatics

Social informatics is problem oriented. Just as the human–computer interaction (HCI) literature reflects the problematic relationships between individuals and computers, and the computer-supported cooperative work (CSCW) literature reflects the problematic relationships between groups of people and computers, the social informatics literature reflects the problems that arise from the bidirectional relationships among social context and ICT design, implementation, and uses. Social informatics research spans levels of analysis, often by making explicit links between particular levels of social analysis and the larger social milieu in which computing takes place. In this way, social informatics is similar to other areas of study that are defined by a problem such as gerontology, software engineering, urban studies, and so forth.

Social informatics research is characterized further by its inclusion of normative, analytical, and critical orientations. The *normative orientation* refers to research whose aim is to recommend alternatives for professionals who design, implement, use, or make policy about ICTs. This type of research has an explicit goal of influencing practice by providing empirical evidence illustrating the varied outcomes that occur as people work with ICTs in a wide range of organizational and social contexts. For example, much of the participatory design research focuses on identifying the nuanced ways in which users come to understand and adapt how they work with information systems.

The *analytical orientation* refers to studies that develop theories about ICTs in institutional and cultural contexts or to empirical studies that are organized to contribute to such theorizing. This type of research seeks to contribute to a deeper understanding of how the evolution of ICT use in a particular setting can be generalized to other ICTs and other settings. One example is Kling's [9] depiction of various perspectives on ICT use in organizations.

The *critical orientation* refers to examining ICTs from perspectives that do not automatically and "uncritically" adopt the goals and beliefs of the groups that commission, design, or implement specific ICTs. The critical orientation is possibly the most novel [10]. It encourages information professionals and researchers to examine ICTs from multiple perspectives, such as those of the various people who use them, as well as people who design, implement, or maintain them. The critical orientation also advocates examination of possible "failure modes" and service losses. Critical approaches provide great insight into how ICT can be better designed (e.g., [6,7]).

Empirical and Theory-Based Focus of Social Informatics

Social informatics work is empirical. The intent is to help make sense of the vexing issues people face when they work and live with computing. This work is always set in the context of social milieus such as work groups, communities, cultural units, societies, and/or organizations.

Social informatics research is often characterized by its use of the wide range of social theories that explicitly engage context in a holistic manner. By social theory we invoke the wide range of perspectives that seek to represent, define, and predict how humans enact and maintain social order, social structures, and social interaction (e.g., [11,12]).[3]

A Socio-Technical Perspective

Social informaticians conceptualize context as comprising interdependent and multilevel networks of socio-technical links (e.g., [13,14]). Strum and Latour [15] emphasize that these links are not merely social, as humans use technologies such as ICT to construct or enforce their view of reality through symbolic and material bonds. Often the literature uses different terms to describe this socio-technical arrangement. No matter the term(s) used, social informatics research is premised on the belief that even common technical components cannot be understood apart from the social and organizational milieu in which they exist. Simply, computing cannot be considered in isolation but must always be studied in specific contexts.

A socio-technical perspective makes clear that people are social actors. That is, people's individual autonomy, their agency, and their behaviors, are shaped by the social

[3] The forms and meanings of social theory are, themselves, a field of vigorous inquiry and there is not space in this chapter to engage in a detailed discussion of what is social theory. For those interested in exploring some of the most widely used social theories, see Ritzer [12]. For those interested in discussions of the roles, meanings, and roots of social theory, see Sica [11].

norms, organizational forces, and (the social and physical) structures that surround them [16]. These structures can be as straightforward as office layout. But, structures also include the uses of computer systems, the inherent organizational structure of data, procedures and interactions, and authority structures based on power and knowledge. Viewing people as social actors makes clear that they are often acting in very constrained, if not sometimes prescribed, ways.

A socio-technical perspective also emphasizes the ensemble view of computing [17]. In this view the elements of computing are seen as enmeshed into the institutional structures of particular situations and the social-actor nature of individuals. Such an institutional appreciation for ICT makes it difficult to abstract "best practices" or decontextualized findings drawn from one site and apply or extrapolate them to a second site.

Transdisciplinary

Social informatics research is being done in many disciplines including information science, communications, sociology, anthropology, information systems, management science, education, and library science, to name some. Often scholars whose work focuses on one domain (such as hospital emergency rooms) do so without knowing that similar work, often leading to similar findings, is being done in another domain (such as software development groups). In this way social informatics is a "transdiscipline:" its literature both spans and links research from disparate fields. Further, although the term "social informatics" may be new, social informatics research is not. Researchers from these various fields have been studying the social and organizational aspects of ICTs for more than 25 years [9]. This work falls under a range of conceptual labels including (but not limited to) the "social analysis of computing or technology," the "social impacts of computing or technology," "information policy," "computers/technology and society," and, more recently, "computer-mediated communication" [18, p. 1]. The sheer number of related fields and the use of a range of terms mean that the research findings and insights have been difficult for scholars and teachers to access [19,20, p. 12]. Moreover, given this dispersion, it is (oddly) possible for a scholar to contribute to the social informatics literature without ever having considered his or her work to be a part of this (or any larger) corpus of similar findings.

A Form of Informatics

The meaning of social informatics rests in part on the broad, evolving, and debated definition of informatics. By informatics we mean the study of information content, representation, technology, and the methods and strategies of its use (see [21]). Informatics is a term commonly used outside of North America to refer to a range of computing research.[4] Although there is an ever-growing number of informatics research areas (e.g., medical informatics, legal informatics, archive and museum informatics, consumer health informatics, bioinformatics, etc), a specific form of social informatics is that work focused on formalized organizational or group boundaries, which we call organizational

[4] See *www.slis.indiana.edu/SI* for more discussion of informatics. This site, maintained by the late Rob Kling, contains a brief history on the emergence of the term and some key contributors. A link to a 1997, NSF-sponsored, workshop on social informatics points to a partial list of additional contributors who attended, commented on, or whose work directly shaped the workshop report. This workshop report can also be found at the Social Informatics Web site.

informatics.[5] Social informatics arose as a descriptor through a series of discussions among like-interested researchers in the early 1990s. Often these conversations were led by or included the late Rob Kling, who maintained one of the most comprehensive social informatics Web sites (see footnote 4) and whose work has been an instrumental part of coalescing social informatics into the interdiscipline I describe in this chapter.

In summary, what then, is social informatics? According to Kling [18, p. 1], "A serviceable working conception of 'social informatics' is that it identifies a body of research that examines the social aspects of computerization. A more formal definition is the interdisciplinary study of the design, uses and consequences of information technologies that takes into account their interaction with institutional and cultural contexts."

What Social Informatics Is Not

Many academic approaches besides social informatics provide theoretical insight and/or commentary on the relationships among ICT's uses and the human condition. In this section we highlight some of these approaches and explain how they differ from our conceptualization of the inclusive literature represented by us as social informatics.

A Theory

Like HCI and CSCW, social informatics is best seen as a large and growing federation of scholars focused on common problems. There is no single theory of social informatics and there is no claim being made that the research in this field is pursuing one particular theoretical notion. Currently many theories are being used by social informaticians and we return to this point in the next section. In the fourth section we point to some contemporary work oriented toward theory building. But, even from the most liberal perspective, social informatics is not a theory.

A Method

Social informatics research is characterized by pluralistic approaches to the conduct of inquiry. It is pluralistic in that it is not method specific. Social informatics researchers employ a variety of methods, ranging from the observational studies [22], secondary data analysis [9], surveys [23], and multiple methods [24]. In this way the social informatics literature differs from fields such as operations research or linguistic analysis that are primarily defined by their methods.

Direct Effects (or Tool) Approach

Direct effects models underlay the earliest and often most simplisitc efforts to anticipate the social consequences of computerization in organizations (see, e.g., [25]). Tool views provide little to social informatics given the relatively simple views of how people interact with the ICTs.

Punditry and Futurizing

In addition, social informatics differs from other nonacademic commentary about ICTs and society. One of the more common forms is the punditry of futurizing: glossy con-

---

[5] We consider organizational informatics a subset of social informatics. For convenience, in the rest of this chapter we use social informatics to denote *both* social and organizational informatics.

ceptualizations of the future impacts of ICT on society with little (or anectdotal) support (e.g., [26]). This, and other forms of futurizing, may often be both thought provoking and popular. But these prophesies are rarely validated by empirical study and are often simplistic or misleading. In this way the public commentary on the value of Web sites such as WebMD® reflect punditry.

Social Informatics Foundations

Three common findings arise from the empirical and rigorous research base of social informatics.

The Roles of the Social Context

The mutual interdependence between ICT and social context frames social informatics research contexts [9,27,28]. By social context we mean a holistic perspective among levels of social analysis, particular characteristics that help to define a level of analysis, characteristics that act as forces on the various levels of analysis, and characteristics that provide the backdrop and perspective from which an understanding of the problem of interest can be made. The exact nature of the social context is intimately related to the problem of interest. This suggests that the characterization of, and factors of interest within, context will vary and the researcher must set out the levels of analysis and factors through either a priori depiction or post hoc description. But all social informatics research will represent social context.

Research that reduces the larger social context to one or two variables, such as level of uncertainty in the environment or some other surrogate, is not typically considered as social informatics. However, factor-based studies that provide a richer picture of context can contribute to social informatics.

As we stated earlier, social informatics researchers explicitly acknowledge that ICTs are conceived, developed, configured, and/or used within a nuanced and interdependent socio-technical system [16]. Thus, ICT are in a relationship of mutual shaping with context [29,30]. For example, the embedded nature of ICTs influences the ways people develop them, the kinds of workable configurations they propose, and how people choose to implement and use ICTs.

Common Social Informatics Findings

Three common findings come from the empirical work in social informatics:

1. ICT uses lead to multiple and sometimes paradoxical effects.
2. ICT uses shape thought and action in ways that benefit some groups more than others and these differential effects often have moral and ethical consequences.
3. Reciprocal relationships exist among ICT design, implementation, use, and the context in which these occur.

ICT Uses Lead to Multiple and Sometimes Paradoxical Effects

Social informatics studies highlight the complex outcomes of ICT use in two ways. First, they show that a particular ICT's impacts are rarely isolated to a desired area, but rather spread to a much larger number of people through the socio-technical links that comprise context. Second, these studies typically highlight unforeseen and unintended outcomes, which, in many cases, may be contrary to the original intentions for the ICT. In summary, these examples serve to illustrate the first common finding of social informatics research: ICT uses have both far-reaching and unexpected outcomes. This implies that we should not assume that it is possible to understand fully the impacts of a particular ICT use. It is likely that any given ICT will shape elements not immediately adjacent to it through connections of socio-technical links. Further, we cannot always expect that ICTs will have the (positive *or* negative) effect we expect them to have.

ICT Uses Shape Thought and Action in Ways that Benefit Some Groups More than Others and These Differential Effects Often Have Moral and Ethical Consequences

The basis of our second common finding is that ICT uses act as sociocognitive structures that shape thought and action. Following Ritzer [12] we understand structure to include both large-scale social structures that shape interaction and micro-structures involved in individual human interaction. The social informatics approach recognizes that these structures shape thought and action in ways that benefit some groups over others and that this structural favoritism often leads to moral and/or ethical consequences.

Reciprocal Relationships Among ICT Design, Implementation, Use, and Context

The third common finding that arises from contemporary social informatics literature is that there is a reciprocal (bidirectional) shaping between ICT and its socio-technical context. That is, social informatics research often leads to discussion of how context shapes ICT or ICT uses and how these ICTs and ICT uses shape their context.

Context and Levels of Analysis in the Social Informatics Literature

We noted earlier in this chapter that social informatics scholars conceptualize context as socio-technical networks of influences. They recognize that these network exist at what Klein et al. [31] call different levels of theory or the "target level at which the researcher aims to depict and explain" (p. 198). In social informatics work this typically includes formal and informal work groups, departments, formal organizations, formal and informal social units such as communities or professional associations, groups of organizations and/or industries, nations, cultural groups, and even whole "societies" [13,14]. Thus, one way of understanding context is to focus on the level of theory and analysis that social informatics scholars portray in their research.

A Social Informatics Perspective on Consumer Health Informatics Research

In this final section we use the principles of social informatics to help reframe some of the ongoing issues and opportunities in consumer health informatics. There seems to be no shortage of issues and opportunities in this area, and here we draw on Eysenbach [32], who notes that the emerging orientation toward evidence-based medicine, increased use of information and communication technologies to get information and deliver services regarding health, and the growing awareness of the need to equalize relationships among health professionals and lay people are tied to cutting healthcare costs. Given these forces, Eysenbach [32] notes four areas of interest to consumer health informaticians:

1. Bringing medical knowledge to consumers
2. Making electronic health records accessible to patients
3. Building decision aides to support consumer's choices
4. Developing quality control mechanisms for health information available over the Internet

Bringing Medical Knowledge to Consumers

As we noted at the chapter's start this is typically conceived as targeting the brain and behavior of an individual. A social informatics perspective suggests that these people are embedded in institutional settings such as families, workplaces, and neighborhoods, with each of these institutional contexts both steering and enabling actions [33]. This social-actor perspective further suggests that this knowledge passing must be tied to a larger discourse (as public health professionals have known for years), must be multichannel, and rarely is connected to formal medical systems or sources of knowledge. This also suggests that application design must embrace the language and idioms being used, requires multiple channels (such as the telephone, Internet links, and perhaps even the television) and needs to be built to enable dialog [a consumer-centric view of interactions, not question answering (a physician-centric view of interactions] [34].

Making Electronic Health Records Accessible to Patients

Two issues are often discussed relative to health records. The first is to make people's medical records more transparent. This, again, is tied to the consumer as an individual. Second, and tied to access, to raise consumer's level of understanding about health-related issues. A social informatics perspective suggests reconceptualizing medical records as also a family or community property [35]. This acknowledges that people are often looking on behalf of others, are sharing within family and other social units, and making collective sense of medical information. Further, a social informatics perspective highlights that there are different contexts of use: those who engage in their medical information in response to emergencies act much differently than do those engaged in long-term care and management of some particular illness. Application designers should focus on balancing private and public access (like a library) rather than as a personal characteristic.

Building Decision Aides to Support Consumer's Choices

By framing decisions as a particular person's personal choice seems central to current thinking in consumer health informatics. It also stands in stark relief relative to relevant contemporary data about how people interact with health information and make decisions [4]. Decision aides are an outgrowth of medical systems and are likely to be as obtuse and off-putting as have been people's interactions with many health professionals (e.g., [6]). A social informatics perspective suggests that this approach is not viable.

Developing Quality Control Mechanisms for Health Information Available over the Internet

Nothing in the literatures on internet usage or human information seeking suggests this is possible [35]. By developing access to information as a quality control issue frames Internet access to medical information as a large-scale problem of people making poor or uninformed choices. This framing neglects the powerful forces of family, friends, and neighbors in both traditional and Internet-driven consumer-health informatics. This was a "problem" with the conceptualization of patient/professional relationships that predates the Internet and quality control efforts are unlikely to remediate a long-standing problem. A social informatics perspective suggests that focusing efforts to develop, facilitate, and enable localized discussions and sharing [36,37].

Two Further Suggestions for Consumer Health Informaticians

An emerging trend in the social informatics literature is the development of theories and models that draw on, and/or extend, social theory to more fully account for the effects of ICT. Consumer health informaticians have the opportunity to contribute to this broad goal while also pursuing more socially relevant and encompassing theories of consumer's health information behaviors.

Second, the expertise with clinical trials provides health informaticians a methodological means to observe the evolution, and contribute to shaping the design of information systems over time. Imagine a trial of two systems: one based on the knowledgeable individual premise that underlies current medical information systems and the other premised on social actor perspectives of users. In the former, its content and advice focused. In the latter, the design is focused on sharing and responding. The efficacy of these systems can be compared. In addition, their subsequent development and operations can be evaluated and assessed over time. Simply, the difference among current views on consumer health informatics and a social informatics perspective of the same issues is both a conceptual and empirical question, and these are the type where our science can help.

In summary, the context-dependency, methodological pluralism, problem-orientation, and transdisciplinary character of social informatics research can help contemporary consumer health informaticians. A social informatics perspective leads to advocating for broad-scale, contextually based research programs in which people are characterized as social actors and the roles of ICT are set within institutionally sensitive contexts. Further, a social informatics perspective focuses our awareness of ICT's varied influences and to provide us a means of engaging in larger-scale discussions of these influences. In this way, social informatics research provides a means of educating practitioners and of extending the research scope of researchers.

References

1. AMIA (American Medical Informatics Association's People and Organizational Issues working group). Available at *http://www.amia.org/working/poi/main*.
2. IMIA (International Medical Informatics Association's Organizational and Social Issues working group). Available at *http://www.imia.org/search.lasso?-database=organizations.fp5&-response=WG_profile.html&-layout=CGI&-sortField=workgroup_SIG&-sortOrder=ascending&-op=bw&type=WGSIG&-maxRecords=1&-skipRecords=13&-search_*.
3. NIST (National Institute of Standards). Hearing on E-health and consumer empowerment: how consumers can use technology today and in the future to improve their health. Available at *http://www.nist.gov/hearings/2001/ehlth.htm* (July 23, 2001).

4. Pew Internet & American Life Project. Health topics searched online. Available at *http://www.pewinternet.org/* (accessed October 6, 2003).
5. Kling R, Scacchi W. The web of computing: computer technology as social organization. Adv Comput 1982;21:1–90.
6. Kaplan B, Farzanfar R, Friedman RH. Personal relationships with an intelligent interactive telephone health behavior advisor system: a multimethod study using surveys and ethnographic interviews. Int J Med Inform 2003;71:33–41.
7. Patterson ES, Cook RI, Render ML. Improving patient safety by identifying side effects from introducing bar coding in medication administration. JAMIA 2002;9:540–53.
8. Etzioni A, Etzioni O. Face-to-face and computer-mediated communication, a comparative analysis. Information Soc 1999;15:241–8.
9. Kling R. Social analysis of computing: theoretical perspectives in recent empirical research. ACM Comput Surv 1980;12:61–110.
10. Agre P, Schuler D. Reinventing Technology, Rediscovering Community: Critical Explorations of Computing as a Social Practice. New York: Ablex, 1997.
11. Sica A, ed. What Is Social Theory? The Philosophical Debates. Malden, MA: Blackwell, 1998.
12. Ritzer G. Modern Sociological Theory, Fourth Edition. New York: McGraw-Hill, 1996.
13. Castells M. The information city: a new framework for social change. In: Wellman B, Bell JK, eds. The City in the 1990's Series (Research Paper 184). Centre for Urban and Community Studies, University of Toronto, Toronto, 1991.
14. MacKenzie D, Wajcman J. The Social Shaping of Technology, Second Edition. Philadelphia: Open University Press, 1999.
15. Strum S, Latour B. Redefining the social link: from baboons to humans. In: MacKenzie D, Wajcman J, eds. The Social Shaping of Technology. Philadelphia: Open University Press, 1999, pp. 116–25.
16. Lamb R, Kling R. Reconceptualizing users as social actors in information systems Rresearch. MIS Q 2003;27:197–235.
17. Orlikowski W, Iacono S. Desperately seeking the "IT" in IT research—a call to theorizing the IT Artifact. Information Syst Res 2001;12:112–24.
18. Kling R. What is social informatics, and why does it matter? D-Lib Magazine 5 (1). Available at *http://www.dlib.org:80/dlib/january99/kling/01kling.html* (1999).
19. Kling R. Learning about information technologies and social change: the contribution of social informatics. Information Soc 2000;16: 217–32.
20. Kling R, Rosenbaum H, Sawyer S. Information technologies in human contexts: learning from organizational and social informatics. Information Today. Available at *http://www.slis.indiana.edu/CSI* (forthcoming).
21. Brookes B. Informatics as the fundamental social science. In: Taylor PJ, ed. Proceedings of the 39th FID Congress: FID Publication 566. New Trends in Documentation and Information. London: ASLIB, 1980, pp. 19–29.
22. Suchman L. Supporting articulation work: aspects of a feminist practice office technology production. In: Kling R, ed. Computerization and Controversy: Value Conflicts and Social Choices, Second Edition. San Diego: Academic Press, 1996, pp. 407–23.
23. Attewell P, Battle J. Home computers and school performance. Information Soc 1999;15:1–10.
24. Crowston K, Sawyer S, Wigand R. The interplay between structure and technology: investigating the roles of information technologies in the residential real estate industry. Information Technology, People; 14:163–83.
25. Negroponte N. Being Digital. New York: Vintage Books, 1997.
26. Toffler A. The Third Wave. New York: Bantam Books, 1991.
27. Argyres N. The impact of information technology on coordination: evidence from the B-2 "stealth" bomber. Organization Sci 1999;10:162–79.
28. Abbott A. Sequence analysis: new methods for old ideas. Annu Rev Sociol 1995;21, 91–113.
29. Orlikowski W, Baroudi JJ Studying information technology in organizations. Research approaches and assumptions. Information Syst Res 1991;2:1–28.
30. Bijker WE. Of Bicycles, Bakelites, and Bulbs: Toward a Theory of Sociotechnical Change. Cambridge, MA: The MIT Press, 1995.

31. Klein K, Dansereau F, Hall RJ. Level issues in theory development, data collection, and analysis. Acad Manage Rev 1994;19:195–229.
32. Eysenbach G. Consumer health informatics. Br Med J 2000;320:1713–16.
33. Kuhlthau C. Inside the search process: information seeking from the user's perspective. J Am Soc Inform Sci 1991;42:361–67.
34. Timmermans S, Berg M. The practice of medical technology, sociology of health and illness. Available at http://www.bmg.eur.nl/smw/m_berg/ (in press).
35. Borgman C. From Gutenberg to the Global Information Infrastructure: Access to Information in the Networked World. Cambridge, MA: The MIT Press, 2000.
36. Bishop A, Mehtra B, Bazeel I, Smith C. Socially grounded user studies in digital library development, first Monday, 5(6). Available at *www.firstmonday.org/issues/issue5_6/* (2000).
37. Hampton K. Grieving for a lost network: collective action in a wired suburb. Information Soc 2003;19:1–13.
38. Hansen M. The search-transfer problem: the role of weak ties in sharing knowledge across subunits. Admin Sci Q 1999;44:82–111.

14 Security of Healthcare Information Systems

Roy Schoenberg

On December 10, 1982, a young man by the name of Michael Fagan was arrested in London after climbing a wall and jumping into the Queen's bedroom at Buckingham Palace. Mr. Fagan seemed to have no violent intent but was arrested for trespassing by the Queen's shocked security guards. In 1993, a young German by the name of Hans Schmidt (a common name in Germany) used his driver's license to open a bank account and issue multiple credit cards in his name. He then forged the card numbers to match those of other people named Hans Schmidt and went shopping for exceptionally expensive jewelry and art pieces. At any sign of danger, he would swap the false card with his own (valid) card and sail to safety. In July 2002, an investment manager at Poalim Bank in Israel took a small (electronically recorded) commission on every transaction she made for her private clients. The eighty-cent commission went unnoticed until a colleague audited her exploding 50-million-dollar savings account.

The criminal nature of these acts is perhaps of little interest to us, but in each of them some form of privacy was compromised. It is easy to perceive a violation of privacy in relation to the queen's bedroom, but the other cases represent merely different degrees of the same violation. Mr. Schmidt violated his fellow Schmidts' privacy by assuming their identities and using those identities to perform actions that were, until that point, at the—other individuals' discretion. The investment manager took the liberty of executing transactions on accounts where transactions were supposedly at the sole discretion of the owner. This action is regarded as an invasion of privacy, despite the fact she *was expected* to manage the transactions in those accounts. Although there is no doubt about the criminal nature of all three cases, they still raise some questions from a security/privacy standpoint. The bedroom incident "sounds" like both a security breach (the security system in Buckingham Palace) and a violation of the Queen's privacy. The investment manager did not breach any security or cross a private perimeter when taking advantage of her clients' bank accounts, but she did bluntly betray the confidence of her clients. Hans Schmidt did not breach security either. He didn't betray any confidence, as it was never extended to him. He did, however, take possession of identities that were the private assets of other people—private in the sense that only those individuals were supposed to hold them (and shop with them). It isn't clear, however, how a security system could effectively protect people's identities. The line between security, privacy, and confidentiality is frequently blurry, and making use of these terms in healthcare is, like everything else, even more confusing [1]. Before we address some of the challenges faced in making computerized systems work appropriately in these areas, it may be useful to bring some clarity to some frequently misused terms.

Definitions—Security, Privacy, and Confidentiality

Security

Definitions of this term vary considerably depending on the context in which the term is used and the authority that formulates the definition (e.g., legal, military, or financial). The notion of security in all cases, however, is based on the *preservation* of someone's right to something and specifically the measures used in order to ensure that this right is not compromised or taken away. In the context of healthcare information systems, we typically do not protect individuals, but rather their health information. We also don't consider every instance of access to this information a breach of security, as it needs to be appropriately accessed by care providers and health administrators. We may therefore regard security as the *process or means* of ensuring that access to, or usage of, protected data is appropriate [2].

Privacy

Whereas security deals with the process and means of appropriate access, privacy deals with the question of what is appropriate [3]. Although the meaning of the word "appropriate" is at best contextual and circumstantial, the term "privacy" is more easily grasped. Privacy relates to what is *not* appropriate under *any* circumstances. Using the same terminology as before, we may say that privacy deals with denying access to or use of protected data to anyone but its owner. In this sense, security reflects the means employed by an institution to prevent anyone other than the patient from accessing his or her private information [4].

Confidentiality

This term is used to define those situations in which some access to personal data is deemed appropriate and the qualifications for such access [5]. As it relates to the notion of privacy, confidentiality is concerned with allowing access to and use of protected data by anyone who is not its owner as long as the data are **not** private. The people or entities allowed access are thus held in confidence by the data owner and it is generally understood that they will access the information for the purpose and in the manner that was intended. The exchange of confidential data is therefore the exception to the notion of privacy. Where access to the information requires no degree of confidentiality, the data are in fact public, the opposite of private.

Disclosure

Disclosure relates to the process by which the owner of private information makes it available to someone else under variable degrees of confidentiality. If the owner of the information requires that none of the data be disclosed to anyone, he or she has effectively defined it as "private." The institution hosting the data should then apply the appropriate means to secure the data so that they are not disclosed. Current legislation (HIPAA) describes in length the manner in which any health entity must acquire and follow the patient's preferences for the internal disclosure of their information [6].

Sensitivity

Many of us use the terms "sensitive" and "private" interchangeably in relation to information. In fact, sensitivity is an attribute of data that is used to determine whether information needs to be "private" or whether it can be disclosed in confidence and to what degree. The degree of sensitivity typically guides the effort needed to either protect the information from access or secure the process of confidential access. To complicate matters somewhat, the same information may be viewed as "highly sensitive" or "not sensitive" in different contexts or at different times.

While the preceding terms are used to define the different aspects of limiting access to information, we may also want to consider their counterparts—the terms that define aspects of access, once granted.

Availability

Availability denotes the consistency with which a system (e.g., a Web site) is ready to perform its function (e.g., make data accessible). A system that is designed to operate with little or no downtime (e.g., by introducing redundancies, mirroring, and monitoring) is regarded as a high-availability system.

Accessibility

This term describes the process by which one can interact with a system. Accessibility relates to the physical distribution of access points as well as the technology used to moderate the access (e.g., dedicated, in-hospital mainframe terminals, Web browsers). The term is often misused to also describe the qualities of the access mechanism, such as ease-of-use and response speed.

Data Integrity

Data integrity refers to the system's ability to ensure that once information has been entered into it, an attempt to retrieve that information will produce the same data that were entered or their intended compilation. If the data retrieved have been erroneously or maliciously altered, a data integrity breach is recorded.

Asking the Right Questions

One of the fundamental challenges in establishing security in healthcare IT environments is the plethora of "moving parts." In many cases, systems represent a combination of preexisting efforts made by different champions in the organization. Each of these efforts carries its own legacy in terms of data, architecture, operational definitions, and security approach. An attempt to consolidate the language used by all the efforts is often an overwhelming task. When the complexity becomes too great, taking a step backwards and asking some abstract questions may help visualize the big picture. Such questions do not define the underpinnings of the system's security, but are nonetheless invaluable in establishing a systematic approach for mapping a proposal for organization. Some of these questions have been included here. They are purposefully phrased broadly, as their answers must be of a qualitative rather than quantitative nature. In answering the first question (What type of information goes through the system?), we should think of answers such as "claim information, scheduling information, and lab results" rather than "results from lab A and the office hours of Dr. X." This will allow us to move forward and understand the sensitivity of the data, its scope, its desired availability, and the security threats that need to be mitigated. You may want to consider the following 10 questions before investing time in implementing security architecture around your system.

1. What types of information are expected to travel through the system?
2. Where are the data generated? How are the data entered and who controls that process?
3. Where are the data stored, and are there multiple or backup copies?
4. Who owns the data and who authorizes access to it?
5. Who needs to access the data and from where?
6. How can we identify and authenticate the participants in this process?
7. What are the repercussions for incorrect access, loss of integrity, or delayed access?
8. What use of the system is regarded as inappropriate (an intrusion)?
9. Who might try and intrude on our system and for what purpose?
10. How can we detect intrusion and what are we willing to do if it is, in fact, detected?

Answering these questions should become more of a habit than a one-time exercise. As the system evolves and expands, so do its uses, its entry points, and its appeal to intruders. Getting a one-time assessment of the threats to a system's security is like reading the newspaper. It is invaluable to keep you on top of things but it has only sentimental value, if any, by the time tomorrow's edition is out.

The Weakest Link

One of the most useful notions in building security into an information system is that of the weakest link in a chain. For example, many organizations spend exorbitant sums on security devices such as firewalls but pay little attention to the methods by which employees can traverse it (e.g., dial-ups or virtual private networks that tunnel the user across the firewall). Clearly, if the credentials for bypassing the security are easily compromised or remain in the custody of people who have left the organization, a security breach is likely to occur, irrespective of the technology protecting the system. Adding an eleventh question to the list, "What's my weakest link right now?" and making a habit of revisiting it at fixed intervals is another valuable practice. A maxim you should keep in mind when hunting for weakest links is that, by definition, as soon as you remove the weakest link, another link becomes the weakest. The hunt is (almost) endless. You must apply judgment when determining at what point hunting the enemy becomes the same as chasing your tail.

Approaches for Assessing Security

As in other projects, taking the first steps is typically the hardest part. This is where many of us consider questions such as: "Where do we start?" and "How can we do this systematically?" and realize "I need professional help here." In reality, there is no one correct answer to these questions. Below is a list of "security probing approaches" that may prove effective:

1. By software and hardware blocks—This approach calls for the initial mapping of all the software packages or programs that take part in the service offered by the

system. The list typically includes an operating system (e.g., Windows), a data source (e.g., an SQL database server), an application technology that allows your programs to manipulate data (e.g., COM+) and the vehicles used to move the data around (e.g., a Web server such as Microsoft's IIS™ or Apache™). Each package typically offers its own access management panels, audit logs, data interfaces (the connection points where it communicates with other applications), and, as we are already accustomed to, an ever-growing list of known glitches and patches. In addition, the map should include the hardware involved in running the software blocks. Dedicated data storage devices (e.g., EMC, SANs, or NAS) have their own security characteristics. Some have modems built in to allow the device to "call the manufacturer" if it detects an operational problem. Others work like a large shared hard drive with their own access management console that can be "hardened" to limit access to the authorized applications. Firewalls, load balancers, and network switches are other hardware components that deserve their own security analysis if this approach is taken. This "horizontal mapping" is especially useful when building a new system from scratch, as it lends itself to the creation of "rules" and "protocols" that can later be reused to govern the implementation of new applications.

2. By application—A slight variation on the aforementioned model (and an approach that is often viewed as complementary) is the review of the system by applications. In this approach, the mapping process targets complete service units (e.g., a scheduling service) and follows them across the software and hardware that enable them. This "vertical approach" is advantageous when securing an existing system, as it allows you to launch secured applications sooner, before other ones have even been reviewed. For example, you may want to review your e-mail system (e.g., Microsoft Exchange™) and then deal with your Web site and the application you use for scheduling. In cases where data sensitivity warrants an especially high level of security, you may want to scrutinize your system using both the horizontal and vertical assessments.

3. By domains—This approach offers clarity when attempting to apply security in large organizations that operate different collections of software and hardware for different purposes. "Domain" refers to an operational unit, such as a clinic, bundled together with its user lists, applications, and in many cases software and hardware. In some cases, domains are used to define perimeters of operations (e.g., development environment, production environment or even intranet, extranet, and Internet). Although there may be similarities between multiple domains in the same organization (e.g., multiple clinics), exempting yourself from the need to review each of them independently may be the equivalent of treating all patients with fever in exactly the same way. Where people are different, so are the domains they work in, irrespective of how "alike" they are supposed to be. The domain map approach is also known as the "star" approach. Each domain has multiple types of software, hardware, and applications (the star arms), and the stars together form the "sky," or the organizational information system environment. Once the domains are listed, you may invoke either the horizontal or the vertical model to assess the threats to them.

4. By logical segments—This fourth approach, which is a relative latecomer in its adoption timeline, is geared toward managing security in Web-based environments. As much of the concentration in consumer-oriented services has moved to Internet applications, this approach may well be the one best suited to identifying and mitigating the most immediate threats faced by most readers [7]. The logical segment approach divides "the world" into three major areas: the server (where your data and applications live—e.g., the Web farm), the network (where your communication with the consumer takes place—e.g., the Internet) and the client (where you allow the consumer

to interact with your application—e.g., a browser). Each of these three segments has a clearly defined role in your service and uses specific applications to fulfill its role. For the purpose of clarity, we will use this logical segment approach in mapping out some potential threats and the possible actions that can be taken to mitigate them.

Server-Side (Application and Data) Security

"Server side" relates to the entire collection of computers and electronic devices that are bound together to deliver the service to the network. Because of the immense diversity in the parts used to operate this collection, it may be valuable to divide the threats into groups.

Bad Programs

These are programs that utilize bad practices in their coding, which may result in a security threat to you once you choose to use them. While it is not within the scope of this book to cover coding practices, some are still worth noting, as they are dangerously prevalent. Applications that store information on disk as a temporary byproduct of their operations (disk cache instead of database) are among them. The assumption that no one would know about these temporary files or attempt to access them is frequently wrong. Hackers or even employees can gain access to the file system long before they can get access to databases, and keeping raw data there just makes their lives easier. Another bad program to watch out for is one that places unencrypted data in the database. Programs that keep crucial credential data in a database as text without encrypting it exist on the assumption that anyone who gains access into the database will not abuse the data there. Many databases allow you to limit the rights available to a user or a program. Using the "master key" (e.g., the "administrator" account in Windows or the "SA" key in an SQL server) to perform all operations is simply bad programming. Some Internet technologies allow a programmer to store frequently used code in modules that can then be "included" in other modules by simply referring to their name. Although this works well for code, this feature is frequently abused to gain database access by placing the access credentials in a file and then calling on it to "open the door" whenever needed. Hacking or copying this file is just as easy. Although most programmers are already aware that allowing files to be uploaded from the Internet into an environment may be risky (and disallow such transactions), few scan the text that gets entered by users. With the evolution of script viruses (viruses that are uploaded as a text program) you may want to watch out for these too. In some cases, part of a service utilizes a program purchased from a vendor. Such programs may take the initiative in communicating information to the vendor, or react to incoming communications that you would otherwise discard. Scanning the communication channels (also known as ports) after introducing a new program to your farm may be well worth the effort. Finally, if you have the time and resources, engage an application security professional (a.k.a. a hacker) to break into your new application and pay him for the results. It's best that the hacker talks to you than to the local newspaper.

Bad People

While hackers may be the first to be considered as bad people, this threat relates to the ones who are already within your organization. Hostile colleagues, clients, and even visitors or temporary contractors are typically given some level of access to your system. If your system offers the ability to connect to the network with a simple laptop and network cable (a Dynamic Host Configuration Protocol [DHCP]-enabled system), anyone who walks through the door (or a thief through the window) can elegantly tap into your valuable data. While it is hard to prevent a disgruntled employee from damaging his own working environment, you may limit the damage in the following ways:

1. Limit the scope of access allowed for each authorized user on your system to the bare minimum he or she actually needs to conduct his or her job.
2. Make a habit of reviewing the list of authorized users on your system and revoking all those who do not require current access. Appropriate management of access lists (and rights) is as important as keeping your firewalls switched on.
3. Monitor and limit the right of users to utilize public resources for purposes that are tangential to their work. Most notably, limit the use of shared storage space for downloaded programs; this may become the eye of the storm when a malicious program is loaded.

Bad Maintenance Practices

You may secure your system from the ground up but fall short when mundane maintenance activity introduces an exception. Databases go a long way toward securing the data they hold, but what happens to the backups? Backup tapes, CDs, or even printouts do not typically receive the same protection as their online counterparts. Almost every operating system runs a hefty log of its activity. HIPAA does an excellent job of defining additional auditing of activity at the application level (e.g., access to records). The logs are a powerful tool for monitoring your system, but they are only as powerful as the habit of reviewing them. Although there are exceptions, most logs collect data that are never used. Most breaches generate an early warning in system logs that is simply never noticed because no one reads the logs. Identifying those audits that are important (e.g., sessions, user access) and setting the method and frequency with which they should be reviewed is advisable. Configuration of the security components you have on your system (firewalls, load balancers, modems, operating systems, databases, Internet servers, and active directories) is without a doubt critical. Although it is not the purpose of this text to detail the specific procedure for tweaking these components (a process called "hardening"), it is worth noting that the configuration you diligently set up yesterday is likely to fall behind what your system is doing today. Two practices are helpful in making sure that you are up to date: First, keep a list of any new service you are introducing or software you are installing as you go, and schedule a session with your best people to review the impact on security generated by the entries in your list before you toss it away and start a new one. Second, use the security probing software available on the market to get a report of your system's standing. It is simple to run and generates a detailed work list for sealing holes you didn't think of. Don't let the report be filed away. Ask "why" about *every* finding until you are satisfied that the concession needs to be made or the correction is in place.

Bad Guests

We have already noted the danger posed by authorized visitors (people) to your network, but here we describe small programs that may be even more dangerous. Viruses represent a significant threat to the availability of your services and to the integrity of your data. Most viruses enter your system via infected files, but their action revolves around disrupting your system or its contained data rather than compromising its privacy protection. You can mitigate much of the danger that viruses present by running up-to-date antivirus software that scans all existing data on your system and also monitors incoming data (specifically e-mail and files) before it actually lands on someone's desktop. One type of virus, known as a Trojan horse, poses a particularly significant threat. Trojan horse programs may enter your system as viruses (or as part of a program you install), but instead of wreaking havoc they operate in stealth mode and use your system and data to serve their remote master. Such programs may lie in wait until they are remotely ordered to wake up and take control of your system (as in denial of service attacks, in which your system suddenly becomes a soldier in an attack on another system) or, worse, communicate information from your system to the Trojan horse's operators. Some antivirus software do a good job of scanning for such programs but a good practice would be to monitor the traffic on your network and identify any unexplained active channels of communication between your system and the outside world. Another point to consider is that, unlike hackers who intrude into your system and gain access to areas or resources they are not supposed to be in, and who can be stopped by a strong guard at the door (e.g., a firewall), Trojan horses (and another variant called worms) work from within and may pose a threat even if you have severed your incoming communication wires.

Bad Passwords

Most of us have heard the (valuable) mantra on the importance of keeping your passwords cryptic and the need to change them frequently. Many, however, are not aware of the fact that most systems come with internal passwords used to allow access to programs that operate within. Typical examples are the "sa" (short for system administrator) password used in a mainstream database server and the blank "administrator" password used in most operating systems as they come out of the box. Even some hardware devices that are used for networking (most notably wireless access points) and Web servers are configured this way. Changing these passwords from their original factory settings is as vital to protecting your system as your own password is. They often represent the weakest link targeted by hackers and other malicious intruders.

Bad Initiatives

We have already touched on the challenge of securing a system that combines many programs from different sources (as most clinical systems do). Behind every program is a programmer, and a programmer's capability to create security back doors should never be underestimated. The ability to create a Web site from almost any desktop, share files and, most importantly, delegate access rights may quickly become the easiest route for an incoming intruder. Making strict policies about what is and is not allowed when people take computing initiatives (frequently to allow them to work from home) is a good starting point. Considering your internal network (intranet) to be as threatening as the outside world and securing your data from it too may be another step in the right direction.

Bad Platforms

Much of the attention in securing systems is directed toward applications that are directly involved in managing data. The other components that allow these applications to function are often overlooked and may represent the weakest link. Old operating systems (such as Windows 95) are now considered easy prey for both human and programmatic threats. Even newer operating systems and antivirus software, as well as devices that have software built into them (also known as firmware), are frequently outdated in their ability to ensure secure operation. The process of upgrading these capabilities and installing vendor updates (patching) must become an integral part of maintaining the system. While newer operating systems and antivirus software often suggest available updates, many devices and applications require you to be the initiator of the process. Make a habit of sweeping your system for components that are out of date and patch them immediately. In cases where physical components are out of date and cannot be updated (e.g., wireless access points with no encryption capability), consider how soon they can be replaced.

Physical Security

Sometimes, the weakest link is not computational at all. If your IT administrator makes heroic efforts to ensure the security of the data on the hard drive, but the drive itself can be removed and taken away by a passerby (e.g., during office cleaning hours), not much has been accomplished. Three general measures apply to maintaining physical security for a small physician's office or a hospital Web farm alike:

1. Lock—Make sure all physical instances of your data (source and backups) and the points where access is gained to it (terminals, etc.) are inaccessible to unauthorized people.
2. Monitor—Watch every time the locked area is accessed. Whether by keeping the key for the door at the receptionist's desk (and keeping a log of entries) or by cameras, biometrics, and man traps in a Web farm, make sure you know each instance of access to and the whereabouts of your data.
3. Anonymize—If all else fails and an intruder does find a way into your sanctum of data, make sure it is unclear where the gold is hidden. Mark your environment (specifically servers, disks, and backup tapes) with names you will recognize but that do not provide an indication of their contents to the intruder. Naming a server "Alabama" is better than "Patient Records Server." Naming a backup tape "LR-11" is better than "Lab Results, November."

Reactive Security

This term relates to the types of measures that can be implemented ahead of time to confine the damage done by an intrusion once it is detected. Most of these measures are in fact written action plans that allow you to act decisively and effectively when time is of the essence and confusion is (typically) at its peak. Generally, such plans are structured as decision trees, where important questions lead to branches that may include actions to be taken and additional questions to narrow down and mitigate the threat at its source. In creating a reaction plan, you must always consider the balance between known damage, ongoing threat, and the impact of threat mitigation on the business operation supported by the system. It's easy enough to turn the system off at the sight of a security breach, but often this is just as damaging to your business as the threat itself. Plan your reactive security in advance. Your coronaries will thank you later.

Network and Transactional Security

In the preceding section we discussed some of the security concerns for operating your application back-end. Once information has been requested and formulated for delivery, your system will send its response out via the network (completing a transaction in doing so). The same process will take place when an end user of your system sends his or her information to you from a data entry point (e.g., a browser). The threats to the information en route differ from those within your servers. The wires are typically on public domain (the Internet). Each packet (the small parcels used to move the information on the Internet) may take a different route to get to its destination and, most importantly, minimal effort is required to intercept the parcels.

Threats

Network and transactional security threats can be divided into the following general groups:

1. Eavesdropping—This threat is equivalent to the mailman reading your postcards. There is no need to actually "steal" the communication in order to read it; all you need to do is listen in. As such, the network poses the same challenges as do phone systems today or as did the radio systems in World War II. The solutions are all based on the assumption that the intruder has successfully intercepted and acquired a complete copy of the information, and are fundamentally the same as they were 50 years ago—make sure that the intercepted information is illegible to the interceptor. Different levels of encryption are now offered on most systems used to communicate data over public networks, and when used appropriately may effectively negate the threat of eavesdropping. (See discussion on encryption later.)
2. Network Impersonation—because communication on networks travels in fragmented and unpredictable pathways, it is much easier to intercept if the intruder pretends to be the rightful recipient. To intercept a communication, the intruder may assume the identity of either the sender or the recipient. Because your system communicates with many individual clients, assuming your identity (rather than that of the end client) is the most lucrative choice from the intruder's perspective. The use of identity certificates, which are issued by trusted organizations (such as Verisign™), ensures the recipient that the communication came from you. Another type of impersonation is IP-spoofing, where the intruder assumes a computer network identity (an IP address) that is reserved for your use. Newer firewalls and routers can automatically drill down on the packet's inner details and call the bluff. You may want to verify that your hardware supports this capacity. More information on IP spoofing can be found at *www.iss.net.*
3. Retransmission—in some cases, an intruder can intercept a transaction of information but doesn't have the capacity to decipher its entire content. Some parts of the message, however, are easily changeable, like e-mail or even mail addresses. After changing the values, the intruder can simply resend the slightly modified communication with the hope that it will trigger the same action on your system as the original was intended to do. This time, however, the intruder is the beneficiary. The result may be an appropriate transaction with compromise of data integrity (see the first section of this chapter). Different solutions are available for maintaining and verifying transactional data integrity, but most rely on the "checksum" model. At the time of the transaction, the system (server or client) calculates a number that is based on important

data elements in the transaction and sends it along with the data. The recipient performs the same calculation on the data received and compares the two numbers. If the numbers are not the same, data integrity has been compromised and the transaction is either cancelled or re-requested. Another methodology uses short-lived tokens incorporated into each transaction. If a token is reused (as in the retransmit process) or is used too late (detecting the time it takes the intruder to introduce the change to the data), the transaction is aborted. Unfortunately, both methods described here require some sophistication to be added to your underlying applications. It is nonetheless helpful to know what to look for when designing a new system or implementing an off-the-shelf one.

4. Denial of service (DOS) attacks—DOS attacks have received a great deal of publicity in recent years. Sites such as Yahoo and CNN went offline for hours as their servers were suddenly overwhelmed by millions of simultaneous page hits coming from around the globe. The source of these attacks is typically numerous naïve home computers that were infected with a Trojan horse (see earlier) and are suddenly instructed by their remote master to hit the target site. DOS attacks do not attempt to hack or intrude on the target system, but rather overwhelm it with service demands that greatly exceed its capacity. The inevitable result is the system's inability to cater to true service demands and the loss of its availability. New firewalls and intrusion detection systems may be able to sense such surges in service request and filter out much of them using request pattern recognition (since all computers are infected with the same Trojan horse, their simultaneous requests tend to be identical in form and content). If your firewall is not designed to withstand a DOS attack, there is little that can be done on the inside of your system to protect it. An innovative solution is to offer your service from two separate Web addresses (e.g., domain names or even IP addresses). If one is under attack, just turn it off and allow your users to receive service from the alternate one. The major drawback of this method is that your users must know of the alternate address in advance. As a solution, it isn't pretty, but neither is a full-blown DOS attack.

Encryption

Believed to be invented by Babylonian merchants in 800 B.C., encryption refers to the transformation of a message from one (legible) form to another (illegible) form in a reversible fashion. The creator of the message uses a key (cipher) to make the message illegible (encrypt it), knowing the reader can use her own key to reverse the process (decrypt it) and read the message. An interceptor of the message who does not have the key cannot read the message unless he finds a way to deduce (decipher) what the key is. The degree of difficulty in deducing the nature of the key is also referred to as its strength, or "cipher strength." New information systems make constant use of encryption protocols. The underlying power of the computers we use today makes the hassle of encryption and decryption almost transparent to the user, but its importance should not be underestimated. The use of encryption in systems that transmit sensitive information over public networks (e.g., e-mail, Internet, wireless networks) is no longer an option; it's a requirement. At the same time, it is important to remember that encryption protects the data only in transit and for as long as its keys are not available to the eavesdropper (see earlier). Many Web-based systems use hardware-based devices to accelerate the encryption/decryption process just before the message is routed onto the Internet or as it comes in. Few systems encrypt communication internally, and we have already named some of the threats we face from within. Like all the other mitigations, encryption is a powerful solution, but be aware that it may or may not solve your weakest link.

1. SSL—"Secure socket layer" refers to the encryption protocol used by most Web browsers. The process requires that the side offering the service (the server) hold a certificate of authenticity and that this certificate be used as the basis for converting all the messages that are exchanged between the service provider and the client. When a communication takes place over an SSL connection (as typically noted by a small golden lock at the bottom of the browser screen), all data moving between the browser and the server (and vice versa) are encrypted and are effectively illegible to an interceptor. You can verify the certificate identity of the server by clicking on the lock icon and can find the strength of the cipher (the number of bits or the length of the key) by reviewing the "about" section of your browser. Cipher strengths of 40, 56, and 128 bits are used by different browsers. The latter is the de facto standard for communicating sensitive information over the Internet and is built into all new browsers (e.g., Internet Explorer 6, Netscape Navigator 7). If your system transmits personally identifiable health information (HIPAA's PHI), you cannot settle for less than 128-bit SSL when communicating over the Web. It is important to note that this prevalent form of SSL ensures the identity of the server only. Any browser that connects to the server can establish a valid encrypted connection, even if the person behind it is not the one who he claims to be. A new variation of SSL (called SSL 3.0) requires that both sides authenticate their identity using certificates. Although this allows much greater certainty that the information is being communicated between the right parties, it requires that the client (e.g., the patient) apply for and install a certificate on his or her browser. Until this process becomes more user-friendly and for the time being, very few organizations require SSL 3.0 as the basis for their services.
2. PKI—Private key infrastructure is one of the most fundamental technologies used in systems that communicate sensitive information over public networks, including those that use SSL over the Internet. Although you don't need to know the underpinnings of the technology, as it is almost transparent to end users, it still warrants some basic introduction. The most compelling notion introduced with PKI is that the keys used to encrypt and decrypt the communication should not necessarily be identical (the keys can be mathematically "asymmetric"). The practical implementation of this notion may work as follows: When another party needs to exchange sensitive information with me (because I asked that it be sent to me or tried to hit a secure Web site), the other party can encrypt the information using a key that I make available in my browser (my public key). Once the other party is done encrypting and sends the information to my browser, I will use my private key (that is, one associated with but not identical to the public key) to decrypt the information. In consequence, anyone can send me encrypted information that can be read only by me. Whenever I log on to my online bank site, asking for a Web page with my account summary, the bank encrypts the data with my public key, thus making sure that I and I alone can read it. PKI splices this technology with the use of certificates (see earlier), digital signatures and key directories to allow rapid and discrete establishment of secure communication between two authenticated parties. The initial step in establishing an SSL connection over the Internet takes advantage of this technology. More on PKI and digital signatures can be found at *http://verisign.netscape.com/security/pki/understanding.html.*
3. Kerberos—Kerberos is another fundamental technology that, like PKI, is well hidden under the surface. Invented at the Massachusetts Institute of Technology (MIT), Kerberos provides a high degree of trust when communicating information inside a

network (rather than on the Internet). Kerberos ensures that the identities of the two parties involved in exchanging information are authentic. Unlike PKI, Kerberos is based on the notion that the two parties share a secret key (an identical, symmetric key). Every transaction between the two sides provides sufficient evidence that the sender indeed has that key, establishing the sender's identity. Kerberos' power is in its ability to demonstrate possession of the secret key (and hence identity) without actually passing it every time and thereby endangering its secrecy. Kerberos has been adopted by Microsoft and became part of its operating systems from Windows 2000 onwards. If your network includes computers running previous versions of Microsoft operating systems (95, 98, Me), consider them a worthy candidate for the title "My Weakest Link." A good introduction to Kerberos can be found at *http://www.microsoft.com/windows2000/docs/kerberos.doc.*

Protocols: HTTP, SMTP, FTP, POP, SOAP

Most of us are not aware of the different vehicles used by the network to communicate our information back and forth. Such vehicles, technically referred to as "protocols," are used simultaneously, as each has a different strength (or ease of use) to accomplish different tasks. We browse the Internet to retrieve information (Web pages) and less frequently send it (via forms on Web sites). We use e-mail to communicate with individuals, but also to send them electronic files in the form of attachments. Some of us use browsers to locate files that are stored somewhere on the network (whether it is on our intranet or the Internet) and download them for our own local use. In recent years, a new breed of applications has allowed us to work locally, on our own desktops, but invoke services on another computer or server that operates elsewhere on the network. The protocols used in each of these instances, namely HTTPS, SMTP, POP, FTP, and Web services (SOAP over HTTPS), carry different security risks you should be aware of if you intend to rely on them heavily to communicate sensitive information. Although it is not in the scope of this chapter to compare the risks between protocols, it is sufficient to note that only two of the four [browser pages exchanged over SSL (HTTPS) and Web services] provide some degree of encryption and protection. As a rule, the use of e-mail for text communication or the use of FTP to exchange files is to be avoided where sensitive information is concerned. While there are tools that allow you to encrypt e-mail or secure FTP services, none of these tools comes bundled with commercially used operating systems and most require significant technical expertise to operate. If you don't intend to add PGP (an e-mail encryption standard anecdotally named—pretty good protection) to your e-mail or buy a secure FTP suite, think of it this way: sending sensitive information via e-mail is like sending your ATM PIN number on a postcard. Placing sensitive files on an FTP server is like stacking your money at home, right behind your front door. You may get away with it, but the odds are not in your favor.

Client-Side Security

Much of the attention in this chapter and in other security reviews is focused on ensuring the safe operation of the systems that serve the information and the networks used to deliver it. The reasoning is clear—this is where intruders will look for the information, and in most cases these are the places intruders can most easily get into. Moreover, the legal obligation of an organization to protect data from improper access typically stops short of the client. Once the data are in the hands of the authorized client, so is the liability for compromising its security. Although this notion may be invaluable in court, the following considerations may help ensure that your sensitive data are secure even after they reach their rightful reader.

- Local cache—Most browsers (and some terminal emulation programs) are configured to "memorize" some of the information they load so they don't need to load it again if it is requested. This "caching" mechanism relates to Web pages themselves (e.g., a page showing lab results), the address for the Web page (the URL line with the access credentials embedded in it as request parameters), or even (as in Internet Explorer) the passwords used in the context of a specific login screen (e.g., to the labs system). This potentially insecure behavior of the browser can be mitigated to a degree with good programming skills. Making sure your system programmatically prevents caching of pages and reminding of passwords, and avoids placing access credentials into URLs, may sound simple, but it will go a long way toward preventing client-side breaches.
- Cookies—Another type of local storage of information on the client side bears the endearing name of "cookies." The term refers to tiny bits of information that are stored locally on the client's workstation and allow the Web site to better personalize its interaction with the specific user. Cookies, like e-mail, are not encrypted and can be easily read by anyone with access to that workstation. If used to store the color preferences of the user, no harm is done, but if used to automate the transmission of login credentials (the most common practice is to auto-suggest the login field), you may end up facilitating the process of intrusion while thinking you are making life easier for your authorized users.
- Session extenders—This is a private case of the local cache but is worth emphasis. The Web operates in what is called "stateless mode." This means the server is not connected to the client browser in any way other than during page transitions, even if the sequence of pages is part of the same operation. To counter this problem, many systems employ sessions—a server-side footprint that carries the memory of the user's previous actions (and in many cases their access authorization) from one page to the next. Sessions are often limited by time and expire if no activity is recorded. Conversely, if an activity is recorded (e.g., when a previous page is resubmitted), the session with all its embedded access rights is revalidated and extended. If a new user on your workstation clicks the "back" button and resubmits one of the pages you worked on an hour ago, there is a good chance that the user will acquire a fresh, fully operational session that will allow him or her to do . . . whatever you were allowed to do. To make things worse, the actions this user chooses to take will be recorded as if they were made by you. Make sure you know the session policy of your system and that it is as restrictive as is practically possible.
- Use of client-side applications (Active-X, Java applets, Flash)—In some cases, it is difficult to create a user-friendly interaction using the Web's stateless ping-pong of static pages (see earlier). Newer browsers allow the embedding of small programs that execute inside the client's browser and generate a much more responsive (attractive) working environment for the client. Although the use of such technologies is greatly encouraged, some operational guidelines must be kept in mind to mitigate some of their inherent security holes. Local applications tend to create a local data footprint that is no longer under your remote control. Some of these technologies (e.g., Flash) are not (yet) configured to take advantage of encryption. Lastly, be aware that the downloaded applications may have a life of their own. They can sometimes

be run outside of the context of the page that was used to download them, or even by another user. If your data serving system interacts freely with its new client-side applications under the assumption it operates within an authorized session, you may be in for an unpleasant surprise.
- Encryption level on older browsers—by now, the use of SSL to encrypt Web-based communication and services has become the rule, rather than the exception. Although implementing SSL capability on your system is straightforward, you should remember that SSL comes in different "strengths" based on the length of the key it uses for encryption (40, 56, or 128 bits). Most new servers take advantage of the stronger cipher and establish a 128-bit SSL connection whenever possible (whenever the browser on the other end supports it too). Unfortunately, just out of the box, the same systems are also likely to serve your sensitive data in 40-bit SSL if that's what the recipient browser is capable of. You must actively configure your system to drop connections that don't support your preferred level of encryption. Non-SSL or 40-bit SSL connections may very well be the weakest link in a system that supports, but does not mandate, state-of-the-art 128-bit SSL.

Allowing Access

Designing, building, and maintaining security in a clinical system is a significant challenge by any standard. Acknowledging the incredible dynamics in the system's operation (new data, new users, new rules, new applications, and new technologies, to name a few) is a good measure of the work involved in rising to this challenge. It is therefore unfortunate that this is only half of the problem. Keeping the wrong people out is sometimes more easily scoped and enforced than managing access for those who are authorized to be in. As in the assessment of physical security, it is a challenge to compile an access management survey that will be applicable in all instances [8]. As before, we can focus on some of the key questions that, given abstract answers, will be helpful in compiling an access policy for the system. Not surprisingly, some of the questions resemble those encountered in assessing security in section one above. After all, we are dealing with two different aspects of protecting the same information. To accomplish this, we will start by assessing the resource (data) that we are trying to control access to, continue by identifying the parties who may need access rights to it, review the general models of access most frequently used in clinical systems, and conclude by considering how access control can be enforced.

Creating an Access Map

Although access management is all about people, it is often the nature of the data that has the greatest impact on the access policy eventually employed. Mapping between data types and possible users can help us determine if access to the system can be governed in a black and white fashion (i.e., all individuals are either granted or denied access) or whether other considerations must be weighed. Some initial questions should include the following:

1. Can we logically group people who need access into collections (user types) that are granular enough to require a single access profile? Are there any crossovers?
2. Can we achieve logical partitioning of the data so that different data partitions can be made accessible to the respective user types?
3. What are the exceptions to this model?

As in the earlier section on security, the answers to these questions are most helpful if given in an abstract fashion. It is somewhat easier to define user types (physicians, nurses, administration staff, technicians, etc.), as we typically use the same metaphors in our daily work. Data collections are not as clearly defined, but once we have the list of users we can employ it to help us with the data. One such approach is to apply what is known in system design jargon as "use cases"—a "thought experiment" simulating how the system will be used by the defined users and the data access they would need in the course of a typical day. If physicians need to access clinical notes, labs, problem lists, insurance information, visit logs and prescription logs, we can then list these six collections and start correlating them to their respective user types. The resulting grid may be extensive, but it's invariably cheaper to have extensive work done on paper than tweaking a system after it is launched. You may want to start the use-case exercise with the following list of user types and extend it according to your needs:

1. Data owner—the patient
2. Data collector—the data storage owner (the clinic or hospital)
3. Data user—the different care providers involved in a care instance
4. Workflow support users—administration staff, utilization reviewers, quality assurance personnel
5. Business associates—HIPAA's version of people you work with but who are not part of your core organization (e.g., pharmacies, labs, claim processing)
6. Application support—IT, vendors, programmers
7. Authorizers—system administrators

Adding an Operational Layer

Mapping possible users into groups and data into partitions and drawing the access correlation between them is a useful first step, but returns at most a static snapshot of your dynamic environment. Because staffing and data change over time, we have to color our access map with some operational patterns:

1. Is there a hierarchy between user types? Do supervisors have all their subordinates' access rights, or are their profiles mutually exclusive?
2. Is the data collection hierarchical (such as access to a parent collection implies/requires access to a sub-collection including lab tests, blood tests, or blood count)? Are there exceptions (e.g., lab tests, blood tests, or CD4 count)?
3. Can the correlation between data and user-type change over time or will the users simply gain designation of additional user types as they need different access? (Alternatively, can the data be moved/copied to the collection that the user is allowed access to?)
4. Are there any other levels of groupings that must be imposed (such as multiple clinics, each having the same access policy for its own collection of users and data, but allowing a provider from one clinic to assume the same role in another)?
5. Are there cases where access to the data may be needed by an external entity (e.g., labs, vendors) that cannot be mapped to a registered user within the system?
6. Do any of the following parameters impact the policy we have created?
   a. Time—is there a notion of "when" access is appropriate or inappropriate?
   b. Location—does it matter if access was achieved from a specific location (e.g., home or office, nurse station, or operating room)?
   c. Frequency—does it matter how frequently a query on the data is made or is this left to the discretion of the authorized user? (Anecdotally, does high frequency of queries made by a user imply abuse of access rights?)

d. Usage—is there a difference between access to the data and usage of the data? Is inappropriate access as dangerous as inappropriate usage (e.g., reviewing the medication list of a patient versus manipulating it)?

Adding Flexibility (Customization versus Administration)

Like high-rise buildings in an earthquake-prone area, any system that does not build some degree of flexibility into its access management rules is likely to collapse. Such flexibility is typically manifested in the administration tools that govern access management, and their ability to handle new data collections, new user types, and new operational (correlation) rules between them. In practice, you will need to make a decision as to the amount of resources that will be invested in allowing the system to change its operational rules *after* you switch it on. In making this decision, it is helpful to make a distinction between two core capabilities:

1. Administration—this represents the ability to extend the current operational rules to new modules, users, systems, and data. The process of adding or revoking users, changing access credentials, reviewing usage patterns, and moving users from one access authorization profile to another are all examples of such functions. Access administration is typically a daily routine and no system is ready for operation without defined tools to accomplish it.
2. Customization—this is the ability to modify or introduce new operational rules and apply them to existing or new objects in the system. An example of customization is the process of defining a new user type (and its access rights) or making a change to the password expiration/validation rules. Unlike access administration, customizing your access model or policies is a rare and demanding process on many levels. Although you may want to identify those areas where customization (such as the addition of a new data source) is expected and validate that the system can reasonably accommodate it, this is the area where *analysis* (of all the possible changes you may want to introduce in the future) may lead to *paralysis*.

Although both customization and administration tools are required for managing access over time, they also introduce an operational concern. Most access breaches are discovered long after they take place. Proper detection, mitigation, and preventive actions can be achieved only if the event is viewed in the context of the access policy that was in place at the time of the event. Making access-policy changes without retaining a complete and thorough audit trail (and often an "undo" function) may be ill advised. The technical term "configuration management" relates to a capability in the system to recall, and in some cases reinstate, its previous operational settings. Having this capability in the area of access management is key to preventing and dealing with access breaches.

Access Authorization Models

Having the technical capability to authorize and manage access (as well as the proper security measures to prevent unauthorized access) is fundamental to running any system with inherent data sensitivities. As expected, the medical environment complicates this challenge further by introducing the unique notion of data ownership. Current legislation emphasizes the right of patients to withhold access to their clinical information from the providers and organizations that created it on their behalf. This emphasis is not merely a clarification of patient rights, but is a fundamental shift from the existing (provider-centric) access model to one that places the consumer in the driver's seat (patient-centric model). Although this trend is only beginning to impact system access architectures in existing healthcare entities, it has created enough momentum to warrant introduction.

The Provider-Centric Model

This model of access (Fig. 14.1) is and has been used by hospitals, physician practices, specialty clinics, and insurance companies for as long as clinical systems existed. In essence, all member-related data are stored as records in a system that is managed by the organization. Ownership of the data, as well as the discretionary decision of who is allowed access to it, is in the hands of the organization. The data are stored primarily to aid the operational activity of the organization so that a physician can, for example, have access to her previous notes on a patient when the patient comes in for a follow-up visit. The access model revolves around the provider in such a way that once her identity is established, she will gain access to all of her patients in the system. To support this model, the system uses an access control list (ACL) that compares the user credentials with the authorized employee list (e.g., of the hospital) and grants or denies access accordingly. From a workflow perspective the model is optimized to support the provider. The provider logs in using her credentials and can work on all data and all modules on all patients until she logs off.

The Patient- (Consumer-)Centric Model

This model (Fig. 14.2) represents the evolution in patient rights that started in the early 1990s and is beginning to formalize in current legislation. The model assumes patients are the sole authorizers of access into their records, irrespective of the physical environment where the data has been generated. This also implies that data aggregation

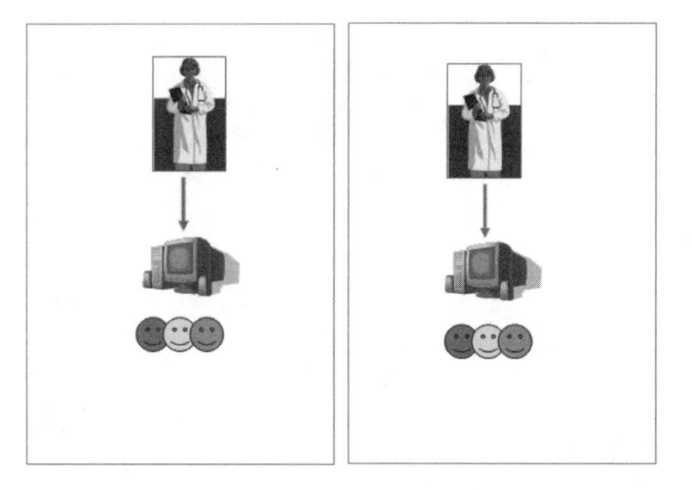

FIGURE 14.1. The provider-centric model. Every provider keeps his or her own patient records. Providers log in once to access all records. One patient may have many records.

will be centered on the patient (through a central trusted data warehouse, possibly operated by the insurer), rather than on the organization that owns the point of care (and the data systems employed in it) [9]. As patients present themselves to providers to acquire care, they will also enable access to their data as needed (e.g., scope, read-only, or read and write). Because the data follow the patient, a more complete record of the continuum of care is attainable while patient privacy is inherently upheld. This model does not require an ACL of authorized providers, as access is given as needed and at the patient's discretion. Beyond privacy, the model holds significant promise in the area of care coordination, prevention of redundant workup, medical error prevention, and cost containment. Unfortunately, the model is extremely obtrusive to physicians' workflows. Their access to a patient record can be established only with the patient's explicit permission and on the system the patient chooses to host his or her data. Even if the patient granted the physician a fixed password to personal records, the physician would have to use different passwords for each patient who comes in for an office visit. Despite the usability flaw, this "personal health record" model is already offered by several commercial and insurance entities with an impressive adoption rate.

The Reconciled Model

Reconciliation of the two models (Fig. 14.3) attempts to grant providers the ability to follow the same workflow they grew accustomed to over the years while still leveraging the benefits and preferential privacy of the consumer-centric model. The difference lies in the method by which access credentials are used and distributed. While maintaining the basic structure of consumer-centric architecture, this model offers providers the ability to store and automatically rebroadcast patient credentials on subsequent visits by clicking on the patient name from their list. The list represents the patients who have given this provider access authorization (using a token such as a password) and can be expanded by the provider as more patients join the panel. Selecting the patient from the list will negotiate the validity of the credentials against the patient-

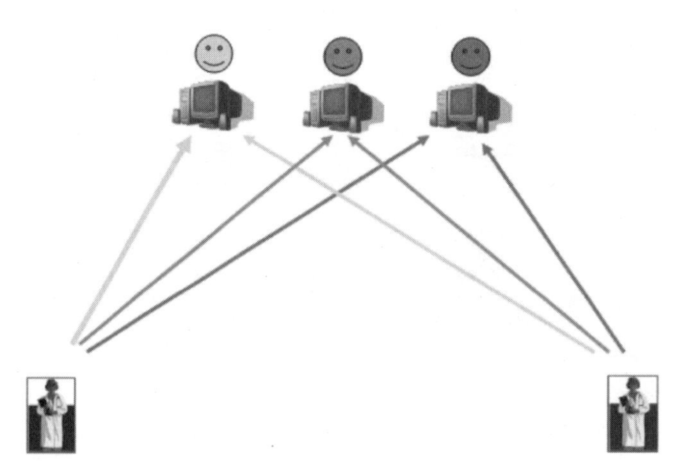

FIGURE 14.2. Patient-centric model. Records are held and controlled by patients. Providers need to use separate logins for each record.

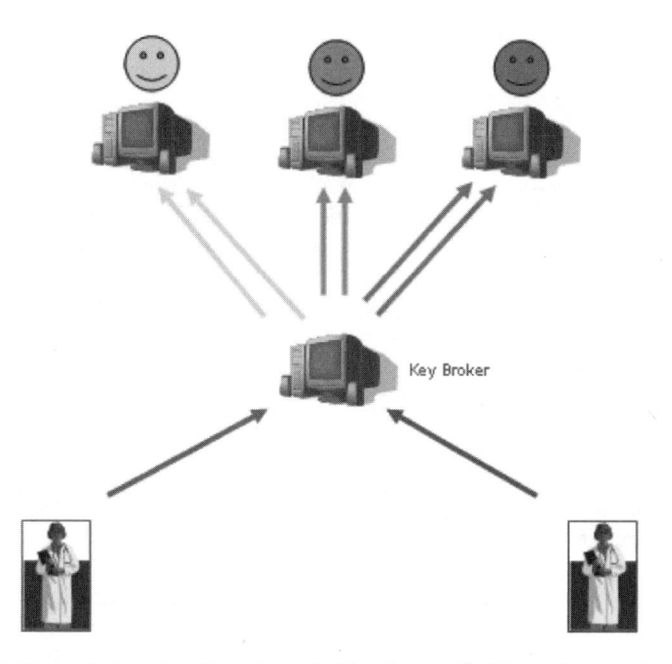

FIGURE 14.3. Reconciled model. Records are held and controlled by patients and providers log in once to gain access to all their patients' records.

centric data store, and if approved, will grant access to the provider. From a physician standpoint, the provider-centric flow of using a single credential to log into a system that offers immediate access to all the patients is preserved. From an operational standpoint, the system remains a true patient-centric environment.

The access paradigm offered by each of these models carries its pros and cons. Introducing change to physician practices has been typically a slow and painful process and casts a shadow on the feasibility of the second and third models, despite their promise. At this time it remains unclear if patient privacy legislation will force such a paradigm shift or whether another model [10,11] will emerge to reconcile the seemingly conflicting interests of providers and consumers in controlling clinical data and access to it.

Access Control

Access Control Lists (ACLs)

In the heart of literally every traditional (provider centric) clinical system lies a list of individuals with their respective access rights in the system. While serving the same purpose, different architectures of ACLs are employed to optimize the service needed in different models of the healthcare environment and their respective clinical systems. The following are some of the most frequently used ACL models.

- A user list—This simplest form of an access list holds the names and passwords of the people who are allowed access. Each person has one credential (e.g., password), and that credential allows full access rights to the entire system. This architecture is the one most easily maintained, and is optimized for environments where all authorized personnel know each other on a first-name basis.

- A pointer list—This two-step variation on the simple list holds two tables, one for the person's identity (name, login, password, ID) and one for the rights that are granted to that person (with the ID field pointing between the two tables). This version allows some degree of differentiation in the scope of access rights granted to each individual (e.g., clinical staff versus administrative staff).
- A role list—geared to handle a large number of authorized personnel, this system offers a three-way association between a person, a role, and the access rights associated with a role. Because every person can have multiple roles and every role can be associated with multiple rights, the system offers a high degree of flexibility.
- A role/domain list—this model adds a fourth layer to the access matrix by qualifying the rights attributed to a role, depending on the domain in which the data or applications are to be accessed. For example, a cardiology consulting physician may have lower access rights on a patient record than the staff physician who ordered the consultation. Although both physicians hold the same role in the system, each has a preferential access to records in his or her domain.

Regardless of the model most appropriate for one specific environment, it is the administration of the list that offers the most strength and, paradoxically, highest vulnerability. The procedures associated with keeping the list up to date and the clear designation of which person this task belongs to are cornerstones to the security of the entire system. Separate procedures must exist for adding people, defining their roles and access rights (depending on the model), removing people or revoking their rights in a timely fashion when necessary, and, most importantly, reviewing the appropriateness of the entire ACL in a repetitive, thorough fashion. Managing the ACL by focusing on its incoming and outgoing traffic (workforce update) is a mistake many ex-CIOs regret to this day.

Identification versus Authentication

Two other frequently confused terms are identification and authentication. The reason for the confusion lies in the fact that many systems use the same credentials to establish both objectives and that the processes themselves "look" like a single-step computational process. Most login screens require a single transaction that grants access based on a username (or login name) and password. Although the two fields are submitted together, they serve different purposes and must have different characteristics. The login name is used to "pinpoint" the person trying to log in on the ACL. The password is then used to authenticate that the person trying to log in is in fact who he or she claims to be by establishing a degree of certainty that the login alone could not ascertain. Identification is therefore the process of establishing a unique (one-to-one) relationship between the person trying to log in and an entity in the ACL, while authentication is the sequence of processes imposed on that individual to establish certainty that this association is in fact correct.

The confusion arises in cases where the process used to establish identity is in itself so robust that it provides the degree of certainty we typically expect from an authentication process. As an example, we can consider an extremely long password—it is likely unique (only one person uses this specific sequence) and, if kept secret, unlikely to be replicated by chance or even maliciously by another person. Merely knowing and typing in the sequence is powerful enough to achieve both objectives. Retinal or iris scans are other examples of powerful unified access tokens. So why so very few systems use a unified token? The answer, ironically, has two parts. In the first place, the low usability associated with very long passwords and the high cost associated with retinal scans make them unpopular for large systems. Second, the preferential performance one gets from a search for a login name in an indexed database table (compared with searching for uniqueness in a binary iris scan pool) makes the two-step process a clear winner.

Establishing Unique Identity

Now that we have established the most important characteristic of the identification key (uniqueness), it is worthwhile to consider some of the associated challenges. Assigning a unique identity number (or sequence) for each person is a good start, but quickly becomes unfriendly when sequences become longer and cryptic. Embedding the sequences in automated-reading tokens such as barcodes in a supermarket solves some of this problem, but the inevitable dependency on barcode reading devices has serious drawbacks (e.g., in phone conversations with a patient). The ability to guarantee uniqueness for an assigned login name can be accomplished by relying on an external, ubiquitous system that is trusted to enforce it. Examples are Social Security numbers or even e-mail addresses. Both are supposedly unique and if the system double-checks to reject duplicate entries (erroneous or malicious entries), both sound like a good bet. The problem is that not every person has an e-mail account and some (certainly citizens of other countries) don't have a Social Security number. Another aspect of the challenge lies in the scope of intended use of the "login" credential. If the login is expected to be unique within a hospital, the medical record number may be sufficient to establish uniqueness, but if two hospitals merge, the same number may now be used to identify two different medical records and a new identification system must be established. Although introducing a new, combined record identification token is immensely complicated, the value is compelling—patient records can now be shared across the hospitals. Expand the scope to a city, a state, or a country and uniqueness becomes a true challenge. Ironically, 2004 legislation introduced a national provider number to tackle the uniqueness problem in ACLs of provider centric systems. The introduction of a national patient identifier (that will streamline patient-centric systems) is still being debated in congress and is controversial to the degree that makes a resolution unlikely in the foreseeable future.

One method used by large healthcare entities to mitigate the problem is called probabilistic identification. The key concept is that using several keys in conjunction can deliver high probability of uniqueness even if each key in itself does not. Combining first, middle, and last names together narrows down the search, but including also gender and date of birth makes the probability of uniqueness good enough for most medical practice utilizations. Probabilistic identification designates an index of certainty, reflecting the number and quality of identity keys used in the search. Because not all keys (e.g., gender) are as useful in narrowing down the possible candidates, such systems often suggest the keys that will be most effective in reaching unique identification within a collection of patients. When uniqueness is established, the system will also point out the index of certainty that the identification is correct (e.g., it is possible to identify a person by a single very esoteric last name, but this is not as complete a proof as identifying him with a conjunction of Social Security number and date of birth).

Authentication

Although most systems use a text sequence (typically a login string) to locate a person in an ACL, great variability is found in the manner of authentication that follows. Passwords (shared secrets of varying number, length, and complexity) are by far the most prevalent authentication method, but are less secure and in some cases even less user-friendly than other means of authentication available today. Of the many nontextual solutions out there, two types deserve special mention.

1. Biometrics—As discussed earlier, such powerful identification methods are often used for authentication in parallel. Better technology (accuracy and speed), plummeting costs, and a shrinking device dimensions have made biometrics the method of choice for environments where high-certainty authentication is critical (e.g., when prescribing chemotherapy to patients). Hardware and software for incorporating fingerprint readouts (automated fingerprint identification systems, or AFIS) into a login process are readily available on mainstream platforms such as Windows® and in newer clinical applications. Iris scans are gaining momentum (as more accurate and potentially less intrusive to workflow than fingerprint devices) but are still too expensive for cross-organizational rollout. Facial recognition, hand geometry, signature vector verification, and voice recognition are the most prominent runners-up, but like iris scans have still to mature into dependable, cost-effective, workflow-friendly technologies.
2. Physical tokens—these are a large group of hardware devices that can communicate stored information at the time of authentication. Possession of such a device by a person indicates that the individual is who he or she claims to be. This method is also known as "two-factor authentication" as it requires both the login (something the user *knows*) and the device (something the user *has*) to complete the authentication process. Notable tokens in this group include smartcards and SecureID®. Smartcards are credit-card sized computer chips that can store information of various amounts and complexity. At the time of authentication, the unique information read from the card is crossed with the person's identity, and the conjunction, if valid (compared with the ACL on the server), is considered a successful authentication. Irrespective of the complexity of the data on the card, all cards require a special reader to extract the information and thus raise usability as well as cost issues for wide-scale deployment. SecureIDs resemble smartcards in size but display a constantly changing number on a small LCD panel embedded on the card. On a SecureID enabled system, the number shown on the card (and keyed in at that same time by the user on any access point) can be authenticated by the main server and establish that the user is in fact holding the card. Because the numbers change randomly and frequently, it is literally impossible to guess (or copy) the code without holding the actual card. Like smartcards, this "proof of possession" is regarded as authentication. Add a biometric to the process and you get a three-factor authentication (a login the user *knows*, a physical attribute the user *exhibits* and a token the user *possesses*).

Delegation of Trust (Single Sign-On Models)

The constant transformation of the healthcare environment poses a major IT integration challenge. Clinics, hospitals, laboratories, and insurance entities associate and dissociate, requiring their systems to support a corresponding continuum of care for their patients. In many cases, it is easier to allow uninterrupted browsing between the systems than to merge the systems (and their idiosyncratic data structures) into one. This process of logging onto one system and transparently gaining access to another (without the need to log in again) is referred to as a single sign-on (SSO) process and can span two or more domains. The trust in the authenticity of the user identity can then take different forms. Depending on the protocols established between the systems, directionality can be limited (e.g., a user can log into system A and browse into B but not from B to A). When the user is passed into the other system, some data may be passed along to indicate the user's role and allow further refinement of the service he or she receives on the second system. In some cases, a report of the activity of the user on the second system is returned to the original system and is recorded for auditing in the user's record. SSOs are primarily used in Internet-based systems, as they typically adhere to the same browser-oriented environment and user-interface conventions. Using URLs (links) to transition between Web pages coming from different servers or even sharing frames on the same Web page makes the browser an SSO-ready environment and drives system integration projects toward Web technology from the start. Several major players in the industry have already introduced systems that allow trust delegation between Web-based applications based on different models of SSO. Microsoft's Passport® and Sun Microsystems' Liberty® project may become the central switchboard for Internet identities following the reconciled patient-centric access model (discussed earlier), but have yet to make an entry into the healthcare arena.

Auditing

HIPAA requires that all activity surrounding patient-related information be audited [12]. The legislation describes in length what the term "related" consists of and what level of analysis needs to be made available based on the audits. Although it is not in the scope of this book to describe the HIPAA roadmap [13,14] (by now, there are probably more publications on this subject than patients), you must consider the impact of such auditing on your system. Because the audits need to allow reconstruction of each access and activity around personal information, the level of detail recorded in each transaction is substantial. The fundamental information you must record for each transaction will include the following:

1. When the transaction took place (and, if different, to what time it was applicable)
2. Who accessed the system and in what role he or she was acting
3. Which patient records were accessed
4. What type of actions were performed
5. What data, within the record, was changed/deleted/added
6. The relationship between this activity and other activities in the same session (if there is a sequence such as rescheduling a treatment)

As a rule of thumb, the system should audit enough information to allow reconstruction, within a reasonable time, of the events that took place and should provide the data needed to mitigate further damage. Unlike firewalls and ACLs that serve as watchdogs and gatekeepers, audits are like security cameras. If you place enough of them in sensitive areas, you will be able to catch infiltrators, but only if you watch the monitors. It is this metaphor that is most useful in guiding your auditing policy: audit all the processes in your system where erroneous or malicious activity may take place and define the routine (possibly computerized) inspection of the logs. While these two rules sound simple, consider this one fact—audit-trails typically consume three to four times the storage space of actual patient data. Implementing a thought-out audit policy may give you the security camera you need, rather than a haystack with an occasional needle.

Conclusion and a "Self-Assessment" Survey

Winston Churchill advocated knowing the enemy is the first step to defeating it. The knowledge and daily vigilance required for maintaining security in a system that manages private and confidential health information follows the same line. This chapter attempts to provide a birds-eye view of the field of battle, even if not actual war tactics. The Web offers a plethora of detailed guides and lessons in each of these areas for those readers who are interested or need a drill (a good starting point can be *www.cert.org* hosted by Carnegie Mellon University). In doing so, it is worth remembering that securing a system is a never ending story and that the main business of the organization is, after all, not security but health care. Like most things in life, balance and sound judgment are the best guides to the proper investment required to secure a system. In some cases, a possible breach may be less harmful than the cost and workflow interference introduced by the security plan. The list below summarizes the questions a security specialist is likely to ask on her first consulting visit to your firm. Asking the right questions is after all where we started off and is thus a good place to conclude. Ask yourself:

1. Do you have a security policy that describes the obligation of the organization to secure its data and assure the appropriateness of its disclosure?
2. Do you have a map of your data assets and how they are used across the organization?
3. Do you have an integrity maintenance plan (a plan that describes the maintenance procedures that need to be taken regularly to ensure the proper function of the security measurements employed in your system)?
4. Do you have an intrusion detection plan (a plan showing how and what data/events need to be monitored to detect an ongoing intrusion or abuse of data)?
5. Do you have an intrusion/incident response plan (a plan describing in detail what actual steps need to be taken in case a certain type of intrusion is detected)?
6. Does your response plan involve compromising patient privacy (e.g., logging into records to ascertain their integrity)?
7. Do you have a disaster recovery plan (a plan describing in detail how the organizational information system can be put back online after an intrusion, or other disaster, forced it to be taken off line or caused corruption of valuable data)?
8. Do you have a communication plan (a plan describing who needs to be notified, what gets communicated, and in what channels in case a breach of security takes place—includes both internal and public/patient oriented messaging)?
9. Is there a clear definition (a list) naming the ones responsible, in your organization, for maintaining the different aspects of security in your system?
10. Do you know your weakest link right now?

References

1. Bodenheimer T, Grumbach K. Electronic technology: a spark to revitalize primary care? JAMA 2003;9:259–64.
2. Austin RD, Darby CA. The myth of secure computing. Harv Bus Rev 2003;81:120–6, 138.
3. Mendelson D. Travels of a medical record and the myth of privacy. J Law Med 2003;11:136–45.
4. Schoenberg R, Safran C. Internet based repository of medical records that retains patient confidentiality. Br Med J 2000;321:1199–203.
5. Russell J. Confidentiality of patients' information must be guaranteed. Br Med J 2003;327:812.

6. Gostin LO. National health information privacy: regulations under the Health Insurance Portability and Accountability Act. JAMA 2001;285:3015–21.
7. Schoenberg R, Nathanson L, Safran C, Sands DZ. Weaving the Web into legacy information systems. Proc AMIA Symp 2000;769–73.
8. Safran C. Health care in the information society. Int J Med Inform 2002;66:23–4.
9. Rigby M, Roberts R, Williams J, Clark J, Savill A, Lervy B, Mooney G. Integrated record keeping as an essential aspect of a primary care led health service. Br Med J 1998;317:579–82.
10. Motta GH, Furuie SS. A contextual role-based access control authorization model for electronic patient record. IEEE Trans Inform Technol Biomed 2003;7:202–7.
11. Wiederhold G, Bilello M, Sarathy V, Qian X. A security mediator for health care information. Proc AMIA Symp 1996;120–4.
12. Asaro PV, Herting RL Jr, Roth AC, Barnes MR. Effective audit trails—a taxonomy for determination of information requirements. Proc AMIA Symp 1999;663–5.
13. Annas GJ. HIPAA regulations—a new era of medical-record privacy? N Engl J Med 2003;348:1486–90.
14. HIPAA reference information Web site: *http://www.hhs.gov/ocr/hipaa/*

15
The National Library of Medicine Reaches Out to Consumers

JOYCE E.B. BACKUS and EVE-MARIE LACROIX

This development, by itself, may do more to reform and improve the quality of health care in the United States than anything we have done in a long time.

—Vice President Al Gore, June 1997 (referring to NLM efforts to provide health resources directly to the consumer)

The National Library of Medicine (NLM) has a history dating back more than a century and a half. From its beginnings as the Library of the Army Surgeon General's Office, it grew to the Army Medical Library (1922), and in 1952 to the Armed Forces Medical Library. By an Act of Congress in 1956, it was named the National Library of Medicine and moved to the Public Health Service of the then Department of Health, Education and Welfare. Throughout its history, NLM has served the information needs of health professionals, developing a scientific and research collection that now numbers more than 7 million items including numerous special collections of prints, photographs, audiovisuals, oral histories, and manuscripts.

Since the early 1960s, NLM has been a leader in applying computer technology to accomplish traditional library functions and improve access to medical information. NLM's MEDLINE® database, the online version of *Index Medicus* launched in 1971, was one of the first large-scale online bibliographic reference databases. MEDLINE now contains more than 12 million references and abstracts from more than 4600 indexed biomedical journals. Quick to take advantage of the reach of the personal computer in the 1980s, NLM developed and launched Grateful Med® in 1985. This desktop computer software package enabled individual subscribers to search MEDLINE at home or in the office at a reasonable cost of $2 to $3 per search. Recognizing the importance of extending access to all health professionals, during the 1990s NLM and the National Network of Libraries of Medicine focused on training individual health professionals to search NLM databases and increased efforts to identify and reach unaffiliated and underserved health professionals. In 1996, NLM introduced Internet Grateful Med, a program for searching MEDLINE via the World Wide Web. The introduction was made at a press conference presided over by Michael E. DeBakey, MD, of Baylor University (and a member of the Library's Board of Regents), and US Senator Bill Frist (R-Tenn.), a surgeon and long-time user of Grateful Med and MEDLINE. Also included in the press conference were patients and families whose lives had been saved or medical situations improved because of physician access to MEDLINE [1].

By 1997, there were about 150,000 subscribers to the NLM system, conducting more than 7 million searches annually. On June 26, 1997, NLM announced that all access to MEDLINE would be free to everyone and without any requirement for registration.

Congress had heard testimony earlier in the year from Dr. DeBakey, who suggested that the Library could provide MEDLINE access to all US citizens, without charge, over the World Wide Web. Dr. DeBakey said that consumers were increasingly turning to the Internet as a source of information to improve their daily lives, including their health. He suggested that NLM might broaden the scope of its databases to include authoritative health information for lay audiences [2].

While conducting the first PubMed search free on the Internet, Vice President Al Gore was prescient in recognizing the impact of making the entire MEDLINE file freely available to anyone, anywhere in the world. Within 1 year of free access to MEDLINE, the number of searches increased from 7 million to 120 million. In addition, whereas MEDLINE had been a scientific information resource used almost exclusively by medical librarians, researchers, and health professionals, about 30% of the searches were done by the general public worldwide [3].

MedlinePlus.Gov

Recognizing that consumers were already frequent users of products geared to health professionals and researchers, NLM made plans to create a product tailored to the needs of the consumer Internet public. Launched in October 1998 with 22 health topics, *MedlinePlus.gov* has grown rapidly to become a comprehensive health information resource for consumers.

NLM had one of the very first US government sites, HyperDOC, which began in 1993 [4]. HyperDOC provided information about NLM's products and services, but was not a direct source of health information. From the day it debuted, visitors entered search statements into NLM's main site seeking health information. One analysis showed that more than 90% of the search statements logged on the main site were for health-related topics and inappropriate for the NLM-services content of this institutional site [5]. Although changes to the main NLM site (*www.nlm.nih.gov*) over the years decreased the proportion of health information search statements, MedlinePlus finally provided a site for users to enter these searches and find appropriate information.

As NLM planned MedlinePlus, its research arm, the Lister Hill National Center for Biomedical Communications (LHNCBC), analyzed a sample of search statements using the Unified Medical Language System (UMLS) [6] and other tools. They determined which health topics and MeSH® (Medical Subject Headings) concepts were the most commonly entered [7]. This matching provided a priority list for creating MedlinePlus topics and features. Staff created MedlinePlus health topics pages of selected, reliable, authoritative links in priority order based on the analysis of consumer health searches. Not surprisingly, the first topics were diabetes, arthritis, AIDS, cancer, heart attack, stroke, fibromyalgia, and depression. The most common feedback from early users of MedlinePlus was for more health topics. The site was launched with 22 health topics and has now grown to well over 600. To address a need for overview information, along with an expressed desire for images, NLM licensed the *adam.com* medical encyclopedia, covering about 4000 medical topics with thousands of images. The analysis also showed that a quarter of the search terms were for specific generic and brand name drug names. Again, to answer this consumer-expressed need for drug information, MedlinePlus added the United States Pharmacopeia Drug Information, Advice for the Patient II in 2000, and the American Society for Health-System Pharmacists MedMaster data in 2002.

In 2000, NLM partnered with the Patient Education Institute (PEI), Iowa City, Iowa, for a pilot test to customize its X-Plain interactive tutorials to NLM's specifications for the Web. The PEI tutorials were a CD-ROM product developed for use in hospitals and clinics, explaining medical conditions and procedures using animated graphics, narration, and interactive questions in easy-to-understand language. The first tutorials were made available in March 2001 [8]. User feedback from the general public, healthcare professionals, and librarians has been overwhelmingly positive, noting that these tutorials meet the needs of low literacy populations, those for whom English is not the first language, those with low vision, and the general population. As a result, MedlinePlus now includes 165 tutorials covering diseases and conditions, tests and diagnostic procedures, and surgeries and treatments.

Although search logs provided an early user profile, subsequent usability tests provided key guidance on the interface. For example, observational usability data informed the simple, alphabetical presentation of the generic, brand, and drug-class names. They are some of the most frequently requested pages on the site and the same design is replicated on other pages. User feedback in many forms has guided MedlinePlus. Health news, a medical dictionary, and functional features such as print format and e-mail, are recent additions, and many others are planned.

MedlinePlus in Spanish

Very soon after MedlinePlus was launched users asked for health information in Spanish and other languages. Librarians, especially public and hospital librarians, as well as health professionals serving Spanish-speaking clientele, expressed the need for the same information in English and Spanish, so that they would know exactly what information they were providing. Focus groups confirmed that often bilingual family members were searching for health information in English and translating it for their Spanish-speaking relatives. After a year's effort, MedlinePlus en español (*medlineplus.gov/esp*) was launched in September 2002, with nearly 500 health topics, a medical encyclopedia, and 30 interactive tutorials (see Fig. 15.1).

Focus groups with Spanish speakers, both unilingual and bilingual, guided the design of MedlinePlus en español. Every Spanish page is directly linked to its English counterpart (where it exists) so that the user can toggle from one to the other. At this writing, nearly all health topics have information in both languages. The 4000 encyclopedia articles and 165 interactive tutorials have been translated so that a user can easily navigate to the equivalent information in the other language. Drug information and Spanish news were added in late 2003, moving toward the goal of achieving a site that is as comprehensive as the English version. NLM also implemented a new search engine from Recommind, Inc., so that users could search effectively in either language. Through usability studies and user surveys and direct feedback, Spanish users have indicated that they would like more images on the Spanish version, a medical dictionary in Spanish, and more health topics in general.

MedlinePlus Technical Background

MedlinePlus began as a database of links with associated metadata. Based on experience with the World Wide Web and with large databases, NLM bypassed the maintenance issues associated with static HTML pages by creating MedlinePlus from a

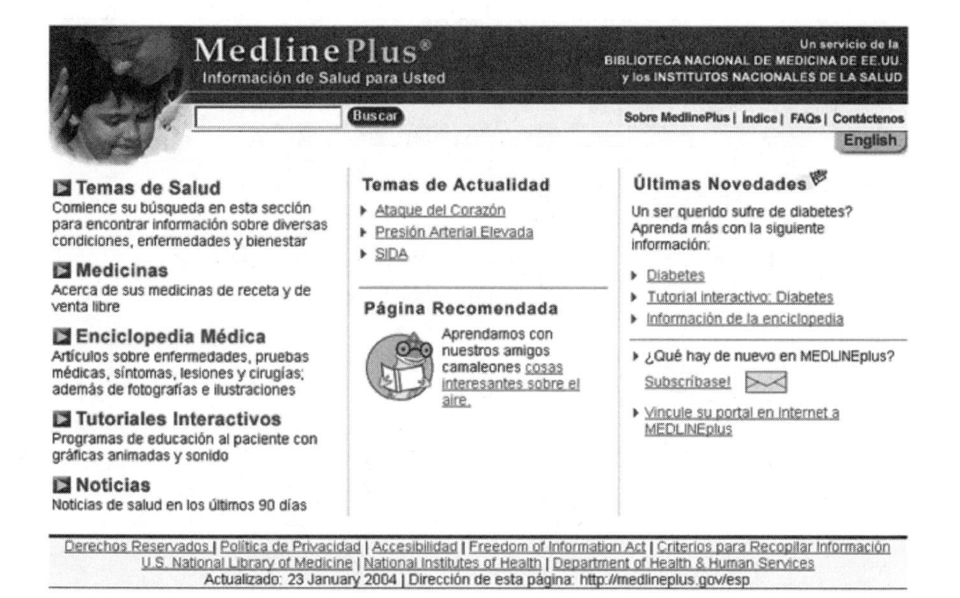

FIGURE 15.1. MedlinePlus en español homepage.

dynamic database [9]. This database houses 15,000 links, which comprise more than 650 health topics pages (see Fig. 15.2) Medical librarians at NLM and at other organizations (under contract to NLM) maintain these links using an NLM developed input and maintenance system that controls workflow, user privilege levels, quality assurance, and global changes. To maintain high standards of quality, the MedlinePlus staff review each link at least biannually and an automated link checker allows staff to repair broken links daily.

As the core resource of MedlinePlus, the health topic pages demand regular vocabulary maintenance. Staff derive the health topic names and the "see references" displayed in alphabetic lists from a variety of sources. MeSH is a primary resource, but consulting other resources such as the search logs, customer service inquiries, language used in full-text consumer-level documents, NLM's UMLS Knowledge Source Server [10] or the Planetree Vocabulary [11] of consumer health library terms provides guidance to language that will be most meaningful to consumers. In addition to naming topics and creating "see references," staff maintain topic groups that refer users from a topic page to other topics of interest. All of this information is maintained in the database and kept up to date with changes in MeSH and the other NLM resources to which it links.

Because it links to other key NLM products, MedlinePlus maintains the vocabulary and software to keep these links current and accurate. Each health topic provides one or more MEDLINE/PubMed searches so that health consumers and others can follow up on the consumer-level information with a live, customized search of the current research and clinical literature. These searches provide brief, clinical, and review articles and the search formulations are updated every 6 months. Where appropriate, health topic pages link to *ClinicalTrials.gov* to provide lists of clinical research studies recruiting participants with that condition. As with the PubMed search, these links

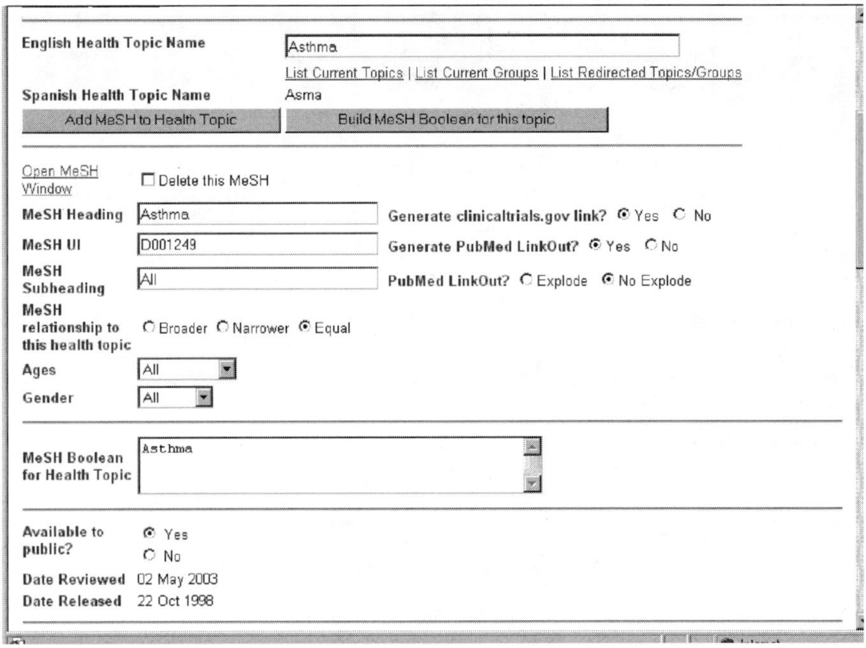

FIGURE 15.2. MedlinePlus health topic management record.

perform a live search each time users click on them, providing consumers with the most up-to-date information possible. Also using MeSH, MedlinePlus maintains links to the LHC's Genetics Home Reference from related health topics pages. These product links are maintained by software that automatically keeps them updated with relevant changes in each system, always linking consumers to the best information regardless of where they initiate their information seeking.

Go Local

From early experience with consumers using MedlinePlus, NLM realized that in addition to the health information provided by MedlinePlus, consumers need information about health providers, facilities, services, and programs where they live. Because local information can be very difficult to find and extremely dynamic, gathering and maintaining this information is best done locally. NLM partnered with the University of North Carolina at Chapel Hill Health Sciences Library and School of Information and Library Science, funding development of a pilot site, launched in January 2003 [12]. *NCHealthInfo.org* is the first "Go Local" site, fully linked to MedlinePlus, that bridges the gap between authoritative health information and local health services. UNC staff have developed and tested methods to identify, select, and organize health services sites and are gathering user feedback from health professionals, consumers, and librarians. Based on the experience of UNC to date, NLM plans to expand the "Go Local" initiative to other states. NLM is building a system to allow other libraries or organizations to focus on selecting and maintaining local information. NLM will be responsible for maintaining the infrastructure and links to MedlinePlus. Organizations in states that already have a site of local health services will be able to map their information to MedlinePlus to create a complete and authoritative health resource for the public in their states.

MEDLINE/PubMed and Consumers

PubMed (*pubmed.gov*) is NLM's bibliographic retrieval system that provides access to MEDLINE. In 1999, PubMed began linking to MedlinePlus through a "consumer health" link on its left-side navigation bar. This link guides users who wish to find information at a consumer level to MedlinePlus. In addition to this general link to the MedlinePlus home page, PubMed also provides links to appropriate health topic pages to read consumer-level information related to the PubMed reference. These links, introduced in April 2000, are part of the PubMed LinkOut feature [13]. Each month, more than 10,000 users visit MedlinePlus from one of these links.

Another PubMed feature of interest to consumers is the "CAM on PubMed" service [14]. This PubMed feature, introduced in February 2001, allows PubMed users to search for articles related to complementary and alternative medicine. Through CAM on PubMed, the public can find references to peer-reviewed articles about various complementary and alternative treatments including acupuncture, herbs, homeopathy, chiropractic, traditional oriental medicine and others. At this writing there are 340,000 citations in the CAM subset.

ClinicalTrials.Gov

Government and industry both sponsor many clinical trials to test promising treatments for medical conditions. Recognizing the benefit to the public of a comprehensive list of these trials, in 1997 Congress included language in a section of the FDA Modernization Act requiring the creation of a clinical trials database, specifically, "A registry of clinical trials (whether federally or privately funded) of experimental treatments for serious or life-threatening diseases and conditions" [15]. In response to this law, NLM released the first version of *ClinicalTrials.gov* in February 2000. The initial release included trials from 21 organizations of the National Institutes of Health (NIH) and has since grown to include trials from many other government agencies as well as those sponsored by the private sector [16].

The development of *ClinicalTrials.gov* as a successful resource for patients, families, and health professionals has depended on overcoming many challenges. The trials records come from a variety of institutions, which requires standardizing and maintaining quality in data elements. The registry is valuable only because it is very up-to-date and complete, but these standards for comprehensiveness and currency require extensive maintenance resources. The LHCNBC, which developed and maintains *ClinicalTrials.gov*, has created a reliable system to address these challenges and update the records daily.

The clean design of *ClinicalTrials.gov* is derived from extensive interviews, community feedback, and usability testing with the user audience (see Fig. 15.3). For example, because feedback showed that some users preferred browsing through information hierarchies and others preferred a more direct search, *ClinicalTrials.gov* provides both navigation options. *ClinicalTrials.gov* maintains links from trial records to MedlinePlus

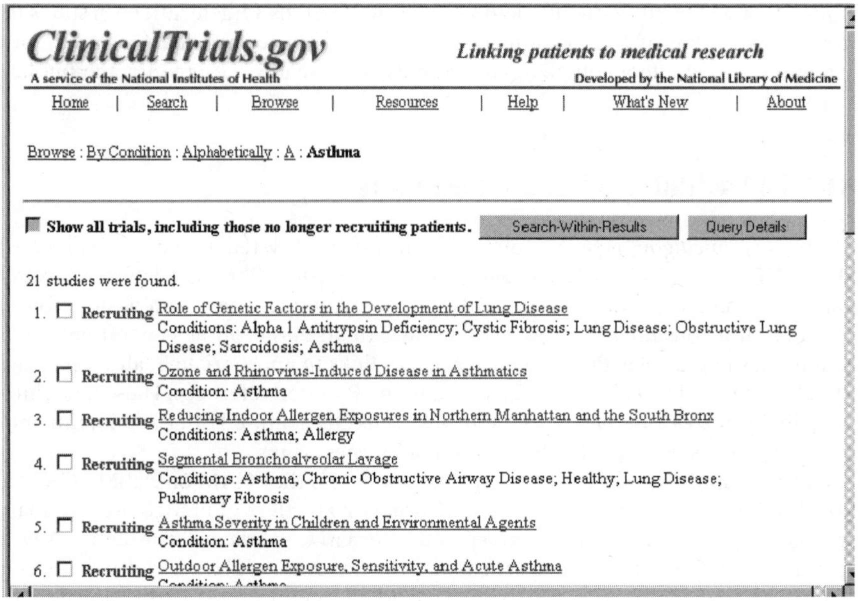

ClinicalTrials.gov
A service of the National Institutes of Health
Linking patients to medical research
Developed by the National Library of Medicine

Home | Search | Browse | Resources | Help | What's New | About

Browse : By Condition : Alphabetically : A : **Asthma**

Show all trials, including those no longer recruiting patients. Search-Within-Results Query Details

21 studies were found.

1. **Recruiting** Role of Genetic Factors in the Development of Lung Disease
Conditions: Alpha 1 Antitrypsin Deficiency; Cystic Fibrosis; Lung Disease; Obstructive Lung Disease; Sarcoidosis; Asthma
2. **Recruiting** Ozone and Rhinovirus-Induced Disease in Asthmatics
Condition: Asthma
3. **Recruiting** Reducing Indoor Allergen Exposures in Northern Manhattan and the South Bronx
Conditions: Asthma; Allergy
4. **Recruiting** Segmental Bronchoalveolar Lavage
Conditions: Asthma; Chronic Obstructive Airway Disease; Healthy; Lung Disease; Pulmonary Fibrosis
5. **Recruiting** Asthma Severity in Children and Environmental Agents
Condition: Asthma
6. **Recruiting** Outdoor Allergen Exposure, Sensitivity, and Acute Asthma

FIGURE 15.3. ClinicalTrials.gov results for asthma.

for consumer-level information on the disease or condition through MeSH vocabulary relationships. As with other user-driven resources, *ClinicalTrials.gov* continues to collect search and use data to make informed decisions about changes and improvements [17].

NIHSeniorHealth

To address the special needs of older consumers, NLM developed NIHSenior-Health.gov in partnership with the National Institute on Aging (NIA). In 2002, the first beta version became available to the public and includes topics of particular interest to seniors. The site accommodates the physical and cognitive changes that NIA research has shown affects seniors' interactions with computers. For example, low vision is a reality for many senior health consumers. To address this need, NIHSeniorHealth uses a large font and provides options for an even larger font, allows users to select a high-contrast bright text on a black background, and even an option to read the text aloud. This "talking" feature does not require a browser plug-in and allows users to click on any paragraph to hear it read in a machine-generated voice.

The navigation of NIHSeniorHealth simplifies browsing for seniors. The pages are one-screen in length with large "next" and "previous page" buttons for easy navigation. All the mouse targets are large for seniors with declining motor control. For clarity, there is lots of white space around the large text. The site reinforces content for this group of users who may have diminished cognitive skills. Quizzes, FAQs, images, and videos all help users in reviewing content for better understanding and recall. Feedback from usability testing and focus groups with seniors and low-vision users has greatly influenced the construction of NIHSeniorHealth. As NIH Institutes continue to contribute content of particular interest to this audience, NIHSeniorHealth is becoming a great place for seniors and low-vision users to start learning about health conditions.

Genetics Home Reference

One of NLM's most recent consumer health resources is the LHNCBC's Genetics Home Reference (*http://ghr.lhc.nlm.nih.gov*). Because genetic conditions can be very complicated, much consumer literature does not cover them in depth. Yet, patients and families affected by genetic conditions often want to know more about the condition. NIH has excellent genetics resources for scientists and healthcare professionals through NLM's National Center for Biotechnology Information and the NIH National Institute for Human Genome Research, but they are not tailored to the consumer. To fill this gap, the LHC has geneticists, genetics counselors, and health science writers creating the Genetics Home Reference. This resource, released in April 2003, describes genetic conditions, risk factors, and other valuable information in language comprehensible to a well-educated lay person. It provides information about the gene, related medical conditions, and tests. It also includes extensive links to MedlinePlus for consumer-level information, to PubMed/MEDLINE for research and scientific articles, to GeneClinics at the University of Washington for laboratories performing specific tests, and other key information resources in genetics. MedlinePlus provides reciprocal links to the GHR so patients, families, and clinicians can follow up on a topic with its in-depth coverage. Based on user feedback, the GHR fills an important need for patients and families affected by genetically related conditions.

Toxicology and Environmental Health

Since its founding in 1967, NLM's Specialized Information Services Division (SIS) has served toxicology and environmental health professionals by creating and maintaining authoritative database and knowledge-base resources. Recently, SIS has released two products especially for the consumer audience, Tox Town (*http://toxtown.nlm.nih.gov*) and the Household Products Database (*http://householdproducts.nlm.nih.gov*). Tox Town looks at an ordinary town or city and points out possible environmental hazards. Tox Town uses color, graphics, sounds, and animation to add interest to learning about connections between chemicals, the environment, and the public's health. Tox Town's target audience is students above elementary-school level, educators, and the general public. It is a companion to the extensive information in the TOXNET collection of databases that are typically used by toxicologists and health professionals.

The Household Products Database links more than 4000 consumer brands to potential health effects from Material Safety Data Sheets (MSDS) provided by the manufacturers and enables consumers to research products based on chemical ingredients. Consumers can identify chemical ingredients and their percentages in specific brands, contact information for manufacturers of a given product, acute and chronic effects of chemical ingredients in a specific brand, and related information in other toxicology databases of NLM.

NLM Research, Evaluation, and Data Analysis

Because a product and its information design must continue to improve to remain useful to its intended audience, NLM continuously seeks feedback in many formats. Consumers provide constant direct feedback through the search terms they enter and pages they choose to view. The anonymous logs of these activities provide valuable insight into the terminology consumers choose to use in their information-seeking. Also, these logs of searches and page use can be correlated to indicate which topics users seek more or less often. NLM uses these data to track trends and make resource and development decisions and guide changes to sites.

In addition to analyzing the data created by those using the systems on a daily basis, NLM collects feedback in many other ways including customer service messages, surveys, usability tests, and a variety of focus group formats. Consumers, health professionals, and others constantly send unsolicited feedback to NLM's customer service system. System developers read and analyze this feedback to better inform changes to the system. NLM has conducted several sample surveys of the users of its consumer-oriented systems over the last few years. From these surveys, NLM gleans demographic data, user satisfaction, and priority areas for improvement.

Outreach

In 1987 the Senate Committee on Appropriations encouraged NLM to develop an outreach program to ensure that all health professionals had access to current, authoritative medical information. The first projects targeted those health professionals serving rural and inner city areas. The report from the review of the first 5 years of projects carried out by NLM and the National Network of Libraries of Medicine (NN/LM) recommended that NLM should consider expanding its current activities in support of consumer health information. NLM's Specialized Information Services (SIS) had shown the positive impact of providing modest funding to local groups to improve information access to community-based organizations, patient advocacy groups, and public libraries working with HIV/AIDS patients [18].

NLM launched a public library pilot project in 1998 to evaluate how to apply its long-developed expertise in collecting, organizing, and disseminating health information to professionals and researchers to serve the general public [19]. Forty-one public libraries or library systems in nine states received training in online health resources and small stipends for consumer health resources, which varied from computers to Internet access to books and brochures. Through this project, NLM and the NN/LM gained valuable advice and guidance, which has been used in the subsequent years toward new and updated products including MedlinePlus and MedlinePlus en español. Through the NN/LM, the Library has funded numerous projects throughout the United States to improve the public's access to health information. These projects have involved a variety of organizations including health science and public libraries and community and faith-based organizations and schools.

NLM now funds a Consumer Health Coordinator in each Regional Medical Library (RML). Coordinators travel around the region demonstrating MedlinePlus, MEDLINE, and other NLM databases and sites to consumers, intermediaries, and health professionals. They also create resources for public and medical librarians to use in reaching out to consumers, coordinate exhibits and training, and provide feedback and advice to NLM on consumers' health information needs.

Summary

Inspired by medical experts such as Dr. Michael DeBakey and with political support from officials such as Vice President Al Gore, NLM began an earnest effort to provide health resources directly to the consumer in the late 1990s. NLM served consumers, first through increased access to its resources for professionals and researchers, then by providing resources specifically geared to the consumer audience. NLM created these resources on the firm foundation of controlled vocabularies, systematic quality control, comprehensive maintenance systems, and user-interface integration to allow navigation between resources. They were developed using feedback from consumers in the form of search logs, surveys, use information, focus groups, customer service feedback, and recommendations from professionals in the health and information fields. NLM will continue to develop and improve consumer access to this information, embracing appropriate technology and ensuring high-quality information resources for patients, families, friends, and the health professionals who serve them.

Acknowledgments. The authors thank Robert Mehnert for his assistance in identifying background materials and editing, and Ruth Hill and Jana Brightwell for significant help in gathering materials and manuscript preparation.

References

1. National Library of Medicine press release April 8, 1996. Internet Grateful Med goes on the World Wide. Available at *http://www.nlm.nih.gov/news/press_releases/igmpr.html* (accessed August 25, 2003).
2. Departments of Labor, Health and Human Services, Education, and Related Agencies Appropriations for 1998: Hearing on H.R. 2264 Before the Subcomm. on the Departments of Labor, Health and Human Services, Education, and Related Agencies of the House Comm. on Appropriations, 105th Cong., 1st Session (1997) (statement of Michael E. DeBakey, MD, Chancellor Emeritus and Professor of Surgery, Baylor College of Medicine).
3. Online usage statistics smashed: free MEDLINE rewrites NLM record book. NLM Newsline 1998;53:1–2.
4. National Library of Medicine programs and services: fiscal year 1994. Bethesda, MD: The Library; 1995. Information Sources Map Project. NIH publication no. 95–256, p. 25.
5. Miller N. Improving the NLM home page: from logs to links. Poster presented at Annual Meeting of the Medical Library Association; 1997 May 26–27; Seattle, WA. Text available at *http://www.nlm.nih.gov/psd/_poster/_poster.html*
6. Fact Sheet: Unified Medical Language System® (Internet). Bethesda, MD: National Library of Medicine. Available at *http://www.nlm.nih.gov/pubs/factsheets/umls.html* (updated July 2003; cited September 15, 2003).
7. McCray AT, Loane RF, Browne AC, et al. Terminology issues in user access to -based medical information. Proc AMIA Symp 1999;107–11.
8. National Library of Medicine site releases the interactive patient education programs X-Plain™. Iowa City, IA: University of Iowa, Patient Education Institute; press release March 28, 2001.
9. Miller N, Lacroix EM, Backus, JEB. MEDLINEplus: building and maintaining the National Library of Medicine's consumer health service. Bull Med Libr Assoc 2000;88:11–17.
10. Fact sheet: UMLS® Knowledge Source Server (Internet). Bethesda, MD: National Library of Medicine. Available at *http://www.nlm.nih.gov/pubs/factsheets/umlskss.html* (updated November 5, 2002; cited September 15, 2003).
11. Schmalz RP, Cosgrove T, Ford C, et al., compilers and eds. The Planetree classification scheme. Version 5.0. San Francisco: Program Planetree; © 1991.

12. MEDLINEplus goes local with NC Health Info. NLM Newsline 2003;58:1–2.
13. LinkOut (Internet). Bethesda, MD: National Library of Medicine, National Center for Biotechnology Information. Available at *http://www.ncbi.nlm.nih.gov/entrez/linkout/* (modified June 18, 2003; cited September 22, 2003).
14. Press Release: NIH Launches CAM on PubMed (Internet). Bethesda, MD: National Library of Medicine; February 5, 2001. Available at *http://www.nlm.nih.gov/news/press_releases/cam_pr01.html* (modified June 14, 2002; cited September 15, 2003).
15. Food and Drug Administration Modernization Act of 1997, Pub. L. 105–115, 111 Stat. 2296 (November 21, 1997). Sec. 113, Information program on clinical trials for serious or life-threatening diseases.
16. McCray AT. Better access to information about clinical trials. Ann Intern Med 2000;133: 609–14.
17. McCray AT, Dorfman E, Ripple A, et al. Usability issues in developing a consumer-based health site. Proc AMIA Symp 2000;556–60.
18. Wallingford KT, Ruffin AB, Ginter KA, et al. Outreach activities of the National Library of Medicine: a five-year review. Bull Med Libr Assoc 1996;84(2 Suppl):1–60. Recommendations for further action; p. 37.
19. Wood FB, Lyon B, Schell MB, et al. Public Library consumer health information pilot project: results of a National Library of Medicine evaluation. Bull Med Lib Assoc 2000;88:314–22.

16
Baby CareLink: Collaborative Tools to Support Families*

CHARLES SAFRAN and DENISE GOLDSMITH

Application of information and communication technologies designed to enhance decision making and communication between providers, patients, and their families will play an important role in supporting the relationship between patient and provider and will assist patients to better understand their illness experience and how their own values affect decision making [1–8]. We call this tight integration of software and people in health care Collaborative Healthware [9–11]. Baby CareLink, an application of Collaborative Healthware, links NICU staff with families of medically complex newborns [12]. Using a Web browser, parents can receive daily updates and track information about their baby's health, see recent pictures of their baby, communicate with NICU staff, access a personalized knowledge base for newborn care, and provide feedback regarding the care process. Following discharge, Baby CareLink can be used to support care coordination, follow-up monitoring, and ongoing communication with parents. Baby CareLink is Collaborative Healthware that supports the relationship between parents and healthcare provider by engaging the family as full partners in the healthcare process.

The birth of a child is a great joy for most families, but for families whose children require care in the Neonatal Intensive Care Unit (NICU) it is a time of great emotional distress. The care of premature infants is truly a miracle of modern medicine. Incubators for premature infants were developed in the 1930s and supported a controlled environment for the infant. For the most part, the prematurity of the lung was the limiting factor to survivability of the infant. Surfactant is a naturally occurring substance produced by the lung to decrease the surface tension in these small air sacks. Only more mature lungs produce this substance. Even modern ventilators with small rapid tidal volumes had problems expanding the small air exchanging units in the lung called alveoli until the 1970s when surfactant was introduced. As doctors attempted to resuscitate smaller and smaller infants, their success rate improved. Concomitant with the introduction of improved ventilation technology was a dramatic improvement in fertility technologies. Pharmaceuticals were developed to help stimulate ovulation and support tenuous pregnancies. Women were also able to receive already fertilized eggs to overcome biological barriers to conception. The result of these advances has been that preterm birth rate has increased 9% since 1990 and 23% since 1981.

---

* This chapter was adapted in part from Safran C. The collaborative edge: patient empowerment for vulnerable populations. Int J Med Inform 2003;69:185–190.

Success, however miraculous, comes at a great cost. Neonatal care accounts for more than 1% of total US health expenditure. More than $18 billion is spent in the United States each year on the care of premature infants; accounting for 25% of total annual expenditures on child and maternal health. The average cost for the birth of a low birthweight (less than 2500 g) baby is $50,000. Premature twins would cost $100,000. Moreover, costs post-discharge for these infants during the first 12 months are 10 to 30 times higher than for healthy, full-term babies.

Today children smaller than 500 g (approx 1 lbs) are cared for in the NICU and have excellent prospects of growing up to be normal adults. About 5% of these small infants die and another 10% have serious disability. The emotional costs for the parents, although hard to quantify, are profound. Parents hope for and expect to bring home a healthy baby. Many parents in their teens, 20s, 30s, and even 40s have had little previous contact with the health system, much less with the type of high-tech medicine they encounter in the NICU. A variety of emotions frequently overwhelms the new parent of a premature infant in the NICU, the central concern, of course, being whether the child will live or die. Parents often describe the experience as an "emotional roller coaster." Families are faced with logistical issues as well. If there are other young children at home, who will care for them when the parents want to be in the NICU with their baby? If a parent has maternity or paternity leave from work, does he or she use this time while his or her baby is in the NICU or several months later when the child can come home? During the prolonged hospitalization parents must assimilate a large body of knowledge relevant to their baby's care. This includes not only information about routine baby care, but also the special needs of their high-risk infant. Their learning is often impeded by fear and anxiety and parents become overwhelmed with information and advice from multiple sources. A study by Brazy [13] showed that during the first week of their baby's life, more than half of parents spend at least 20 hours seeking information. Even after 4 weeks of hospitalization, more than one third of parents perform the equivalent of a half-time job seeking information about and for their child. In addition, and perhaps more alarming to parents, the need for information and problems with its access do not end when the baby goes home. Skills and knowledge gained at one point may be lost or forgotten in the whirlwind that can exist during the early days following discharge. Almost 40% of babies discharged from the NICU return to an emergency room, and half these visits are generally recognized as medically unnecessary. Like most areas of health care, NICU care has great local and regional variation. Although the average stay for a preterm infant is about 3 weeks, gestational age or birthweight are among the best determinate of length of stay for any particular infant. First, the child has to be medically ready. Most infants progress from an early intensive care phase to the feeding and growing stage. Once in this second phase, it is only a matter of time until parents can take their child home. Clearly the infant needs to meet some medical criteria before going home, but the judgment of the clinicians about the parents' and community's readiness is the second factor determining the date of discharge.

Baby CareLink History

Baby CareLink was developed at Boston's Beth Israel Hospital as part of a federal initiative to evaluate telemedicine's impact on clinical care. Starting in 1997, a team of neonatologists led by Jim Gray and neonatal nurse specialists led by Grace Pompilio worked with the teams of informaticians at the Center for Clinical

Computing to develop an Internet-based application to support families with infants in NICUs.

Six major areas of clinical content and resources were part of the original Baby CareLink including a daily clinical report, a message center, a see your baby section, a family room, a clinical information section, and a section focused on preparation for discharge to home. The daily report is webpage that provides clinical updates about a baby's clinical care and status. The message center is a secure WWW-based messaging system through which parents can share confidential communications with members of the NICU staff. Baby CareLink also contains a context-sensitive messaging throughout the CareLink site to allow parents to easily compose messages related to the content they are viewing. The see your baby section is a pictorial daily journal comprised of images captured by the staff with a consumer grade digital camera. Baby CareLink also provides a mechanism for allowing families to share these photos outside of the confines of the CareLink security architecture. By changing a picture's status through the WWW-based interface, parents can post pictures to a password protected WWW where their families and friends can see their baby. The family room provides a potpourri of supports including answers to common questions, information about services available to families, links to WWW-based resources, and an online library for browsing available print and video resources. "The Kid's Corner" provides a collection of information and support materials specifically geared for older siblings of our patients. "The Emotional Side of the NICU" allows parents to both read about the issues that confront families of high-risk newborns and view high-quality digital video of NICU families discussing how they coped with their NICU experience. The clinical information and care section describes the issues present at various stages in a baby's NICU stay including when a baby is first admitted, as a baby stabilizes and family members becomes more active participants in their baby's care, and the period prior to discharge when families prepare to take over all of their baby's care at home. The "NICU-Pedia" provides an online encyclopedia of clinical conditions, tests, treatments, and medications relevant to the care of high-risk newborns. The preparing for discharge section is an on-line discharge teaching module where parents can view multimedia modules describing the knowledge and competencies they must acquire prior to discharge. This module is constructed so that NICU clinicians can individualize the content for each baby's needs using a simple WWW interface. It also allows parents and clinicians to track acquisition of knowledge.

A randomized controlled clinical trial of this early Baby CareLink was conducted between November 1, 1997 and March 30, 1999 and published in the journal *Pediatrics* [12]. This study showed Baby CareLink significantly improved family satisfaction with inpatient care and definitively lowers costs associated with hospital to hospital transfer. The study suggested the use of Baby CareLink supported the educational and emotional needs of families and facilitated earlier discharge to home.

In July 1999, a commercial version of Baby CareLink was developed for national use by Clinician Support Technology (CST). CST's early version of Baby CareLink did not support two-way videoconferencing.

Baby CareLink Today

CST Baby CareLink provides parents, clinicians, and care managers with innovative Internet-supported tools that foster an environment where parents become more active and empowered in their baby's care. Providing parents with timely information establishes a common framework for understanding developmental milestones and reinforces discharge education. All content in CST Baby CareLink is written in easy to understand English and Spanish. CST incorporates multimedia, voice-over and Web technologies to make complicated information more understandable for all parents, even those with low reading, computer, or health literacy.

CST Baby CareLink helps grow a better parent: one who is more comfortable, confident, and competent in caring for their fragile newborn. These parents are more likely to take their infants home sooner and less likely to utilize valuable emergency room resources for routine care issues. From anywhere, using an Internet browser, parents can access an individualized knowledge base for newborn care, receive daily updates, and track information about their baby's health and progress. Parents can communicate with the NICU team through a secure messaging center and receive prescribed educational modules.

Baby CareLink offer a comprehensive, organized platform for families to document issues for discussion with their primary physician, track their infant's progress toward developmental milestones, and maintain accurate, up-to-date immunization records. Parents can access a knowledge base particular to infants who experienced a NICU stay and who may have ongoing medical problems and/or an anticipated developmental timeline that differs from that expected with a full-term healthy infant. Early recognition by parents of a delay in reaching critical milestones helps ensure that an infant's potential is maximized. In addition, parents are provided with the early warning signs that could indicate if their baby may need to be seen by a physician. This helps parents identify potentially serious clinical problems before they progress and lead to emergency care and/or re-hospitalization. This information can be delivered at predetermined intervals such as during flu and allergy seasons to serve as a reminder. Collaborative Healthware applications can make the challenges associated with taking a baby home from the NICU a bit easier for parents and for the clinicians who care for them.

CST Baby CareLink has evolved to a solution for broader aspects of maternal–child care to support the family from the beginning pregnancy though the first year of life. Baby CareLink has content and tools for parents, tools for clinicians, and tools for care managers.

Content and Tools for Parents

The content for parents starts with pregnancy and supports the parents' educational and emotional needs though their child's first year of life. Topics might include fitness and lifestyle, nutrition, growth and nutrition, infant safety, and immunization. For the medically complex infant requiring care in the NICU, Baby CareLink currently has the following modules:

1. **Clinical Dashboard** is the opening portal to all the functions of Baby CareLink. From this page a parent can easily see if there are messages, a new educational prescription, or a clinical update concerning their child's health.
2. **Welcome to the NICU** is a description of the NICU setting, visiting policies, hospital information, and important phone numbers.
3. **The Meet the Staff** page allows parents to see a photo and identify members of the NICU team.
4. **The See Your Baby** page is a secure, patient-specific photo gallery that can be easily updated by the NICU team.

5. **The Message Center** is a secure messaging center, linking individual families to their baby's entire care team.
6. **Clinical Information** is a complete NICU reference library, including an encyclopedia and glossary.
7. **Caring for Your Baby** is a comprehensive parent guide to baby care, safety, and development.
8. **The Family Room** is a comprehensive resource center with information on books, emotional issues associated with the NICU experience, Web links, and sibling games.
9. **Preparing for Discharge** provides individualized discharge teaching tools for parents. Parents can submit questions online and clinicians can monitor progress and keep a record of completion.
10. **My Journal** allows parents to keep track of questions they may have about Baby CareLink educational materials, take notes on material relevant to their baby, and/or to bookmark selected Web pages for future reading.

More than 1500 topics are covered and are written in English and Spanish at a sixth-grade reading level. To accommodate different learning styles, the content is delivered in multimedia using text-to-voice and video clips.

Tools for Clinicians

Clinicians can prescribe and track educational modules for parents, are supported by rule-based care, and discharge planning forms and documentation. Like parents, clinicians use the message center to communicate with families.

Tools for Care Managers

Care managers have tools that help in the transition home, provide for ongoing assessments, and have access to the same message center as do the clinicians and parents, thereby fostering collaboration.

The Digital Divide

Unfortunately, there has always been a gap between those people and communities who have access to the newest technology available and those who do not. The term "digital divide" is used to refer to this gap. While there are conflicting reports on the extent of the divide most agree that a divide does exist. *A Nation Online: How Americans Are Expanding Their Use of the Internet* [14] reports on the rapidly growing use of new information technologies such as the Internet across all demographic groups and geographic regions.

More than half of the nation (54%) is now online and the rate of growth of Internet use in the United States is currently two million new Internet users per month. The profile of computer and Internet users demonstrates that the rise in computer and Internet use is spread across a wide range of the population. Internet use is increasing for people regardless of income, education, age, race, ethnicity, or gender [14].

While Internet use continues to rise among people who live in lower income households, family income remains the main indicator of whether a person is likely to use a computer or the Internet. Individuals who live in high-income households are more likely to be computer and Internet users than those who live in low-income households [14]. Internet use has also increased across all races and groups. White Americans continue to be the largest segment of the population using computers despite the fact that growth in Internet use rates was faster for blacks and Hispanics. Between August 2000 and September 2001, Internet use among blacks and Hispanics increased at annual rates of 33% and 30%, respectively. Whites, Asian Americans, and Pacific Islanders experienced annual growth rates of approximately 20% during these same periods [14].

For families who depend on Medicaid support, the emotional, social, and economic toll of serious illness is magnified not only by circumstance, but also by stereotyped preconception. For instance, Medicaid mothers who have preterm infants in Neonatal ICUs (NICU) are younger, have attained lower levels of education, may have had less prenatal care, and have more children at home than do mothers who have paid for in vitro fertilization. However, the circumstance of being poor and receiving support from Medicaid does not imply that a parent lacks the motivation or intelligence to use e-Health applications. On the contrary, a mother of a sick child is a powerful advocate for her child's health regardless of socioeconomic status. Collaborative Healthware can be a valuable and effective approach for this medically underserved and disadvantaged population that makes up such a large proportion of those families with low birthweight or medically complex newborns requiring NICU care.

Many medically fragile infants have complex chronic medical problems that place them at higher risk for postdischarge mortality, childhood morbidity from acute and chronic illnesses, and long-term developmental/educational difficulties. Those infants who are born into socioeconomically disadvantaged families are faced with even greater risk because they lack the financial resources and adequate social and emotional support they need. Providing Medicaid parents with the resources of Collaborative Healthware will enhance the early identification of critical issues facing families prior to and on integration into the community with a medically complex infant.

Despite the fact that compliance with postdischarge programs may help prevent adverse outcomes for their infant, many Medicaid families have a hard time following up with recommended medical care and developmental services. Collaborative Healthware applications can be used to support care coordination, follow up monitoring, and facilitate ongoing communication with parents and care partners. Early identification of issues facing families on integration into the community avoids costly readmissions and helps to decrease the stress associated with caring for a premature or low-birthweight newborn.

Use of Baby CareLink

As of the beginning of 2004, Baby CareLink operates in 13 hospitals in 8 different states. In three of these states, Baby CareLink is being deployed as part of a State-Medicaid initiative. More than 4000 infants were registered in the system in 2003. These parents are logging onto Baby CareLink more than 6000 times per month and viewing more than 30,000 Baby CareLink Web pages each month.

Thirty-eight percent of the time parents access the educational material such as "caring for you baby" or "preparing for discharge." Thirty-four percent of the time, parents look at pictures of their infants. Twenty-eight percent of the time parents use the collaborative tools to receive personalized information from the clinical staff or to send messages back to the clinicians.

Case Reports

One infant was diagnosed with gastroschisis. The infant was delivered prematurely and scheduled for a secondary repair at the nearby Children's Hospital a few weeks after birth. The parents were bilingual, although Spanish was their spoken language at home. The parents were lent a laptop computer through the lending program so they could have access to Baby CareLink. They expressed the value of looking up information in Spanish so that they could better understand it. They were able to complete several of the discharge learning modules from home, and their baby went home a few weeks after his repair.

Premature babies are in the hospital for so long their parents cannot always remain in the area for their entire length of stay. Some parents opt to return to work while their baby is hospitalized and take their maternity leave once their baby comes home. One family from Wyoming was unsure of how they would care for their baby, and felt guilty that they couldn't remain in Denver to be with their baby. Both parents had access to a computer at work, and used the message center to communicate with the NICU team. The NICU team was able to provide updates on their baby's condition and assign discharge learning materials to the parents. The parents felt like they were doing something for their baby and were preparing for their infant's homecoming. This boosted the parents' confidence. The parents reviewed the educational materials and asked questions through the message center showing the NICU team that they had really read and thought about the materials.

For one infant with an extended hospitalization because of extreme prematurity, the mother visited almost every day. While in the NICU, she logged on to the site and read everything available. She entered chat rooms with other NICU parents, asking for suggestions about helping her baby to learn to bottle-feed. It was uplifting to see her find other resources outside of the NICU that she could use in supporting her baby's care. She utilized this resource effectively, giving the additional information to her baby's care team. Her baby's course was uncomplicated and the baby went home as soon as possible with a very confident young mother.

Discussion

Baby CareLink represents a new class of tools and applications in health care that we have termed "Collaborative Healthware." These tools enable patients and their families to be full participants in the care process. The introduction of programs such as Baby CareLink has the potential to change clinical processes. Parental discharge teaching, which was previously concentrated on the day of discharge, is now initiated earlier and provided over a more extended period of time using Baby CareLink. Parents are more motivated to learn and prefer the autonomy and ability to control the pace of their learning using the computer system on their own. Clinicians review with the parents any questions they have after reading the assigned Baby CareLink learning modules and assess their comprehension of the material. As a result of the targeted, personalized education, parents ask more informed questions and understand their challenges much better. Clinicians believe that parents who use Baby CareLink are more confident about caring for their children and are prepared to take the infants home sooner.

Clinicians adopt programs such as Baby CareLink in different ways. Some sites have not enabled parent-to-parent chat, and one site does not allow parent to clinician email.

On the other hand, several sites use Baby CareLink as their principal method to provide and document discharge education and learning. Baby CareLink has been used in teaching hospitals, rural hospitals, and inner-city hospitals. In each environment, parents from all socioeconomic backgrounds and prior Internet experience have embraced tools designed to help them help their infants.

The evaluation of clinical systems such as Baby CareLink represents a continuing challenge. The initial evaluation of Baby CareLink [12] involved a randomized clinical trial. Such an evaluation is complex, difficult, and expensive. Moreover, really clinical systems such as Baby CareLink are constantly changing and improving based on customer suggestions and good suggestions from a clinical advisory board. The underlying technology of Baby CareLink tries to provide "just-in-time" information to the parent. Providing the right information at the right time might change a child's care, but measuring this impact is quite difficult. Baby CareLink has delivered more than one-quarter million pictures of premature infants to their families while only 80,000 pages of discharge learning material. Does this mean that the pictures are more valuable than the educational material? Ultimately, each component of Baby CareLink provides part of a framework that allows patients and their families to better collaborate with their care teams. For some, this strengthens existing relationships and for others technology facilitates new linkages.

Collaborative Healthware supports the relationship between healthcare provider and patient by engaging the patient and their families as full partners in the healthcare process. In a collaborative partnership, patients expect that their clinicians will provide information and guidance. Patients expect that their clinicians will educate them and their families on illnesses, available therapies, potential outcomes, and complications, so that decisions can be made based on the patient's individual preferences [2,15–17].

More often patients are presented with opportunities to actively participate in decisions that affect their lives and well being [3,6,8,18]. While patient preferences for participation in clinical decisions vary greatly [1,2,4], the desire for information about their health and health care is high [19]. Patients want information that addresses their individual concerns and conditions as well as interactive tools to manage their health and disease [20,21]. Providing patients with enhanced health related information favorably affects their trust in, relationship with, and confidence in their healthcare providers [22].

Collaborative Healthware solutions allow the development of prescribed healthcare communities that facilitate effective connectivity among participants. These solutions provide better access to information for patients, better distribution of expertise throughout the healthcare system, improved collaboration and coordination of care, and improved quality of care. The enabling technologies of Collaborative Healthware solutions are based on secure sharing of information and knowledge in a cost-effective manner.

Technology can play an important role in restoring relationships between patients and the healthcare system. Technology can facilitate improvement in quality, cost, and patient satisfaction. Properly applied Internet technology can be used successfully as a platform on which to deliver interventions to patients that significantly enhance the outcomes of care [23].

References

1. Benbassat J, Pilpel D, Tidhar M. Patients' preferences for participation in clinical decision making: a review of published surveys. Behav Med 1998;24:81–8.

2. Brennan PF. (1999). Health Informatics and community health: support for patients as collaborators in care. Methods Inform Med 1999;38:27–48.
3. Brennan PF, Ripich S. Use of a home care computer network by persons with AIDS. Int J Technol Assess Health Care 1994;10:258–72.
4. Brennan PF, Strombom I. Improving health care by understanding patient preferences: the role of computer technology. JAMIA 1998;5:257–62.
5. Eng T, Gustafson D, eds. Wired for health and well being: the emergence of interactive health communication. Washington, DC: US Department of Health and Human Services, 1999.
6. Ferguson T. Online patient-helpers and physicians working together: a new patient collaboration for high quality health care. Br Med J 2000;321:1129–32.
7. Gustafson DH, McTavish F, Boberg E, et al. Empowering patients using computer based health support systems. Quality Health Care 1999;8:49–56.
8. Gustafson DH, Hawkins RP, Boberg EW, et al. (2001). Chess: ten years of research and development in consumer health informatics for broad populations, including the underserved. Medinfo 2001;10:1459–563.
9. Goldsmith D, Safran C. Collaborative healthware. In: Nelson R, Ball MJ, eds. Consumer Informatics: Applications and Strategies in Cyber Health Care. New York: Springer-Verlag, 2004.
10. Goldberg HS, Morales A, Gottlieb L, Meador L, Safran C. (2001). Reinventing patient-centered computing for the twenty-first century. MedInfo. 10 (Pt 2):1455–8, 2001.
11. Safran C. The collaborative edge: patient empowerment for vulnerable populations. Int J Med Inform 2002;1–6.
12. Gray J, Safran C, Weitzner GP, Steward JE, Zaccagnini L, Pursley D. Baby CareLink: using the Internet and telemedicine to improve care for high-risk infants. Pediatrics 2000;106:1318–24.
13. Brazy JE, Anderson BM, Becker PT, Becker M. How parents of premature infants gather information and obtain support. Neonatal Netw 2001;20(2):41–8.
14. US Department of Commerce. A nation online: how Americans are expanding their use of the Internet. *http://www.ntia.doc.gov/ntiahome/dn/* (2002).
15. Ferguson T. Consumer health informatics. HealthCare Forum 1995;28–33.
16. Mandl KD, Kohane IS, Brandt AM. Electronic patient-physician communication: problems and promise. Ann Intern Med 1998;129:495–500.
17. Slack VW. Cybermedicine: how computing empowers patients for better healthcare. Medinfo 1998;1:3–5.
18. Porter SC. Patients as experts: a collaborative performance support system. Proc AMIA Symp 2001;548–52.
19. Tang PC, Newcomb C, Gorden S, Kreider N. Meeting the information needs of patients: results from a patient focus group. Proc AMIA Symp 1997;672–6.
20. Kaplan B, Brennan PF. Consumer informatics: supporting patients as co-producers of quality. JAMIA 2001;8:309–16.
21. Goldsmith D, Silverman LB, Safran C. Pediatric Cancer CareLink: supporting home management of childhood leukemia. Proc. AMIA Symp 2002;290–4.
22. Tang PC, Newcomb C. Informing patients: a guide for providing patient health information. JAMIA 1998;5:563–70.
23. Goldsmith D, Safran C. Using the web to reduce postoperative pain following ambulatory surgery. Proc AMIA Symp 1999;6:780–4.

17 CHOICEs: Patients as Participants in Shared Care Planning at the Point of Care

Cornelia M. Ruland

Recent years have seen a proliferation of health information and self-help communication on the Internet, together with a growing trend toward empowering patients to take a more active role in their own health care [1,2]. There is evidence that patients want to be informed about their medical conditions and to participate actively in their own care [3]. Access to health information can enable patients to be more active participants in treatment processes [1,4]. Customized computer-based support systems provided to patient over the Internet such as "CHESS" [5,6] and "HeartCare" [7,8] have been shown to increase confidence in patients' decision making, improve health status, reduce social isolation [7–9], and significant effects on self-reported quality of life, social support, participation in health care, negative emotions [6,10,11], and reduction in symptoms and depression [12].

Although Internet-based support can provide important assistance for consumers and patients who seek health information from home, this does not automatically change patient care for patients who enter the healthcare system. Patients may be well informed about their conditions and treatment options and explicit about their preferences; however, unless they are treated as partners and patient preferences are acknowledged as important by their clinicians and integrated into actual patient care, it may have little impact on the actual care patients receive. In reality, patient problems are often still identified from the perspective of healthcare providers and their assumptions about what care is in the patient's best interest, without verifying these assumptions with the recipient of care, the patient. Therefore, systems are needed at the point of care that facilitate shared decision making (SDM) between patients and their healthcare providers. Such systems can assist in systematically eliciting patients' perceived health problems and preferences and in selecting treatment and care consistent with patient preferences.

This chapter discusses shared decision making tools at the point of care in the context of consumer health informatics and their state of the art. To illustrate such a tool, CHOICEs (**C**reating better **H**ealth **O**utcomes by **I**mproving **C**ommunication about Patients' **E**xpectations) is used as an example of a computerized support system that assists clinicians at the point of care in shared decision making and patient preference-adjusted illness management of cancer patients.

The Need for Shared Decision Making Systems at the Point of Care

A rapidly growing amount of literature has addressed the importance of shared decision making between health providers and patients, working collaboratively to select treatment and care that includes patient preferences [13–16]. Along with a strong focus on evidence-based patient care, there is an increasing awareness that an important piece of evidence to support clinical decision making is missing in the absence of patients' perspectives of their health problems and preferences for treatment and care. Evidence-based patient care and SDM are, at least in theory, viewed as models for good clinical practice [17,18].

The underlying assumptions for these efforts are that illness, treatments, and outcomes have value dimensions to patients that are highly personal. The vast differences in values patients place on clinical outcomes make an individual approach to patient care particularly important. To make the best care decisions from the perspective of the individual, patients must be asked in the clinical encounter to participate in the decision process about their care [17,19,20].

A number of studies have demonstrated that healthcare providers often do not know how patients experience their health problems and symptoms, nor can they infer what patients value, or assume what care decisions are in the patients' best interest [21–25]. Patients may have their own ideas about the nature, causes, severity, and consequences of their problems. In addition, cultural beliefs, values, and practices affect patients' perceptions of illness and preferences for treatment. Even people with similar disease and functional limitations vary considerably in their tolerance and attitudes toward symptoms [26]. Also, what healthcare professionals perceive as excellent outcomes may not be experienced in the same way by the patient. Wennberg et al. found that nothing in the objective reality of the patient, such as clinical history, physical findings, laboratory scores, urine flow, or symptom level, strongly predicted the degree to which patients were bothered from benign prostatic hyperplasia and had aversions to the risks of surgery [27,28]. In a recent study among cancer patients [29] many of the symptoms that were most frequently reported by patients were usually not included in routine assessments, and there were large variations in patients' reports of the frequency, severity, and degree of bother of these symptoms. Therefore, patients and clinicians can benefit from the assistance that tools to support SDM at the point of care can provide.

It is the experience of illness that brings people to the healthcare system. People do not come primarily for diagnosis and treatment; they come to be made well, made whole, and to recover a sense of health and well-being [13]. Lack of shared understanding about the patient's subjective concerns and the more objective approach to diagnosis and treatment by healthcare providers can lead to poor clinical management, poor care, and poor compliance. Professional care providers need, therefore, to understand, acknowledge, and integrate patients' perspectives of their needs into clinical decision making. This has become even more imperative in the Internet age, when more and more patients come well prepared and articulate about their needs to the healthcare system and are expecting that their preferences and health perspectives will be acknowledged. If the healthcare system does not adjust to these changing patient roles and expectations, for example, by introducing ways to increase patient–provider communication and SDM, discrepancies between patients' expectations and health care, poorer patient outcomes, and patient dissatisfaction may result.

What Is Shared Decision Making?

In the clinical, health services, and methodological literature, terms such as evidence-informed patient choice [17] and shared decision making are used to describe the process of involving patients, in appropriate ways, in treatment/screening decisions and care planning. The goal is to inform patients by the best available evidence about options and potential benefits and harms, and help them consider their preferences [16,30–32]. The concept of patient preferences capitalizes on the need to modify treatment and care to the particular values and experiences of the individual. Patient preferences can be defined as the appraisal by an individual regarding the relative desirability of entities, such as health states, treatment, outçomes of treatment/care such as symptom relief, or other aspects of health or health care [16].

The model in Fig. 17.1 displays key elements of SDM. SDM requires at least two core players: the patient and the healthcare provider. However, other factors may also influence healthcare decisions such as the patients' families, the cultural context, or societal priorities. The model recognizes the importance of patients as sources of information about their own values and preferences for patient care as well as research evidence to inform clinical decision making.

Communication and information exchange between patient and healthcare provider are crucial elements of SDM. Appropriate clinical decision making requires the consideration and sharing of two important knowledge aspects: (1) knowledge about facts, such as the patient's diagnosis, symptoms, and problems; available treatment options; and associated risks and likelihood of outcomes and (2) information about values, such as the desirability of these outcomes and how one values various aspects of health. Many patients have personal knowledge and experience about living with an illness, about how it affects their personal life and well being, and about their values and preferences. For a clinician to be able to plan individualized, evidence-based patient care consistent with patients' values and preferences this information needs to be communicated by the patient.

For patients to participate in SDM, they need to understand their illness condition, what the available treatment/management options are, as well as the likelihood of various outcomes of treatment according to research evidence. The patients need this information to be able to consider options and outcomes in light of their own values and preferences. Therefore, research evidence and clinical expertise needs to be com-

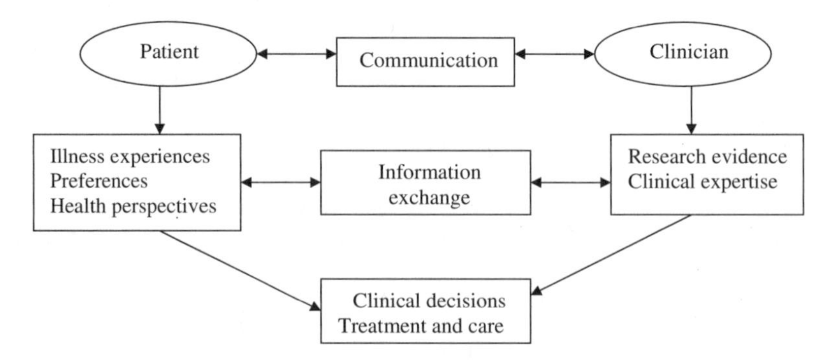

FIGURE 17.1. Participants in and elements of shared decision making.

municated between clinicians and patients. SDM tools can support such patient–provider communication and information exchange.

Support Systems for Shared Decision Making

There are two major types of systems to support SDM that include the elicitation of patient preferences: (1) systems that are primarily designed to assist patients in difficult decisions and that are usually referred to as Decision Aids (DAs) and (2) support systems for preference-adjusted illness management that are designed to assist clinicians in including patients' illness experiences and preferences into patient care of chronic or serious, long-term illness over time.

Decision Aids

The primary purpose of DAs is to help people make specific and deliberate choices among options by providing (at a minimum) information on the options and outcomes relevant to the person's health status [31]. Factors that should be considered in a treatment/screening decision are outlined, often in the context of the individual patient's characteristics. DAs are meant to be adjuncts to clinicians' counseling, so that patients can understand the probable benefits and risk of treatment options, consider the values they place on benefits versus risks of health outcomes, and participate actively with their clinician in selecting treatments that best address the patients' individual values and needs [30,32]. Studies evaluating DAs have reported higher scores on cognitive functioning and social support [11], more active and satisfying participation in decision making [30], better scores on general health perceptions and physical functioning [34], improved knowledge, and reduced decisional conflict [31,35].

DAs differ from the traditional patient education programs that primarily provide information, advice, and support with regard to already prescribed treatment [30]. DAs are appropriate when decisions are difficult, for example, under conditions in which more than one treatment alternative is available, or when outcomes are uncertain or there are major differences in outcomes or complications. Furthermore, they are beneficial when decisions require making tradeoffs between near- and long-term outcomes, when a choice can result in a small chance of a grave outcome [15] or the values for the benefits relative to the risks are more variable or unknown [32,36]. Also, DAs are useful in situations where patients may be very risk aversive or attach unusual importance to certain possible outcomes. In contrast, treating a patient with urinary tract infection with antibiotics is the recommended treatment where no other equally effective alternative exists [37]. For these kinds of more straightforward, less problematic decisions there is no need to employ a DA.

However, DAs have been confined primarily to the relatively narrow segment of decisions about single episodes of screening/treatment choices. Also, similar to Internet support for patients, DAs are designed mostly for use from home and less at the point of care, and there is evidence that DAs have been difficult to integrate into busy clinical practices [18]. Yet clinicians often encounter situations in which a major task is not how to select one treatment versus another, but how to attend simultaneously to multiple problems in a manner that gives priority to those that matter most to the patient, which may change over time along with changes in patients' symptom and health status. This is often the case in management of a chronic illness associated with multiple, complex symptoms and functional problems for patients and that clinicians need to attend to simultaneously. For example, a patient may suffer from acute stroke that causes impaired functioning, involving loss of coordination skills and problems eating; he or she may be at risk for falling, may have problems dressing, may be worried how he or she will be able to manage at home with three flights of stairs, or whether he or she will be able to return home at all. It is these types of problems that are experienced and valued differently by individual patients.

Support Systems for Preference-Adjusted Illness Management

While a recent Cochrane review identified 87 DAs to support patients in treatment or screening choices, where 24 DAs were tested in randomized clinical trials [35], much less work has been devoted to the development of computer-supported systems to assist clinicians in eliciting and integrating patients' illness experiences and preferences into symptom/illness management of seriously or chronically ill patients. It is only recently that systems have been developed that assist clinicians in eliciting and integrating patient preferences into the processes of illness management over time [29,33,38]. These types of systems are particularly relevant because a large part of health care is directed toward management of chronic illness that often affects multiple, value-laden dimensions of patients' personal lives. Support systems for patient preference-adjusted illness management are, therefore, somewhat different from those designed to assist in making treatment choices. They provide patients and clinicians with the salient symptoms and problems associated with a specific health condition based on research and clinical evidence, and a method for helping patients to establish the importance they place on their problems and outcomes to denote their preferences for treatment and care. CHOICE is such a support system to assist clinicians in preference-adjusted illness management of cancer patients and is described in the following section.

CHOICEs

CHOICEs includes (1) a comprehensive patient assessment tool for cancer-specific symptoms, functional problems, and preferences along physical, psychosocial, emotional, and spiritual dimensions and (2) a SDM/Care Planning component that highlights in an easy-to-use format for clinicians which symptoms patients are experiencing, including their severity, degree of bother, and importance to patients. This information can be used to discuss with the patient an appropriate plan of treatment and care in hospital as well as in ambulatory settings.

The CHOICEs application builds on experiences from previous studies and beginning cumulative evidence of the effectiveness and feasibility of such systems to improve patient-centered care. Two previous studies on a palm-top–based support system for preference-adjusted care of rehabilitation patients have shown significant effects on congruence between patients' problems and patient care and on patient outcomes of functional status and preference achievement [33,38]. Similar to this earlier system, CHOICEs for preference-adjusted symptom management of cancer patients was developed based on a thorough and critical review of the evidence-based literature to identify problems, specific symptoms, and functional limitations commonly encountered by cancer patients. This search and literature review included the healthcare bibliographic databases as well as the World Wide Web (WWW) for clinical guidelines, educational material, workbooks, measurement tools, and other relevant material. It resulted in a preliminary list of symptoms and functional problems for potential inclusion in the CHOICEs assessment. An expert focus group with specialists in cancer care (physicians, nurses, social workers) met in parallel. They critically reviewed the clinical evidence abstracted from the literature and the WWW for relevance, comprehensibility, completeness/level of detail, and supplemented with expert opinion. Particular attention was paid to describe symptoms and problems in simple, understandable, nonmedical lay language. The focus group also critically reviewed the design and interface during the development of the CHOICEs application. A preliminary version was pilot tested among 15 cancer patients who were asked to complete and evaluate the assessment for clarity of meaning, appropriateness, wording, completeness, redundancy, and format, and add comments [29]. These evaluations provided suggestions for revisions that were then discussed in the expert focus group before final revisions were made.

The current CHOICEs application is contained and administered on a touch-pad, tablet computer. It supports complex branching, so that only relevant questions are asked, and conditional tailoring, so that questions and summary reports are tailored to a subject's previous responses [29].

When using CHOICEs on the tablet computer, patients are presented with a series of questions and select their answers with a pen on the touch screen. After an introduction screen that introduces patients to CHOICEs and explains its purpose, patients are first asked two questions about their perceived overall health and Health-Related Quality of Life (HRQoL) on analog scales (range 0 to 100).

Thereafter, patients are asked to identify among 19 problem categories those that apply. If a patient is not sure whether a problem area applies to him or her, he or she can look up the specific associated symptoms/problems associated with that category by touching the info-button next to it. For example, given that a patient had selected problems with "eating and drinking," "bowel and bladder," and "mood and feelings" on the previous screen as applying to him or her, the more detailed list of symptoms is triggered from which the patient again selects those that apply, for example, taste changes, nausea, lack of appetite, and so forth under "eating and drinking." Then patients are asked about the degree of bother from their selected symptoms. In this manner patients are not troubled with many detailed questions that are not relevant to them, while focusing particularly on those symptoms and problems that are difficult.

Finally, patients are asked to rate the importance of their problems as priorities for treatment/care on analog scales from 0 to 100 (patient preferences). This allows clinicians to pay particular attention to those problems that are most important to patients to be addressed by their provider. After the patient is finished, an assessment summary is displayed in which patient problems are rank ordered by importance to patients, and that can be printed and used by the clinician and patient to jointly plan appropriate care.

Effects of CHOICEs and Similar Systems on Patient Care

There is beginning evidence about the usefulness and feasibility of use of support systems in clinical settings such as CHOICEs [29,33,38]. In a recent study 52 outpatients undergoing cancer treatment (mean age: 56.6 years; 59% women) used CHOICEs for assessment of their perceived HRQoL, symptoms, and functional problems, including severity, bothersomeness, and preferences for treatment/care, on a touch-pad computer in the outpatient waiting room prior to being seen by their physician or nurse [29]. This information was processed, printed, and given to the clinician in the subsequent consultation in the experimental group, but not in the control group. While equivalent at baseline, there was significantly greater congruence between patients' problems and symptoms and those addressed by their clinicians in the experimental group. Patients had few problems with the touch-pad computer, and CHOICEs received high scores on ease of use and usefulness by patients [29]. Comparable effects were found for a similar system for preference-adjusted symptom management in rehabilitation patients [33,38]. Two clinical trials with patients from acute care for the elderly and rehabilitation units demonstrated significantly higher congruence between nursing care and patient preferences and better outcomes of preference achievement and functional status when the system was used [33,38]. A multisite RCT that follows 220 hematological cancer patients for one year is currently underway to test the effects of CHOICEs for cancer patients on patient care as well as on patient outcomes in a larger study. The aforementioned studies demonstrate that a system such as CHOICEs can effectively help clinicians eliciting patients' symptoms and are a useful and feasible strategy to improve patient-tailored illness management for cancer patients.

Furthermore, CHOICEs extends previous SDM tools in two significant ways: (1) it is designed to support clinicians in eliciting and including patients' reported symptoms and preferences at the point of care; and (2) it extends SDM tools from supporting patients in single episodes of treatment/screening choices into the realm of symptom management for cancer patients over time. Extending SDM tools into symptom management of serious/chronic illness is important and was supported in the aforementioned study by the fact that almost all symptoms available in CHOICEs were selected by at least one patient. Large variations in patients' reports of frequency, severity, and degree of bother of these symptoms indicated that clinicians cannot automatically anticipate what symptoms and problems patients are experiencing or what patient care is in their best interest. Therefore, clinicians can benefit from the assistance that support systems such as CHOICEs can provide.

An interesting observation that deviates from most findings in the SDM literature was the effects on patient care of the CHOICEs intervention. Studies examining the adoption of SDM tools to support patients in treatment or screening decisions have reported clinicians' reluctance to use such tools, primarily because of their concern that this may add additional tasks for which they do not have time [18]. Attention to the workload, time requirements, feasibility, and acceptability are important factors to consider when introducing new SDM tools in clinical practice. Systems such as CHOICEs may be easier to implement than other types of SDM tools that have been primarily designed to support patients while at home. From the beginning its purpose was to support clinicians, and, therefore, particular attention was paid to streamline the CHOICEs application into the workflow of clinical practice. When patients were seen by clinicians in this study, assessments of their symptoms and problems that usually are part of the consultation were already completed beforehand. Thus, clinicians had this information ready when they saw their patients and could use it actively together with their patients.

In summary, although Internet support can provide patients with health information and self-help tools as important means to empower and prepare them for active participation in decisions regarding their health care, this does not automatically change the health care they receive. Healthcare institutions and clinicians need to adapt to changing patient roles and expectations and treat patients as partners in clinical decision making. Methods and tools are needed that facilitate SDM at the point of care. This chapter discusses SDM tools and methods and how they can be implemented into clinical practice. The example of CHOICEs is used for illustration, a support system that assists clinicians in eliciting cancer patients' illness experiences and preferences at the point of care. With the help of such systems clinicians can easier engage in partnerships with their patients and integrate patients' perspectives and preferences into patient care. The novelty of systems such as CHOICEs, however, requires considerably more work in this field. A particular interesting line of research would be to develop systems for preference-adjusted illness management for a wider range of patient populations other than rehabilitation and cancer patients and test the effects on patient care and outcomes.

References

1. Jimison HB, Sher PP. Advances in presenting health information to patients. In: Chapman GB, Sonnenberg FA, eds. Decision Making in Health Care. Cambridge, UK: Cambridge University Press, 2000.
2. Brennan PF. Health informatics and community health: support for patients as collaborators in care. Methods Inform Med 1999;38:274–8.
3. Degner LF, Sloan JA. Decision making during serious illness: what role do patients really want to play? J Clin Epidemiol 1992;45:941–50.
4. Greenfield S, Kaplan SH, Ware JE, Yano EM, Frank HJ. Patients' participation in medical care: effects on blood sugar control and quality of life in diabetes. J Gen Intern Med 1988;3:448–57.
5. Gustafson DH, Hawkins RP, Boberg EW, et al. CHESS: ten years of research and development in consumer health informatics for broad populations, including the underserved. Medinfo 2001;10:1459–563.
6. Gustafson DH, Hawkins R, Pingree S, et al. Effect of computer support on younger women with breast cancer. J Gen Intern Med 2001;16:435–45.
7. Brennan PF, Moore SM, Calewell B. Using WebTV to deliver health information into the home: experiences, successes, and regrets. Proc AMIA Symp 1999;1203.
8. Brennan PF, Caldwell B, Moore SM, Sreenath N, Jones J. Designing HeartCare: custom computerized home care for patients recovering from CABG surgery. Proc AMIA Symp 1998;381–5.
9. Brennan PF. The ComputerLink projects: a decade of experience. Stud Health Technol Inform 1997;46:521–6.
10. Gustafson DH, Hawkins RP, Boberg EW, Bricker E, Pingree S, Chan CL. The use and impact of a computer-based support system for people living with AIDS and HIV infection. Proc Annu Symp Comput Appl Med Care 1994;604–8.
11. Boberg EW, Gustafson DH, Hawkins RP, et al. CHESS: the comprehensive health enhancement support system. In: Brennan PF, Schneider SJ, Tornquist E, eds. Information Networks for Community Health. New York: Springer-Verlag, 1997;171–88.
12. Moore SM, Brennan PF, O'Brien R, Visovsky C, Bjournsdottir G. Customized computer home support improves recovery of CABG patients. Circulation (Suppl) 2001;104(II):533.
13. Gerteis M, Edgman-Levitan S, Daley J, Delbanco TM. Through the patients' eyes. Understanding and promoting patient-centered care. San Franciso: Jossey-Bass, 1993.
14. Kasper JF, Mulley AG, Wennberg JE. Developing shared decision-making programs to improve the quality of health care. QRB Qual Rev Bull 1992;18:183–90.
15. Kassirer JP. Incorporating patients' preferences into medical decisions. N Engl J Med 1994;330:1895–6.
16. Holmes-Rovner M, Llewellyn-Thomas H, Entwistle V, Coulter A, O'Connor A, Rovner DR. Patient choice modules for summaries of clinical effectiveness: a proposal. Br Med J 2001;322:664–7.
17. Hope T. Evidence-Based Patient Choice. London: Kings Fund, 2000.
18. Holmes-Rovner M, Valade D, Orlowski C, Draus C, Nabozny-Valerio B, Keiser S. Implementing shared decision-making in routine practice: barriers and opportunities. Health Expect 2000;3:182–91.

19. O'Connor AM, Drake ER, Fiset V, Graham ID, Laupacis A, Tugwell P. The Ottawa patient decision aids. Eff Clin Pract 1999;2:163–70.
20. O'Connor AM. Patient education in the year 2000: tailored decision support, empowerment, and mutual aid [editorial; comment]. Qual Health Care 1999;8:5.
21. Wenrich MD, Curtis JR, Ambrozy DA, Carline JD, Shannon SE, Ramsey PG. Dying patients' need for emotional support and personalized care from physicians: perspectives of patients with terminal illness, families, and health care providers. J Pain Symptom Manage 2003;25: 236–46.
22. Shannon SE, Mitchell PH, Cain KC. Patients, nurses, and physicians have differing views of quality of critical care. J Nurs Scholarsh 2002;34:173–9.
23. Higgins PA. Patient perception of fatigue while undergoing long-term mechanical ventilation: incidence and associated factors. Heart Lung J Acute Crit Care 1998;27:177–83.
24. Hiltunen EF, Puopolo AL, Marks GK, et al. The nurse's role in end-of-life treatement discussions: preliminary report from the SUPPORT project. J Cardiovasc Nurs 1995;9:68–77.
25. Reilly CA, Holzemer WL, Henry SB, Slaughter RE, Portillo CJ. A comparison of patient and nurse ratings of human immunodeficiency virus-related signs and symptoms. Nurs Res 1997;46:318–23.
26. Nease RF, Kneeland T, O'Connor GT, et al. Variation in patient utilities for outcomes of the management of chronic stable angina. Implications for clinical practice guidelines. Ischemic Heart Disease Patient Outcomes Research Team. JAMA 1995;273:1185–90.
27. Wennberg JE, Barry MJ, Fowler FJ, Mulley A. Outcomes research, PORTs, and health care reform. [Review]. Ann NY Acad Sci 1993;703:52–62.
28. Fowler FJ, Jr., Barry MJ, Lu-Yao G, Roman A, Wasson J, Wennberg JE. Patient-reported complications and follow-up treatment after radical prostatectomy. The National Medicare Experience: 1988–1990 (updated June 1993). Urology 1993;42:622–9.
29. Ruland CM, White T, Stevens M, Fanciullo G, Khilani SM. Effects of a computerized system to support shared decision making in symptom management of cancer patients: preliminary results. J Am Med Inform Assoc 2003;1–7.
30. Molenaar S, Sprangers MA, Postma-Schuit FC, et al. Feasibility and effects of decision aids. Med Decis Making 2000;20:112–27.
31. O'Connor AM, Rostom A, Fiset V, Tetroe J, et al. Decision aids for patients facing health treatment or screening decisions: systematic review. Br Med J 1999;319:731–4.
32. O'Connor AM, Fiset V, DeGrasse C, et al. Decision aids for patients considering options affecting cancer outcomes: evidence of efficacy and policy implications. J Natl Cancer Inst Monogr 1999;25:67–79.
33. Ruland CM. Decision support for patient preference-based care planning: effects on nursing care and patient outcomes. J Am Med Inform Assoc 1999;6:304–12.
34. Goldstein MK, Clarke AE, Michelson D, Garber AM, Bergen MR, Lenert LA. Developing and testing a multimedia presentation of a health-state description. Med Decis Making 1994;14:336–44.
35. O'Connor AM, Stacey D, Rovner D, et al. Decision aids for people facing health treatment or screening decisions (Cochrane Review). Cochrane Database Syst Rev 2001;3:CD001431.
36. Eddy DM. A manual for assessing health practices and designing practice policies for explicit research. Philadelphia: American College of Pysicians, 1992.
37. Goldstein MK. Applying utitily assessment at the beside. In: Chapman GB, Sonnenberg FA, eds. Decision Making in Health Care, Cambridge, UK: Cambridge University Press, 2000.
38. Ruland CM. Handheld technology to improve patient care: evaluating a support system for preference-based care planning at the bedside. J Am Med Inform Assoc 2002;9:192–201.

18 MedCERTAIN/MedCIRCLE: Using Semantic Web Technologies for Quality Management of Health Information on the Web

GUNTHER EYSENBACH

The Semantic Web

What Is the Semantic Web?

The Semantic Web is a vision: the idea of having data on the web defined and linked in a way, that it can be used by machines—not just for display purposes, but for using it in various applications. (*http://www.semanticweb.org/introduction.html*)

This chapter examines how the World Wide Web might evolve in the near future, from an "information jungle" environment with largely narrative, human-understandable information, to a global knowledge repository, where much of the information is machine readable and directly processable by computers, enabling the use of advanced knowledge management technologies to steer consumers to trusted health information. This vision has been called the "Semantic Web" by its inventor, Tim Berners-Lee, who from the beginning had envisaged the Web to be a worldwide, distributed knowledge base rather than a medium with primarily narrative information targeted only for human consumption, as the web presents itself today [1–3]. The "Semantic Web" can be thought of an extension of the present Web, with Web authors publishing an additional layer of machine-processable data beneath the visible layer of human-readable information. It is essentially an attempt to create a global, decentralized knowledge base, represented as a "semantic net" that is woven by a large heterogeneous community of "authors." A semantic net is a knowledge representation method with a long history in Artificial Intelligence ever since first introduced by Quillian back in the late 1960s [4]. Semantic nets use the idea that the semantics (meaning) of a concept comes from its relationship to other concepts. In other words, information—a collection of unrelated facts—becomes knowledge if it is contextualized by making links to related concepts explicit. In a semantic net, the concepts can be graphically depicted as nodes, and the relationships (links) between the nodes can be illustrated as labeled arcs. Turning the current World Wide Web into a global semantic net requires that (at least some) individuals and organizations who currently publish information on the Web will publish additional machine-processable documents (e.g., using XML) which describe the concepts and their relationships with other concepts (which may be defined on other Web sites) unambiguously, so that software can aggregate this knowledge and draw inferences. The idea of the MedCERTAIN project and its successor organization MedCIRCLE, an international nonprofit collaboration of consumer health information gateways and health Web sites, is that members of the collaboration make standardized machine-processable statements about health Web sites and health information providers using a common agreed-on vocabulary with agreed-on semantics, so that applications can aggregate, "understand," and use this meta-information, for example, to match it against individual consumer needs, and to help consumers to make informed choices. This is the basis for decentralized quality management on the Web, without a single organization being in charge of "accrediting" health Web sites in a "top-down" fashion [5].

It could be argued that on today's Web people are already expressing relationships with other chunks of information in a "machine-processable" way by using hyperlinks. However, hyperlinks are semantically ambiguous; that is, they can imply many different kinds of relationships, such as a reference ("see also"), an endorsement ("recommended reading"), or sometimes even something completely else, for example, pointing to contradictory information. In addition, a hyperlink usually links from a word or text phrase (which may be semantically ambiguous, in that others may use the same word but mean a different concept) to another Web page (which also is ambiguous, as it is not clear which concept is meant, that is, does the relationship refer to the individual behind that Web site, the topic discussed on the Web site, etc.). The sentence, "For further information see *http://www.healthfinder.org*" may be understandable to humans, but a piece of software cannot easily figure out which relationship between which entities this statement implies, unless some natural language processing software is employed. Indeed, Meric [6] has reported that there is no correlation between the number of links pointing to a site and "quality" as defined by health professionals (although it is debatable whether this gold standard of "quality" is the correct criterion). It is also obvious that an expression of trust or quality should not be simply binary (trust yes/no, quality yes/no), but needs to be more explicit in why and which aspects are trusted. The need for a more expressive "vocabulary" and language to express the meaning of relationships between sites (but also people, organizations, etc.) is obvious.

In contrast, on the Semantic Web, statements such as "see-also" or relationships between actors on the Web (such as "is-member-of" or "has-certified") [7] would be published in an unambiguous, machine-processable way, and can be processed by software that can draw inferences from the knowledge chunks provided on different Web sites.

Building standards and tools for the Semantic Web is currently one focus of the activities of the World Wide Web Consortium (W3C), which describes the aim of its activities as follows: "The goal of the Semantic Web is to develop enabling standards and technologies designed to help machines understand more information on the Web so that they can support richer discovery, data integration, navigation, and automation of tasks. With the Semantic Web we not only receive more exact results when searching for information, but also know when we can integrate information from different sources, know what information to compare, and can provide all kinds of automated services in different domains from future home and digital libraries to electronic business and health services" [8].

Metadata

One prerequisite for the Semantic Web is that authors of Web sites and Web documents provide richer machine-processable information, essentially metadata. Metadata are "data about data." The vision of using standardized metadata on health Web sites can be compared with food labels: Similar to producers of food, who have to display ingredients on standardized labels, telling consumers, for example, the amount of fat and sodium contained in their products, health information providers on the Web should use standardized labels to disclose certain facts about their information, so that consumers can make informed decisions [5,9,10]. Until 1999, there had been many different ways to link metadata to Web documents, for example, using META tags in HTML or using PICS (Platform for Internet Content Selection) for self- and third-party descriptions of information. Although PICS was developed primarily with description and rating adult Web sites in mind, a vocabulary to describe and "label" health Web sites was developed in 1997 [11,12]. The W3C subsequently unified different approaches and the result of these efforts is the Resource Description Framework (RDF)—the current standard based on XML (extensible Markup Language) to transport metadata and a major pillar of the Semantic Web [13–15]. One feature of RDF is that (other than, for example, the HTML META-tag) it allows people to describe concepts and resources other than a Web document. In contrast, by using the HTML META-tag and a set of keywords the developer implicitly makes a statement about the document or Web site (but often it is not even clear whether the keywords refer to the document or the entire Web site), but cannot make more broad statements, for example, about other resources or concepts, as with RDF. Further, RDF provides a mechanism for giving unambiguous meanings to metadata keywords. In contrast, keywords used in META tags are essentially just ambiguous "words" that have no meaning (semantics) for software as they are not linked to other concepts. Words can be ambiguous in that they may have different meanings. For example, the word "virus" can refer to a computer virus or a biological virus. RDF provides a mechanism to define what kind of "virus" is meant by referring to the RDF statement or site where this concept is defined [again, through its relationship to other concepts, for example "virus (as defined in this statement) is-a software," linking the word software again to another RDF document on the Web that defines "software," etc.], thereby creating "meaning."

As noted earlier, RDF can be expressed in XML syntax [15]. Although RDF is basically an XML file, the difference between an RDF document and a "plain" XML document is significant: Whereas XML-Schemas only tell computers (and us) how, for example, an application form for a driver's license *looks like*, RDF is able to explain to a machine what a driver's license *is*, by providing the meaning of the concepts used in a driver's license. This is done by providing the relationships of the concepts to other concepts. As the RDF developers point out, RDF is a simple frame system, that is, a format for knowledge representation, where objects (concepts) and their relationships to each other are specified. The RDF specification does not contain a reasoning system; this needs to be built on top of it.

Unfortunately, the uptake of providing metadata on the Web—even in its simplest, nonsemantic form, the META tag—has been slow so far: Web content is still largely devoid of metadata labels [13] and a critical mass of metadata has to be generated before applications can be developed making use of it. The MedCERTAIN/MedCIRCLE projects (explained in detail later) developed some open source tools for health information providers to enter disclosure information deemed ethical (see Chapter 4, this volume) as machine-processable metadata. The health information provider does not need to understand RDF—all he or she needs to do is to fill in a questionnaire for self-disclosure and description, and his or her answers will be translated into metadata [16]. Finally, existing tools for creating knowledge bases, such as Protégé-2000, can be used to create RDF statements [17], and future Web editors may provide additional functionalities to model knowledge and build knowledge bases.

Application Scenarios

If the vision of the Semantic Web becomes reality, this will have a profound impact on how people will interact with the Web and obtain information. The first and most obvious change will include the markedly improved abilities of search engines to conduct accurate and relevant searches on the Web, and to guide users to trusted and relevant health information. Search engines will not only better "understand" what a user is looking for, but also what the Web pages they are indexing are about. They can, for example—if a user looks for "SARS in Canada"—recognize that the user is likely looking for information on severe acute respiratory syndrome rather than the South African Revenue Service, and then list only those Web sites that contain information about the disease and not the Revenue Service. The results will even include links to relevant Web pages that do not use any of the search terms—for example, if a Web page contains the word SRAS (for syndrome respiratoire aigu sévère), it will be found as well, because the search engine looks for semantic rather than syntactic matches, and the Web crawler has previously "understood" the context in which the word has been used and what the Web page on which it appeared is all about.

The idea of the MedCERTAIN/MedCIRCLE approach (described later) is that results in search engines will be better "ranked" not only by relevance but also by "quality," for example, the degree of how trusted a health resource is in a community.

Accessibility and quality issues of health information on the Web are especially hot topics in the medical literature and subject of hundreds of empirical "descriptive infodemiology" [18] studies. These studies mostly suggest that it is hard for consumers to find high-quality health information among a flood of dubious or commercially driven information [19]. Surveys such as the Pew Internet Survey also show that 86% of consumers are concerned about getting low-quality health information on the Web [20]. While empirical studies now provide more than sufficient evidence on the inadequacies of the current Web, there is a surprising lack of debate in the medical world discussing the possibilities of technology to address these problems—presumably as many of the current developments in the field are unknown or remain not understood. The current MedCRICLE Collaboration for Internet Rating, Certification and Labelling of Health Information, a global collaborative network of health information gateways described in detail later, is working toward this aim by enriching the current Web with machine-processable evaluation and trust data.

Knowledge Translation for Consumers on the Semantic Web

From Information to Knowledge

The Web as it exists today has played a significant role in fostering consumerism in health care [21,22]. The current Web provides an abundance of information, but giving "information" to a patient is certainly not enough. The ultimate goal is to enhance "knowledge": the information has to be put into context, the concepts have to be explained and defined, and their relationships to other concepts and to personal information (e.g., in the health record) have to be made explicit. This is the difference between "information" and "knowledge." The Semantic Web enhances the possibility of supporting "knowledge translation" for consumers, the translation of information into knowledge. Doctors who are confronted with "Web-informed" patients often complain that patients often find irrelevant information on the Web—information the patient (and the clinician) have to sift through and evaluate, and that is often not applicable to the individual situation [23]. Many patients do not even know the correct names of their diagnoses and are therefore unable to enter the correct terms into search engines. The vision for the future is that people will use their Web-based personal health record as a starting point that may be enriched by all kinds of information gathered by intelligent agents from trusted sources on the Web that are specifically relevant to the patient [24]. For example, if the Web-based health record contains a certain diagnosis, and on the same day the *British Medical Journal* publishes new research results published about this disease, the agent (which would be a part of the electronic health record software) could automatically generate a link to that article. It doesn't matter if the *British Medical Journal* article uses a different terminology than the doctor in the health record, as the agent will be able to link the terminologies. The Web-based electronic health record would be a dynamic entry point and knowledge management platform for patient and health professionals alike. Challenges, described in detail elsewhere, include privacy and disintermediation [25].

Using the Semantic Web for Steering Patients to Best Quality Health Care

Perhaps most challenging for healthcare providers is the prospect that people will use the Web not only to locate the least expensive used car in their neighbourhood, but also to search for the best quality healthcare providers, taking into account their own preferences and decentralized data from different sources such as hospital report cards, specialized providers of healthcare performance data such as *healthgrades.com*, and—perhaps most significantly—also based on ratings given by fellow patients with the same conditions and similar demographic background [26]. The Semantic Web makes relationships between things explicit and computable, and therefore further increases the transparency for consumers, much as the current Web has already made it easier to compare prices and offers, revolutionizing other areas such as the travel industry. The Semantic Web will make it even easier to compare things, as software can, for example, map different terminologies and aggregate decentralized knowledge dispersed all over the Web. For example, software agents would roam the Web and return information on who has the best offer of a certain car model in a given community. Similarly, software could be used to aggregate experiences of people with all kinds of health services and products, including, for example, their experience with over-the-counter or prescription drugs, hospitals, or individual physicians. While today patients use primarily mailing lists, newsgroups, and chat rooms to exchange anecdotal and narrative information and experiences about health products, services, and providers, patients could publish their experiences about virtually anything and everything in RDF on homepages—from experiences with a new dishwasher to experiences with healthcare professionals, hospitals, or drugs. Patients could rate their treatments and services directly in the Web-based electronic health record and feed them (in anonymized form) into the Semantic Web (e.g., hospitals and doctors provide RDF dumps of their patients on their sites), so that agents can aggregate this information. Such "knowledge" evolving on the Web could also be used systematically for post-marketing surveillance efforts to monitor the ongoing safety of marketed drugs on a global scale.

Overcoming Quality Issues as Opportunity

When people write and talk about the Semantic Web today, they mainly stress the advantages for information retrieval. However, the Web is an information space that reflects not just human knowledge but also human relationships; thus the Semantic Web can also represent trust relationships among people and organizations.

"Trust management" is a prerequisite for successful knowledge management on the web. Without the possibility for people to filter information or for agents to make semiautomated decisions on which knowledge chunks, ontologies, or sources to trust, the jewels on the Web will be lost in a "noise" of imperfect, cheaply produced or commercially motivated, biased information.

Although central authorities to regulate, control, censor, or centrally approve information, information providers, or Web sites are neither realistic nor desirable [5], health professionals are still interested in making systems available that direct patient streams to the best available information sources.

MedCERTAIN and MedCIRCLE

The author of this chapter has argued for many years that on a decentralized, electronic medium such as the Web, a global metadata infrastructure is the most appropriate answer to the current debate on the "quality of health information on the Web." One has to think along the lines of a collaborative "Semantic Web of trust" when it comes to the question on how consumers can be steered (or can steer themselves!) to the best available health information on the Web [5,7,12,27,28]. A "Collaboration for Critical Appraisal of Health Information on the Web"—a loose community of health information providers and health gateways using metadata to describe and annotate health Web sites—had been proposed as early as in 1997, and mentioned in two seminal articles in 1998 and 1999 [5,12]. Today, such a collaboration is known as the MedCIRCLE Collaboration, a loose nonprofit umbrella organization for health information gateways and health Web sites, inspired by the model of the Cochrane Collaboration. Membership is open to any organization using a standardized metadata vocabulary to express evaluative and descriptive statements about health information resources. The basic idea is that quality management on the Web should be based on a collaborative model with many actors (including health professionals and consumers) being able to say different things about anything in a machine-processable way (i.e., using metadata). This would enable software to analyze the trust relationships and would enable "downstream filtering" at the client computer or positive selection of trusted content using agents, instead of relying on upstream filtering approaches such as kitemarks [5] or even such well-intended but misguided proposals for (ab-)using top-level domains to centrally approve health information providers [29]. It would also allow search engines to rank their results according to quality and trust criteria of the individual user.

A metadata vocabulary for this purpose, MedPICS [based on the W3C PICS (Platform for Internet Content Selection Standard)] was first proposed in 1997, and also contained metadata elements that could be used by third parties to express evaluative statements about other sites [12]. The MedPICS proposal later led to the MedCERTAIN (2000–2001) and MedCIRCLE (2002–2003) projects, both of which aimed to implement such metadata on health Web sites and third-party organizations. With the PICS standard being superseded by XML/RDF [13], the projects became early "Semantic Web" projects, using RDF to transport and exchange metadata. As the

PICS standard became obsolete, MedPICS was renamed into HIDDEL (Health Information Disclosure, Description and Evaluation Language) [16]. Unlike other initiatives in this field, such as Health on the Net Foundation (HON), Centre for Health Information Quality kitemark (CHiQ), URAC Health Web Site Accreditation program, MedCERTAIN is *not* a traditional "kitemark" (i.e., seal of approval) project, but instead tried to develop an infrastructure and common ontology to link existing approaches, to make them interoperable, and to generate a critical mass of health-related descriptive and evaluative metadata on the Web. Unfortunately, the ideas behind MedCERTAIN/MedCIRCLE are not easy to communicate and the projects were consistently and repeatedly misunderstood and misrepresented as a "kitemarking" or third- party certification program [30], while the main goal—to develop and demonstrate a decentralized Web-of-trust infrastructure using of metadata—were not widely understood.

The constant misunderstandings concerning MedCERTAIN were one reason to change the project name to MedCIRCLE (Collaboration for Internet Rating, Certification, Labeling and Evaluation of Health Information), stressing the collaborative idea. The Collaboration involves a wider medical community to assess health information, demonstrating the power of collaborative and interoperable evaluations in a Semantic Web environment.

Figure 18.1 illustrates the operational model of health information providers collaborating in the MedCIRCLE. MedCIRCLE members are primarily trusted health information gateways, government portals, medical societies, accrediting organizations,

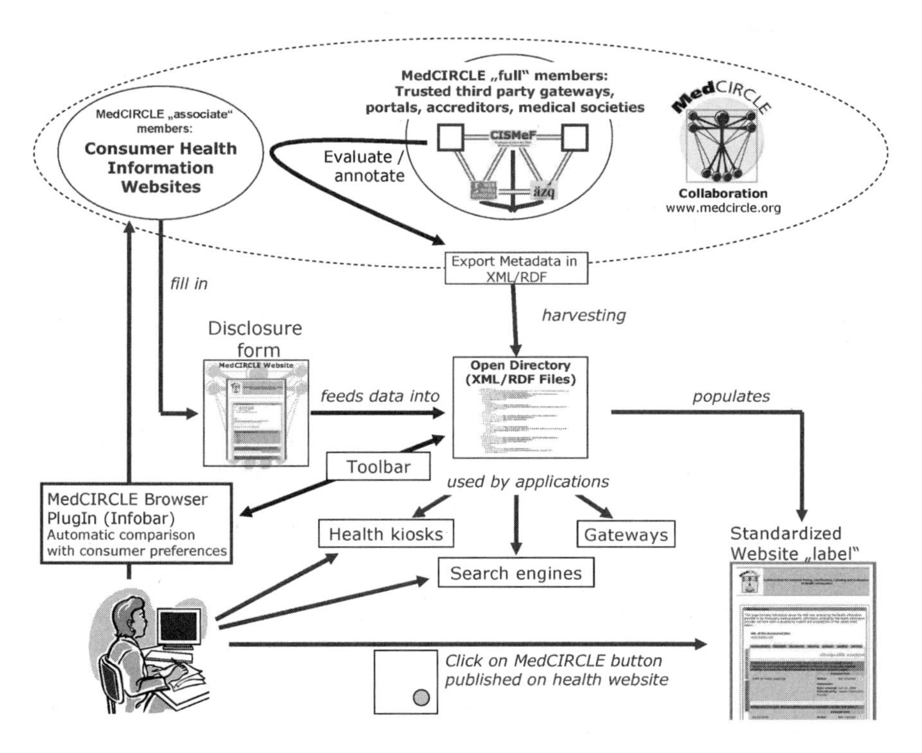

FIGURE 18.1. Operational model of the MedCIRCLE collaboration.

and libraries. What they have in common is that all are "third parties" that are in the business of describing, annotating, or making statements about other organizations, health information providers, or consumer health Web sites. For example, a medical society offering "recommended links for consumers" is a "gateway." Rather than offering unspecific hyperlinks to "recommended sites," the gateway can semantically enrich the endorsements by using a standardized vocabulary HIDDEL (Health Information Disclosure, Description and Evaluation Language) [16], expressed in XML/RDF, to report evaluation results in detail. Similarly, an organization in the business of "accrediting" health Web sites would use the vocabulary to express accreditation results. Among the current MedCIRCLE members are, for example, three major European gateway sites for consumer health information, two of which are backed by official professional physician associations. Other health subject gateways, accreditation, or rating services are encouraged to join the Collaboration simply by implementing HIDDEL on their gateways. The hope is to eventually establish a global Web of trust for networked health information.

As illustrated in Fig. 18.1, MedCIRCLE members export HIDDEL/XML/RDF data into an Open Directory. In addition, participating consumer health information Web sites can export disclosure and self-descriptive data into the Open Directory. Data in the Open Directory can be used by various applications and other Web sites under an Open Directory license, that is, free of charge, as long as the originator of the data and MedCIRCLE are acknowledged, and the integrity of the data is left intact. For example, MedCIRCLE gateways can display the data of other MedCIRCLE members, search engines can use data to rank their results, health kiosks can use the data to facilitate access to trusted Web sites, and client-side software, for example, browser plug-ins or "toolbars," such as the MedCIRCLE infobar (Fig. 18.2), can make use of the data.

Conclusion

"Consumer health informatics" is the emerging science at the crossroads of health informatics and public health that deals with investigating determinants, conditions, elements, models, and processes to design, implement, and maximise the effectiveness of computerised information and telecommunication and network systems for consumers [31]. Nobel laureate economist Herbert A. Simon (quoted in Coiera's paper on "information economics" [32]) once stated that "Information consumes the attention of its recipients. Hence a wealth of information creates a poverty of attention, and a need to allocate that attention efficiently among the overabundance of information sources that might consume it." One of the central topics of consumer health informatics is how to guide consumers to quality health information. Technology for producing and distributing information is useless without some way to locate, filter, organize, and summarize it. In that sense the Semantic Web remains a double-edged sword. The main opportunities lie in the fact that consumers will have even better possibilities to find, aggregate, and appraise health information than today. On the other hand, one might fear that this may lead to a further overreliance on external information, a process of disintermediation between patients and healthcare professionals, and erosion of the patient–physician relationship. Such concerns may not, however, stop the development of the Semantic Web, as the possibilities for e-commerce can be mind-boggling, in that search engines such as Google may evolve into marketplace managers and personal assistants to find, buy, and sell articles on the Web [33]. As health infor-

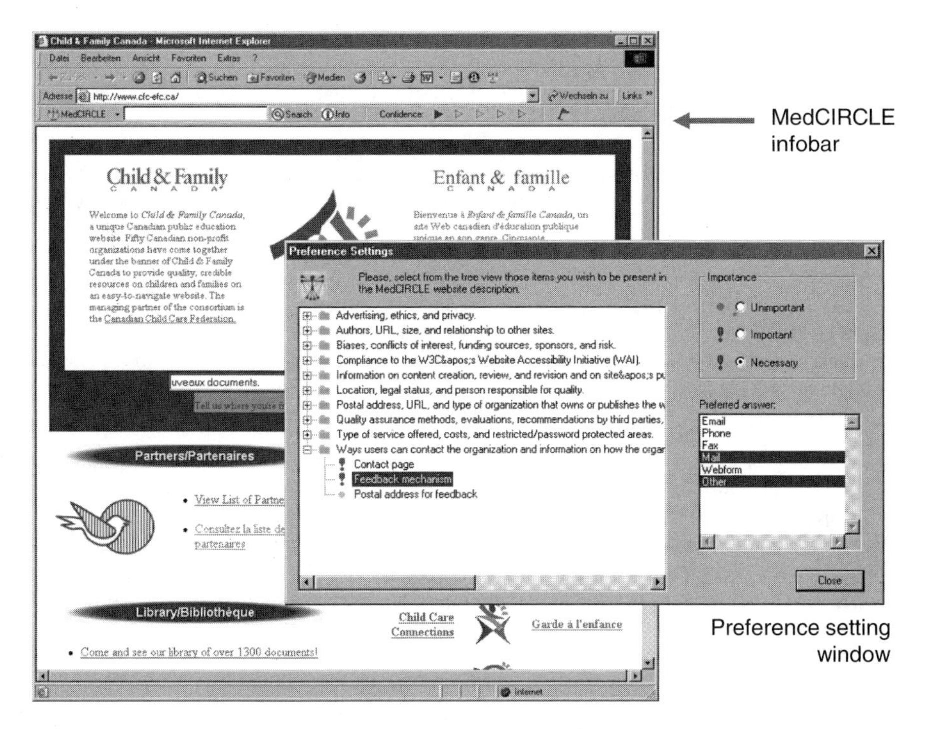

FIGURE 18.2. The MedCIRCLE infobar, a browser plug-in displaying a confidence score based on the user's preference setting concerning the presence of certain quality criteria, and what MedCIRCLE members say about the accessed health Web site.

mation is still some of the most sought after content on the Web, constituting of about 4.5% of all queries in search engines [34], people will not stop short of using these technologies for health products and services, researching the attributes and reputation of health products and services with a far greater sophistication than on today's Web. The World Wide Web as it exists today might be just the beginning of yet another consumer health informatics revolution.

References

1. Berners-Lee T. Weaving the Web. San Francisco: Narper, 1999.
2. Berners-Lee T, Hendler J, Lassila O. The Semantic Web. Sci Am 2001;284:34–43.
3. Berners-Lee T. Information Management: A Proposal. CERN, 1989.
4. Quillian MR. Semantic memories. In: Minsky MM, ed. Semantic Information Processing. Cambridge: MIT Press, 1968, pp. 216–70.
5. Eysenbach G, Diepgen TL. Towards quality management of medical information on the internet: evaluation, labelling, and filtering of information. Br Med J 1998;317:1496–500.
6. Meric F, Bernstam EV, Mirza NQ, et al. Breast cancer on the World Wide Web: cross sectional survey of quality of information and popularity of websites. Br Med J 2002;324:577–81.
7. Eysenbach G. An ontology of quality initiatives and a model for decentralized, collaborative quality management on the (semantic) world-wide-web. J Med Internet Res 2001;3:E34.
8. Koivunen MR, Miller E. W3C Semantic Web activity. In: Proceedings of the Semantic Web Kick-off Seminar in Helsinki, Finland, November 2, 2001.
9. Eysenbach G, Köhler C, Yihune G, Lampe K, Cross P, Brickley D. A framework for improving the quality of health information on the World-Wide-Web and bettering public (e-)health:

the MedCERTAIN approach. In: Medinfo 2001, Proceedings of the Tenth World Congress on Medical Informatics Amsterdam: IOS Press, 2001, pp. 1450–4.
10. Eysenbach G, Yihune G, Lampe K, Cross P, Brickley D. Website labels are analogous to food labels [Letter]. Br Med J 2001;322:794.
11. Eysenbach G, Yihune G, Lampe K, Cross P, Brickley D. Quality management, certification and rating of health information on the Net with MedCERTAIN: using a medPICS/RDF/XML metadata structure for implementing eHealth ethics and creating trust globally. J Med Internet Res 2000;2:2E1.
12. Eysenbach G, Diepgen TL. Labeling and filtering of medical information on the Internet. Methods Inform Med 1999;38:80–8.
13. Swick RR, Brickley D. PICS Rating vocabularies in XML/RDF. *http://www.w3.org/TR/rdf-pics* (2000).
14. Klyne G, Carroll JJ. Resource description framework (RDF): concepts and abstract syntax. *http://www.w3.org/TR/2003/WD-rdf-concepts-20030123/* (accessed February 12, 2003).
15. Lassila O, Swick RR. Resource description framework (RDF) model and syntax specification. *http://www.w3.org/TR/REC-rdf-syntax/* (1999).
16. Eysenbach G, Köhler C, Yihune G, Lampe K, Cross P, Brickley D. A metadata vocabulary for self- and third-party labeling of health web-sites: Health Information Disclosure, Description and Evaluation Language (HIDDEL). Proc AMIA Symp 2001;169–73.
17. Noy NF, Sintek M, Decker S, Crubezy M, Fergeson RW, Musen MA. Creating Semantic Web contents with Protege-2000. IEEE Intell Syst 2000;16:60–71.
18. Eysenbach G. Infodemiology: the epidemiology of (mis)information. Am J Med 2002;113:763–5.
19. Eysenbach G, Powell J, Kuss O, Sa ER. Empirical studies assessing the quality of health information for consumers on the world wide web: a systematic review. JAMA 2002;287:2691–700.
20. Fox S, Rainie L. Pew Internet and American Life Project. The Online Health Care Revolution: How the Web helps Americans take better care of themselves. 2000. *http://www.pewinternet.org/pdfs/PIP_Health_Report.pdf.*
21. Eysenbach G. Consumer health informatics. Br Med J 2000;320:1713–16.
22. Eysenbach G, Jadad AR. Evidence-based patient choice and consumer health informatics in the Internet age. J Med Internet Res 2001;3:e19.
23. Potts HW, Wyatt JC. Survey of doctors' experience of patients using the Internet. J Med Internet Res 2002;4:e5.
24. Eysenbach G. Theme issue for medics and health informed public. What the future might hold for the BMJ in 2013. Br Med J 2003;326:166.
25. Eysenbach G. The Semantic Web and healthcare consumers: a new challenge and opportunity at the horizon? Int J Healthcare Techology and Management 2003;5:194–212.
26. Bates DW, Gawande AA. The impact of the Internet on quality measurement. Health Aff (Millwood) 2000;19:104–14.
27. Eysenbach G, Yihune G, Lampe K, Cross P, Brickley D. MedCERTAIN: quality management, certification and rating of health information on the Net. Proc AMIA Symp 2000;230–4.
28. Eysenbach G, Diepgen T, Lampe K, Brickley D. EU-project medCERTAIN: certification and rating of trustworthy and assessed health information on the Net. Stud Health Technol Inform 2000;77:279–83.
29. Frenk J. Proposal to ICANN for health Internet Top Level Domain. ICANN. 2000. *http://www.icann.org/tlds/health1/WHO-C-SO-Proposal.htm.*
30. Purcell GP, Wilson P, Delamothe T. The quality of health information on the Internet. Br Med J 2002;324:557–8.
31. Eysenbach G, Jadad AR. Consumer health informatics: health information for consumers in the Internet age. In: Edwards A, Elwyn G, eds. Evidence-Based Patient Choice. Oxford: Oxford University Press, 2001.
32. Coiera E. Information economics and the Internet. J Am Med Inform Assoc 2000;7:215–21.
33. Ford P. This is August 2009: How Google beat Amazon and Ebay to the Semantic Web. *FTRAIN.com*. (2002).
34. Eysenbach G, Kohler C. Healt-Related Searches on the Internet. JAMA 2004;291:2946.

19
The MI-HEART Project

Rita Kukafka, Yves A. Lussier, and James J. Cimino

Among various factors associated with increased mortality of coronary heart disease, excessive patient delay (PD) in seeking medical care during acute myocardial infarction (AMI) has been shown to play an important role [1]. Two thirds of the delay from onset of symptoms to treatment is patient related, and one quarter is hospital related [2]. Clinical studies have repeatedly shown that most patients do not seek medical care for 2 hours or more after symptom onset for AMI [3–7]. Their prolonged PD precludes or limits the rational utilization of potentially lifesaving procedures, as timely delivery of optimal therapy for AMI is crucial [8]. It is well documented that a significant reduction in PD would increase the proportion of patients eligible to receive reperfusion or interventional therapies and possibly also reduce the out of hospital deaths [5,8].

Many factors contributing to an increase in PD, such as denial of symptoms of AMI, self-treatment, asking a family member or physician for advice [9,10], inappropriate coping mechanism, hampering health beliefs, and so forth, have been identified [5,11]. Modifiable factors include somatic and emotional awareness [12,13], perceived threat [14,15], health beliefs [10,16], knowledge about AMI symptoms [16,17], and relevant decision making [18,19]. Self-treatment and asking a family member or physician for advice are noteworthy modifiable factors demonstrated to delay arrival to the emergency by an hour or more. Nonmodifiable factors associated with increased delay pertain to patient history, the context in which symptoms arise, the symptoms presenting during AMI, and sociodemographic factors.

PD can be costly considering that the first hour immediately after a heart attack is the crucial time when thrombolytic therapy can significantly improve the victim's chances for survival. Although the efficacy of thrombolytic therapy has been known for years, only a fraction of those experiencing an AMI receive this treatment. If time can be reduced from the onset of heart attack symptoms to allow for the delivery of appropriate therapy, lives could be saved and long-term cardiac damage avoided. It is difficult to imagine a more striking example of how information, particularly information provided using innovative technologies, can save lives.

The Myocardial Infarct Health Education Aimed at Rapid Therapy (MI-HEART) Project, funded by the National Heart Alert Program (NHAAP), used such novel technologies to examine ways in which a clinical information system can favorably influence the appropriateness and rapidity of decision making in patients suffering from symptoms of AMI. When designing the MI-HEART project, it was understood that persons who experience symptoms need to be informed on how best to respond. However, when patients experience symptoms that may be indicative of a heart attack, their reaction is very complex. Developing an intervention to modify this response required an understanding of the process so that important variables that contribute to the decision are identified. It is only then that information can be effectively *tailored* to each individual's psychological state on the factors that contribute to patient decision making. Tailoring information to an individual's characteristics, needs, and interests increases the personal relevance of intervention messages, which in turn results in an increase in the effectiveness of an intervention [20–22].

Therefore in phase one of the MI-HEART project, we developed a conceptual model that allowed us to isolate and measure specific factors that contribute to patient decision making. In phase two of the project, we conducted a randomized trial that examined the following hypothesis, based on the model and using the existing clinical information system at New York Presbyterian Hospital: *educational tools that make use of information from a patient's medical record will exert a favorable influence on measurable parameters of the patient's cognitive processes, suggesting that they are more likely to perform appropriately in an acute situation.*

Development of the Conceptual Model

The model for patient decision-making incorporates several behavior models (Health Belief Model [23], Social Cognitive Theory [24]) and includes somatic and emotional awareness, perceived threat, expectations of symptoms, self-efficacy, and outcome expectations to explain the response of an individual to his or her symptoms. We used formal behavioral theories, an extensive review of published empirical investigations, and qualitative methods to guide the selection of these factors. Table 19.1 provides a summary of variables in our model, their theoretical origin, and a brief description.

Based on this set of variables, we assembled our model [25], shown in Fig. 19.1, by expanding on previous medical and health behavior models used to reduce delay in seeking care for AMI [26,27]. Whereas most previous research examined variables separately, our model presents a framework to consider how these variables might be interrelated in explaining the act of decision within the context of moderating variables.

According to our model, we can consider patients to be in some cognitive state prior to an educational intervention and in some second state following the intervention.

TABLE 19.1. Modeling patient response to AMI summary of variables.

Variable	Description
Somatic and emotional awareness	Individuals ability to identify inner experiences of emotion and body sensations
Perceived threat[a]	Individuals perception of his or her risk of getting an AMI
(vulnerability/seriousness)	Feelings concerning the extent of harm that could result from an AMI
Expectations of symptoms	Individuals ability to match the signs and symptoms to their concept of how a heart attack should feel
Response efficacy	Individuals estimate that their behavior will lead to a certain outcome
Self-efficacy	Individual's confidence in his or her ability to take action by performing the behaviors necessary
Symptom context	Consultation with others (spouse, co-worker); decision to consult a physician, time and place of symptom onset
Sociodemographic/ health history	Demographic and health history type variables, e.g., history of diabetes, angina, age, sex, etc.

[a] Based on the Health Belief Model, the combination of vulnerability and seriousness is labeled *perceived threat.*

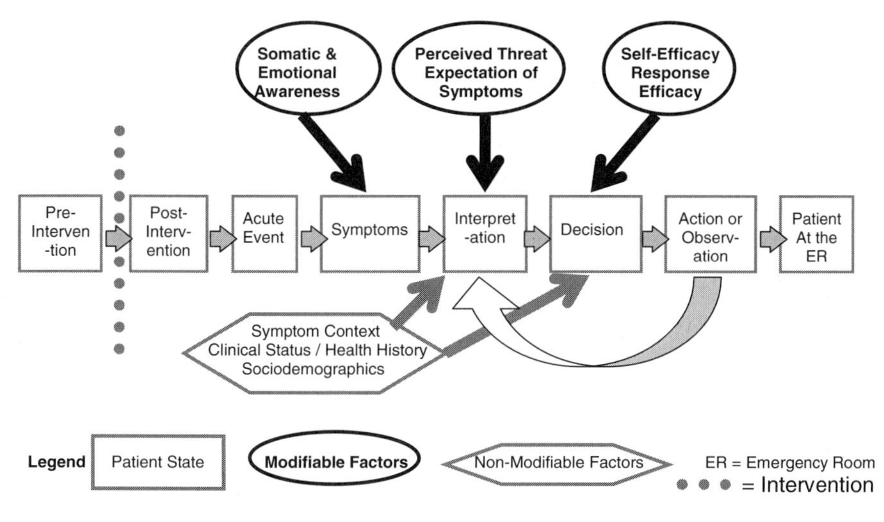

FIGURE 19.1. Model of patient response to an AMI.

When an actual event occurs (the physiological episode), external stimuli (e.g., chest pain) cause the patient to enter the **Symptom Phase**. Symptoms from the episode may be experienced with varying degrees of sensitivity related to the *somatic and emotional awareness* levels of the individual. Low somatic and emotional awareness are characteristics that tend to diminish the perception and/or reporting of cardiac symptoms, thereby leading to excessive delay in seeking medical attention [28]. Published studies concur that subjects who report higher levels of bodily and emotional awareness were more likely to seek treatment for symptoms of AMI earlier [29]. Patients unable to identify their symptoms are not likely to attend to them and may respond only when the symptoms cannot be ignored. Accordingly, the disruptive qualities of symptoms will determine whether the patient pays attention to or ignores symptoms. Providing that symptoms are attended to, the individual enters into the **Interpretation Phase**. In this phase, symptoms attended to are ascribed to a cause by the individual, for example, indigestion, nothing important, or cardiac. This labeling process requires that the signs and symptoms attended to be put within an understandable framework. Few patients are able to determine rapidly that their signs and symptoms represent a heart attack. Rapid self-diagnosis is more likely to occur when the individual is able to match these signs and symptoms to their concept of how a heart attack should feel [30]. We label this variable *expectation of symptoms* in our model referring to the matching of signs and symptoms to the patient's preconceived prototype of what symptoms should feel like. Knowledge of chest pain is recognized as an important heart attack symptom; however, knowledge of the complex constellation of heart attack symptoms is deficient in the US population, especially in socioeconomically disadvantaged and racial and ethnic minority groups [31].

Knowledge alone is insufficient to motivate action, and may be insufficient to cause the patient to ascribe familiar symptoms to AMI. In addressing other cognitive and emotional consequences of symptoms attended to in the previous stage, the individual may perceive a *threat* from the prototypical meaning of symptoms. Because the act of decision process involves the labeling of these deviant patterns of symptoms, that is, assessment of the imminent health threat, our model proceeds to adopt the value-expectancy notion contained within the Health Belief Model suggesting that the notion of threat has its greatest impact in this initial decision [32]. The Health Belief Model suggests that the labeling of deviant health patterns and response to symptoms is influenced by the person's beliefs about how susceptible he or she is to a heart attack or other heart trouble, how serious the illness is, and how effective specific actions will be in reducing the perceived threat. It is the individual's *perception of vulnerability* to heart attack coupled with the individual's *perceptions of seriousness* of heart attack that combine to form belief about an imminent health threat. Perceived levels of threat affect the ability to correctly ascribe symptoms to a cardiac origin. If the threat is perceived as irrelevant or insignificant, then there is no motivation to take action. If the interpretations of the symptoms are as noncardiac, the action taken may be inappropriate. Perceptions of threat compiled by the individual suggest that the individual employs two types of memories: episodic, which are autobiographic memories from the individual's past experiences and include affective responses, and semantic memories which reflect more abstract and conceptual information about symptoms provided by healthcare associations, for example, the American Heart Association's warnings of a heart attack [33]. For some individuals, arousal from the threat is so intense that they become unresponsive to the symptoms. These individuals may present with a presumably silent AMI, or be among those who die outside the hospital with sudden cardiac deaths. The Interpretation Phase ends when the individual has a label or hypothesis as to the meaning of the symptoms and proceeds to the **Decision Phase** to address the demands in terms of developing an action strategy. Once into the Decision Phase, *response efficacy*, that is, beliefs about the effectiveness of the recommended response, and *self-efficacy*, that is, beliefs about one's ability to perform the recommended response and confidence in labeling symptoms [34], determine whether the patient will become motivated to accept or reject the proposed action plan. Within this study "accept" defines the decision to go to the emergency room for medical care whereas "reject" defines the decision not to go to the emergency room. High perceived efficacy (i.e., people feel able to perform an effective recommended response and confident that they are responding correctly) coupled with high perceived threat (i.e., people believe they are vulnerable to a significant threat) promote the "accept" response.

The development of the conceptual model was an essential first phase to guide the development of a tailored technology-based program to reduce patient delay. By isolating and explaining the reasons why people delay, we were able to design tailored and theoretically grounded strategies, resulting in a more effective intervention and evaluative tools that better affect patient decision-making.

The next phase two was directed at three specific accomplishments: creation of tailored educational messages, development of a computer-based system for delivering the messages, and a pilot study to measure the impact of messages.

Creation of Tailored Messages

The importance of creating tailored messages cannot be underscored enough. Prior research consistently demonstrates that tailored messages have a significantly greater effect on patients' behavior than generic messages [20,35–38]. Tailored messages are information intended to reach one specific person, based on characteristics unique to that person. It is information technology that allowed us to deliver the tailored messages through ubiquitous technology windows. These seamless communication channels enabled the recipients of our project to be reached with patient-specific messages using a one-by-one technique.

To create the tailored messages, it was necessary to collect and retrieve information for each individual on each variable contained in the cognitive model. At New York Presbyterian Hospital (NYPH), existing clinical information systems provided this capability for some variables. Additional patient data on the decision-influencing variables specified in our model not contained in the patient medical record were collected for our project using an online tailoring questionnaire.

While similar in design to a tool used to collect baseline data in a research study, the distinguishing feature of the tailoring questionnaire is the close-ended nature of the questions. In order to create all possible tailored messages before the assessment takes place, the response choices to each question must be known. There is benefit to abstracting data from the medical record when it exists because it reduces user burden, the time it will take for an individual to complete the questionnaire. MI-HEART participants received the online assessment questionnaire immediately after they logged on to the Web site, and were blocked from education content until all questions are answered.

The assessment questionnaire provided the framework for developing tailored messages. Because questions in the assessment questionnaire were developed to address the most important variables underlying patient decision making, the process was fairly straightforward. Managing the process involved the following steps: (1) write down each question contained in the assessment tool; (2) for each assessment question, list all its response choices; and (3) create unique content that would be appropriate for a person who gave each particular response to the assessment question. Response items for each question in the assessment tool then guided the development of educational strategies. To illustrate, one series of questions measured self-efficacy, and the response item was calculated as "low." Content was then designed to enhance self-efficacy by showing a graphic of a person similar to the user successfully performing the desired behavior. Skill building exercises and clearly elucidating the model users' success and skill acquisition were other strategies used to enhance self-efficacy. This type of learning, referred to as vicarious experience [39], is effective because visualizing people similar to oneself perform successfully typically raises efficacy beliefs in observers that they themselves possess the capability to master comparable activities. They persuade themselves that if others can do it, they too have the capabilities to raise their performance.

To increase outcome expectations, educational content was designed to demonstrate the relationship between the behavior and outcome and provided opportunities for users to experience specific outcomes as a result of the decision he or she has made. In the MI-HEART project, we used the process of *microtailoring* [40] to enhance the individualization of content by allowing an even greater amount of tailoring to occur in the messages themselves. Table 19.2 shows this tailoring methodology related to *expectation of symptoms. The expectation of symptoms* variable is defined as a person's ability to match the signs and symptoms to his or her concept of how a heart attack should feel. We used microtailoring for this variable because we know that certain characteristics of an individual may affect the types of signs and symptoms experienced. A description of this reasoning follows. Because heart attack symptoms may differ among persons with varying characteristics, the message content for this variable would be most relevant to each individual if it varied to match these characteristics. The decision as to what are the relevant characteristics was made using clinical

TABLE 19.2. Tailoring of messages with regard to expectation of symptoms.

	Patient profile								
		No Angina				Angina			
	No	More than two risk factors				Regardless of risk or no risk factors			
Nitroglycerin	Regardless	No	No	Yes		No	Yes	No	Yes
COPD	Regardless	No	Yes	No	Yes	No	No	Yes	Yes
Expectation of symptoms:									
Low	Message A	Message B	Message C	Message D	Message E	Message F	Message G	Message H	Message I
High	Message J	Message K	Message L	Message M	Message N	Message O	Message P	Message Q	Message R

judgment, standardized guidelines [41], and published research. The following considerations were used.

First, angina was regarded as a relevant characteristic because the symptom sets for patients with angina that could be warning signals for AMI are different than for the general population. Persons with angina or more than two cardiovascular disease (CVD) risk factors need to be aware of symptoms that may lead to unstable angina. Second, foreknowledge of chronic obstructive pulmonary disease (COPD) and CVD risk factors were regarded to be relevant characteristics, as persons with this condition are likely to experience unstable angina and angina equivalent such as shortness of breath, symptoms with potential to be confounded with the symptoms of COPD. Third, having an active prescription for nitroglycerine was regarded as a relevant characteristics because these individuals need to be informed that shortness of breath and chest pain that does not go away after taking nitroglycerine are considered to be warning signals as specified by the AMA. Fourth, scoring high or low on the expectation symptom variable itself was regarded to be a relevant characteristic because the framing and content of the message for persons with high levels must be designed specifically to avoid redundancy, while content for persons with low levels must be provided in detail. Thus, Table 19.2 distinguishes 18 messages based on a combination of the relevant characteristics [42].

The distinguishing feature enabled by Web technology is that it is possible to deliver a tailored mix of educational content directed simultaneously at motivation, beliefs, and skills—the multitude of determinants that affect a single behavior. Because we know that behavior change does not come about by providing a single uniform message, this feature has strong advantages over mass communications that are directed to everyone but no one in particular. Even individuals who need to make similar behavior changes are likely to differ on factors that influence their health behaviors. One individual may not feel at risk for developing a specific disease and thus may not perceive the need to be screened for that disease. This individual should have different content than someone who avoids the screening procedure because he or she fears finding out that he or she has the disease. It should also be noted that while tailoring has distinct functionality well suited to facilitate behavior change, developers need to carefully consider that even the benefits of tailoring interventions depend heavily on which kinds of behavioral determinants and individual characteristics are targeted. Sophisticated tailoring to weak or irrelevant determinants and individual characteristics will yield poor results.

Development of the Web-Based System for Delivering the Messages

Developing the Web-based system for delivering the messages required that a wide number of issues be addressed including user interface, security, database, and clinical trial management software.

User Interface

A dedicated Web portal, *www.mi-heart.com*, provided the access to the MI HEART messages. We spent a great deal of time developing and testing the user interface to ensure that it would be usable by a wide variety of patients, including those who might have chronic medical conditions such as arthritis (of the hands) and diabetes mellitus (with visual impairment). The user interface consisted of left buttons that trigger sub-buttons on the top of the screen. The center of the screen contained the tailored or nontailored educational material that was dynamically generated to correspond with the participant's group assignment in the randomized trial. The two-level hierarchy of buttons was required to provide "oversized accessible text sizes" on the buttons and limiting the information overload. Test users were videotaped during an extensive usability trial of all sections of the site and corrections to the design were conducted accordingly.

Security

Although no identifying data were available to users of the system, users' health data were shown in messages given to the tailored users. We therefore sought an intermediate level of authentication, using an ID and password. A "cookie" maintained the active session parameters and timed out after 10 minutes without user-initiated actions.

Database

The application consisted of one Access database (miheartdb.mdb) containing several distinct tables. TblUser contained the "study group identification" (tailored IT, non-tailored IT, non-tailored paper), while tblUser_Answer contained the answers of the patients to the tailoring questionnaires. The tailored messages for symptoms and actions were contained in the knowledge-base: cfsymptom2.mdb. It consisted of several tables interoperating according to 14 observations of the past history to produce 212 different guidelines. The other tailored components of the education were programmed as independent Coldfusion files evoked according to the absence, the presence, or the unavailability of one observation of the patient history. They consisted of individualized text, images, and sound tracks. The sound tracks contained individualized recommendations from physicians. A Web-based instrument for prediction of coronary heart disease risk was implemented according to the Framingham algorithm and messages were tailored to the patient according to the calculations.

Clinical Trial Management Software

A clinical trial management and administration module was developed to enroll and monitor the progress of enlisted patients. This component also provided valuable data to analyze usage between the trial groups. Multiple alerts and progress reports were made available throughout the project.

The Pilot Study to Measure the Impact of Messages

We describe the pilot study that was conducted in the final phase of the MI-HEART project with particular attention to the issues and caveats that may be useful to others embarking on a similar effort. The pilot study utilized a three-group randomized controlled design with pre- and post-intervention measures to determine the impact of the tailored messages. Following consent, all participants completed on online tailoring questionnaires and were then randomized into one of three groups: (1) tailored Web-based, (2) nontailored Web-based, or (3) nontailored paper-based. After completing the questionnaire, participants in the Web-based intervention groups had access to the intervention online. The paper-based intervention group received the educational materials by mail.

Participants were recruited from physicians' offices, advertisements, online resources, and promotional materials, for example, brochures and flyers. Potential participants interested in the study were sent a letter asking them to provide consent and consent from their physician. Physicians were also asked to confirm eligibility according to predetermined AMI risk criteria.

Baseline Data

Of the participants who enrolled in the study ($N = 94$), most were male (71%), married (77%), Caucasian (89%), with college or professional/postgraduate degrees (68%). The mean age was 57 years (SD = 10 years), 20% had yearly incomes between $50,000 and $74,000, and 35% had yearly incomes over $75,000. Fewer than 20% reported their health as excellent, 44% good, and 21% fair or poor. Thirty-five (35%) had had a heart attack, with a total of 60% told by a physician that they have a heart condition. Seventy-eight percent (78%) reported being told by a doctor or other health professional that their blood cholesterol is high, 70% were told that their low-density lipoprotein (LDL) or "bad" cholesterol level was high.

When asked, "If you had arm pain or numbness, shortness of breath, and sweating, how likely would you:

	Very likely
Contact spouse, friend, co-worker	63%
Contact physician	49%
Call 911	36%

Alternatively when asked, if you had chest pain, how likely would you:

Contact spouse, friend, co-worker	42%
Contact physician	34%
Call 911	31%

More often participants reported they would contact their spouse, friend, or co-worker when experiencing arm pain or numbness than if they had chest pain. Interestingly, more would contact their physician or call 911 with arm pain or numbness compared to what they would do if they experienced chest pain.

Changes in Self-Efficacy Scores

We have reported to date on one key construct contained in our model: self-efficacy [43]. Results of the randomized controlled study show trends in improved self-efficacy scores for all groups at 1-month follow-up, with sustained significant increases in scores only for the Web-based tailored intervention. According to our hypothesis, we anticipated that the tailored intervention would more favorably influence self-efficacy scores; however, new questions arise as to why the tailored intervention was the only group to sustain the effect at 3 months.

Analysis of "Hit-Count"

The Web-based delivery of our intervention allowed us to look at the usage logs to determine if there were differences between tailored and nontailored groups in the frequency the system was used. Usage was determined by "hit-count," the number of times the user selected a specific Web page to view. Note that the user could have performed many actions on one specific Web page, for example, print the contents of the page, scroll, and select audio clip. In this analysis, a repeated action on a given Web page still counts as one. The mean "hit-count" in the tailored groups was significantly higher than in the nontailored group, 21.8 and 12.4, respectively ($t = 2.09, p < .005$).

Discussion

Results of a randomized controlled study show trends in improved self-efficacy scores for all groups at 1-month follow-up, with sustained significant increases in scores only for the Web-based tailored intervention. According to our hypothesis, we anticipated that the tailored intervention would more favorably influence self-efficacy scores; however, new questions arise as to why the tailored intervention was the only group to sustain the effect at 3 months.

One possible explanation could be related to exposure. The logs on "hit-count" show that use of the tailored intervention was significantly greater when compared to the nontailored Web group. Of course, we have little to say about the paper-based group, as these data were not logged.

Previous studies have already alluded to reasons why tailored interventions are more effective than nontailored or generic type information. Because tailoring provides each person only the information selected for his or her characteristics, the messages contain less redundant information. People are therefore more likely to pay attention to the essential relevant information. Attention to the message is of essential importance for the health message to have an impact. Few previous studies were able to assess usage as we have done in this study, because most have used a paper-based delivery system. Based on the data we report here, exposure as defined as "hit-counts" may shed light as to why tailored interventions have a greater impact. One plausible explanation is that tailored interventions may not only increase attention, but also increase the cognitive effort that people are willing to invest in reading, comprehending, and processing a message.

Implications of Lessons Learned and Future Directions

The number of participants we recruited to the study was fewer than we had planned for. Although the final number recruited enabled data analysis to yield significant impact on selected outcome measures, the main caveat here is that even well researched and developed systems can and will be underutilized. An information resource that provides knowledge on health issues, particularly health promoting issues that are generally not the main concern of most intended users, requires thoughtful interventions to overcome low motivation. One possible solution is to intertwine the health promoting technology into everyday life patterns and other applications as much as possible. Bringing the user into incidental contact with the intervention may motivate interest in a health-promoting topic that may otherwise be of low salience.

A second issue relates to the digital divide. Our participants were primarily Caucasian, male, and well educated. Although we attempted to address many issues of access including developing the educational content to an appropriate literacy level, we faced what appeared to be downright resentment by individuals we attempted to recruit but were unwilling to participate because they were antagonized by yet another resource moving onto the Web. These participants may have had a computer with Internet access at home or at a nearby library. Their concerns, however, extended beyond the hard-wire access and their unease prevented them from reaching the point where they could appraise the usefulness of the content. The caveat here is for developers of new technologies to build into their interventions theoretical and empirically tested methods and implementation planning frameworks that account for the social and cultural factors of the digital divide, not just the technical factors [44,45].

The MI-HEART project required the development of three software components: a customizable user interface, an application for producing tailored messages, and a system for managing and monitoring research subject data. Each of these components has been designed to be reusable for other purposes and current projects are under way, or proposed, that will make use of them.

Acknowledgments. This work has been supported by National Library of Medicine Contract (NO1-LM-3534), and NLM Training Grant LM07079.

References

1. Gurwitz JH, McLaughlin TJ, Willison DJ, et al. Delayed hospital presentation in patients who have had acute myocardial infarcation. Ann Intern Med 1997;126:593–9.
2. Weaver WD. Time to thrombolytic treatment: factors affecting delay and their influence on outcome. J Am Coll Cardiol 1995;25(Suppl.):3S–9S.
3. Gurwitz JH, McLaughlin TJ, Willison DJ, et al. Delayed hospital presentation in patients who have had acute myocardial infarction. Ann Intern Med 1997;126:593–9.
4. GUSTO Investigators. An international randomized trial comparing four thrombolytic strategies for acute myocardial infarction. N Engl J Med 1993;329:673–82.
5. Lambrew CT, Bowlby LJ, Rogers WJ, et al. Factors influencing the time to thrombolysis in acute myocardial infarction. Arch Intern Med 1997;157:2577–82.
6. Cox JL, et al. AMI Therapy: determinants and effect on short-term non-fatal outcomes of acute myocardial infarction. Can Med Assoc J 1997;156:497–505.
7. Meischke H, Ho MT, Eisenberg MS, et al. Reasons patients with chest pain delay or do not call 911. Ann Emerg Med 1995;25:193–7.

8. Califf RM, Newby LK. How much do we gain in reducing time to reperfusion therapy? Am J Cardiol 1996;78(Suppl 12A):8–15.
9. Bleeker JK, Lamers LM, Leenders IM, et al. Psychological and knowledge factors related to the delay of help-seeking by patients with acute myocardial infarct. Psychother Psychosom 1995;63:151–8.
10. Theisen ME, MacNeill SE, Lumley MA, et al. Psychological factors related to unrecognized acute myocardial infarction. Am J Cardiol 1995;75:1211–13.
11. Lambrew CT. Factors influencing the time to thrombolysis in acute myocardial infarction. Arch Intern Med 1997;157:2577–82.
12. Kenyon LW, Ketterer MW, Gheorghiade M, Goldstein S. Psychological factors related to prehospital delay during acute myocardial infarction. Circulation 1991;84:1969–76.
13. Kenyon LW, Ketterer MW, Gheorghiade M, Goldstein S. Psychological factors related to prehospital delay during acute myocardial infarction. Circulation 1991;84:1969–76.
14. Dracup K. Australian patient's delay in response to heart attack symptoms. Med J Aust 1997;166:233–6.
15. Schmidt SB, Borsch MA. The prehospital phase of acute myocardial infarction in the era of thrombolysis. Am J Cardiol 1990;65:1411–15.
16. Clark LT, Bellam SV, Shah AH, Feldman JG. Analysis of prehospital delay among inner-city patients with symptoms of myocardial infarction: implications for therapeutic intervention. J Natl Med Assoc 1992;84:931–7.
17. Johnson JA, et al. Influence of expectations about symptoms on delay in seeking treatment during a myocardial infarction. Am J Crit Care 1995;4:29–35.
18. Alonzo A. The impact of the family and lay others on care-seeking during life-threatening episodes of suspected coronary diseases. Soc Sci Med 1986;22,12:1297–311.
19. Lambrew CT. Factors influencing the time to thrombolysis in acute myocardial infarction. Arch Intern Med 1997;157:2577–82.
20. Kreuter M, Strecher V, Glassman B. One size does not fit all: the case for tailoring print materials. Ann Behav Med 1999;21:1–9.
21. Dijkstra A, DeVries H. The development of computer-generated tailored interventions. Patient Educ Couns 1999;36:193–203.
22. Kreuter MW, Farrell D, Olevitch L, Brennan L. Tailoring Health Messages: Customizing Communication Using Computer Technology. Mahwah, NJ: Lawrence Erlbaum, 1999.
23. Rosenstock IM. Historical origins of the health belief model. Health Educ Monogr 1974;2:328–35.
24. Bandura A. Social Foundations of Thought and Action: A Social Cognitive Theory. Englewood Cliffs, NJ: Prentice-Hall, 1986.
25. Kukafka R, Lussier YA, Patel VL, Cimino JJ. Modeling patient response to acute myocardial infarction: implications for a tailored technology-based program to reduce patient delay. Proc AMIA Symp 1999;570–4.
26. Simons-Morton DG, Goff DC, Osganian S, et al. Rapid early action for coronary treatment: rationale, design, and baseline characteristics. Acad Emerg Med 1998;5:726–38.
27. Meischke H, Ho MT, Eisenberg MS, Schaeffer SM, Larsen MP. Reasons patients with chest pain delay or do not call 911. Ann Emerg Med 1995;25:193–7.
28. Taylor GJ. Toward the development of a new self report alexithymia scale. Psychother Psychosom 1985;44:101–99.
29. Kenyon LW, Ketterer MW, Gheorghiade M, Goldstein S. Psychological factors related to prehospital delay during acute myocardial infarction. Circulation 1991;84:1969–76.
30. Scherck KA. Recognizing a heart attack: the process of determining illness. Am J Crit Care 1997;6:267–73.
31. Goff DC Jr, Sellers DE, McGovern PG, et al. Knowledge of heart attack symptoms in a population survey in the United States: the REACT trial, rapid early action for coronary treatment. Arch Intern Med 1998;158:2329–38.
32. Rosenstock IM, Strecher VJ, Becker MH. Social learning theory and the health belief model. Health Ed Q 1988;15:175–83.

33. Alonzo AA, Reynolds NR. The structure of emotions during acute myocardial infarction: a model of coping. Soc Sci Med 1998;46:1099–110.
34. Strecher VJ, DeVelllis BM, Becker MH, Rosenstock IM. The role of self-efficacy in achieving health behavior change. Health Educ Q 1986;13:73–91.
35. Rimer BK, Glassman B. Tailoring communications for primary care settings. Methods Inform Med 1998;37:171–8.
36. Brug J, Glanz K, Van Assema P, Lol G, Van Breukelen GJ. The impact of computer tailored feedback and iterative feedback on fat, fruit, and vegetable intake. Health Education and Behavior 1998;25:357–71.
37. Dijkstra A, De Vries H, Roijackers J. Long-term effectiveness of computer-generated tailored feedback in smoking cessation. Health Educ Res 1998 Jun;13(2):207–14.
38. Skinner CS, Campbell MK, Rimer BK, Curry S, Prochaska JO. How effective is tailored print communication? Ann Behav Med 1999;21(4):290–8.
39. Bandura A. Social Foundations of Thought and Action: A Social Cognitive Theory. Englewood Cliffs, NJ: Prentice Hall, 1986.
40. Kreuter MW, Farrell D, Olevitch L, Brennan L. Tailoring Health Messages: Customizing Communication Using Computer Technology. Mahwah, NJ: Lawrence Erlbaum Associates, 2000.
41. Braunwald E, Mark DB, Jones RH, et al. Diagnosing and Managing Unstable Angina. Quick Reference Guide for Clinicians, Number 10. AHCPR Publication No. 94-0603:1994.
42. Lussier YA, Kukafka R, Patel VL, Cimino JJ. Formal combinations of guidelines: a requirement for self-administered personalized health education. Proc AMIA Symp 2000;522–6.
43. Kukafka R, Lussier YA, Eng P, Patel VL, Cimino JJ. Web-based tailoring and its effect on self-efficacy: results from the MI-HEART randomized controlled trial. Proc AMIA Symp 2002; 410–4.
44. Kukafka R, Johnson SB, Linfante A, Allegrante JP. Grounding a new information technology implementation framework in behavioral science: a systematic analysis of the literature on IT use. J Biomed Inform 2003;36:218–27.
45. Bishop AP, Mehra B, Bazzell I, Smith C. Participatory action research and digital libraries: reframing evaluation. In: Bishop AP, Van House NA, Buttenfield BP, eds. Digital Library Use Social Practice in Deign and Evolution. Cambridge, MA: The MIT Press.

20 CHESS: 10 Years of Research and Development in Consumer Health Informatics for Broad Populations, Including the Underserved*

David H. Gustafson, Robert P. Hawkins, Eric W. Boberg, Fiona McTavish, Betta Owens, Meg Wise, Haile Berhe, and Suzanne Pingree

Introduction

This paper reviews the research and development around CHESS (The Comprehensive Health Enhancement Support System) developed and tested by the Center for Health Systems Research and Analysis at the University of Wisconsin. The review will place particular emphasis on what has been found with regard to acceptance, use and impact of such systems by high risk and underserved groups.

Consumer Health Informatics Systems

Consumer Health Informatics Systems (CHIS) include patient-oriented interactive computer-based programs that provide- information, decision, behavior change and emotional support for health issues [1,2]. Many of these systems track patient status and concerns. That role may grow as computers share patient information with providers.

CHIS operate on telephones, palm and Internet appliances, personal computers and public kiosks. Initially, CHIS were stand-alone systems. For example, our BARN system initially used Apple II computers placed in school libraries to help teens prevent smoking, drug abuse and sexual activity [3].

In the 1980s, these stand-alone systems began to add modems allowing users to communicate with each other and experts [4]. When the Internet could rapidly transmit information, many CHIS migrated to it. However, some continue in a stand-alone format because they need more speed and processing than is available on the Internet.

CHIS services can range from simple applications such as a single article or discussion group to ones offering many services including information, communication, analysis, personalized web pages and computer based games designed to promote behavior change.

* Reprinted with permission from *International Journal of Medical Informatics* 2002 Nov. 12; 65(3):169–177.

A growing body of research evaluates impact of such systems in decision support [5–8] and educational roles [9–14]. A number of important findings have been made. For example, CHIS have been found to elicit more honest information than can clinicians and that information, when presented to the clinician, can significantly improve patient care [15,16]. Moreover a number of studies have found that depressed patients prefer computer over human interviews [17–19].

Our early research found that BARN (while initially designed to prevent health risk behaviors) was more effective in meeting the needs of those facing crises [20] and also was quite effective in reaching hard-to-reach audiences [21]. It was then that we changed our focus from developing and testing computer systems for primary prevention to using them to help people facing life threatening illness with a particular emphasis on underserved populations [22]. Hence our research around the resulting system (CHESS) has been a primary source of empirical studies on the acceptance, use and impact of CHESS with particular attention to underserved populations [23,24].

CHESS

First developed in 1989, CHESS has been tested in several research studies and is now Internet-based. CHESS programs are based on needs assessment surveys typically involving several hundred patients and families. Users test relevance and readability of content created by clinical experts. Patients access CHESS through home-based computers. Many organizations offering CHESS lend computers to patients who do not have their own.

When users log on to CHESS they enter a code name and password to prove they are legitimate users. From the main menu (one example of which is shown in Fig. 20.1)

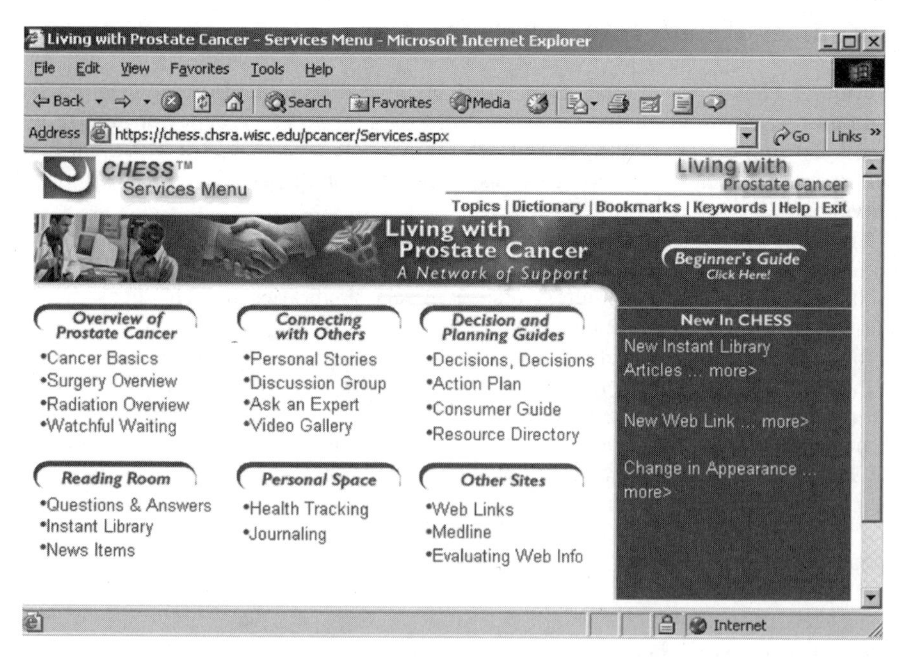

FIGURE 20.1. A CHESS main menu.

they choose a topic, pick a key word or enter into a service of interest. The services are described below using the prostate cancer module as an example.

Information Services.

Questions and Answers include brief answers to 400 frequently asked prostate cancer questions. *Instant Library* links users to over 200 full-length articles drawn from the scientific and popular press available. *Consumer Guide* describes 150 services to help users visualize what it will be like to receive the service and learn to identify a good provider, and be an effective consumer. *WebLinks* connects users to other high quality websites specific to prostate cancer. *Resource Directory* describes local and/or national services and ways to contact them.

Communication Services offer information and emotional support. Patients and families use bulletin board style *Discussion Groups* to share information and support. Separate groups (e.g. for patients, partners, prayer) are limited to 50 and professionally facilitated. *Ask an Expert* provides confidential responses to questions by specialists at NCI's regional Cancer Information Service. Responses are depersonalized and made available in *Open Expert.*

Journaling provides a private place where users write their deepest thoughts and feelings about prostate cancer in a timed, controlled environment. *Personal Stories* show how people cope with prostate cancer. Professional writers interview patients and family and prepare stories to reflect priorities set by our needs assessment studies. *Video Gallery* shows prostate cancer patients and their spouses describing how they coped with the disease and treatment. Video is also used in other services (e.g. *Overview* and *Decisions*) to supplement text and graphics.

Analysis Services help users think through key issues. These collect data from users, process it and provide feedback). CHESS *Assessments* focus on specific issues of importance to prostate cancer patients (e.g. depression). *Health Tracking* collects data on health status every two weeks and displays graphs showing changes over time. CHESS uses that information to guide people to material relevant to their situation. CHESS does not currently share this information with clinicians although it could. *Decisions* helps users make important treatment decisions. Video clips show prostate cancer patients talking about their decision. Alternatively, they can use a decision analysis to learn about options, values, and consequences of choices. *Action Plan* employs a decision theory model build, evaluate and improve their behavior change strategies. A *Cognitive Behavior Therapy* program to address depression has been developed and is being tested.

While CHESS is quite comprehensive there are services it does not offer. CHESS could collect key health tracking data whenever a user logs on and triage the user to specific services. CHESS could monitor system use to guide users to particularly helpful but so far unused services. It could automatically collect and use health information (e.g. blood sugar level) to tailor messages or send information to clinicians. CHESS does not force people to use particular parts of the program, relying instead on providing information and support in several formats that allow the user to pick to presentation that best fits their learning style.

CHIS that focus on primary prevention or even chronic disease management have the challenging task of creating or maintaining "tension for change". CHESS focuses on life threatening diseases, such as a recent diagnosis of cancer, HIV and coronary artery disease where people are already motivated to obtain information and support.

To better understand CHESS we will contrast it with typical access to the Internet. (1) The Internet is a vast but unfocussed repository of cancer information of varying quality. CHESS is a non-commercial system, owned by the University of Wisconsin, whose content and presentation is developed and updated by clinicians and patients. CHESS Research Consortium members [Dana Farber Cancer Institute, Fletcher Allen Health Care, Hartford Hospital, Harvard Pilgrim Health Care, Evanston Northwestern Health System, St. Paul's Hospital (BC), and the University of Wisconsin] contribute to its content, design and testing. (2) The Internet provides support through chat groups involving many people, some of whom can be pretenders. CHESS limits discussion and chat group access to a comparatively small number of approved people in a facilitated environment. (3) The Internet's interfaces vary substantially between programs and can be cumbersome. CHESS provides one easy-to-use interface that takes users to important materials within its own boundaries and to specific pages within other websites without having to learn to navigate each site. (4) The most important strength of CHESS may be its closed, guided universe of information and support options; an integrated package where everything points to everything else, instead of requiring search and discovery.

CHESS is one of the most thoroughly studied CHIS, including three randomized clinical trials [25–28] and several field tests [29,30]. Five randomized trials are currently examining the CHESS impact on decision-making, behavior change and quality of life. We will review some key study results below.

The Digital Divide

A study by the National Telecommunications and Information Administration (NTIA) [31] found that only 25% of people over age 55 have computers compared to 50% for younger adults. Only 13% of people over age 65 use the Internet and 64% have no interest in using it. NTIA also found that the gap between white and other non-Hispanics and the other two groups has widened since 1998 [32].

Rural areas are also disadvantaged regarding the Internet. Only 2% of rural people with elementary educations access Internet versus 4% in the central city. Many features that enhance the effectiveness of CHIS will use broadband. While 56% of cities over 250 000 have DSL and 65% have cable moderns, less than 5% of towns under 10 000 have them [11].

There are many faces to the digital divide including race, poverty and disability. But the prime indicator is poverty. The NTIA studies found that about 3% of Hispanics and black non-Hispanics with incomes below $15 000 use the Internet compared to 25% of the same ethnic groups with incomes between $35 000 and $75 000. Again, the gap seems to be increasing.

With the limited resources available to solve society's problems, does it make sense to use them to close the digital divide? Would health behavior change? Would health improve? Would costs be reduced? The paper will examine what CHESS research tells us about these questions.

Acceptance and Use of CHIS

Measuring use of CHIS is a complex process. The *number of hits* indicates how often a person enters a site but does not indicate how long the user spent on the site and what they were doing while there. A person who lands on a site by accident and leaves immediately is counted as equivalent to a person spending hours in the site. Measuring the minutes spent in a program (or in a service) indicates intensity of use. But, some services are properly used in seconds; others require minutes. Moreover, this measure is complicated because we do not know whether a person is using the site for those minutes or eating lunch. How the service is used is important. A person who spends 45 min on a live chat group discussing his/her fears gets one set of benefits. A user gets different benefits by first reviewing frequently asked questions about pain, then reading articles on pain, then writing to an expert on pain, and then raising cancer pain in a discussion group. Measuring delay is important. But the Internet, especially from a modern, can have large delays and make people stop using it.

In our research use of CHESS is measured by the number of services used beyond a minimum time threshold and minutes of use within a service.

One key finding is that many stereotypes are wrong regarding who will accept and use CHIS. When CHIS were first developed many wondered whether age, gender and race would affect acceptance and use. CHESS studies suggest that underserved use CHESS as much as more affluent Caucasians. One randomized trial, with 204 HIV patients, found little association of total use with any demographics [33]. Another population-based study attempted to recruit elderly Medicare women with breast cancer to CHESS. Those 51 women (mean age 73) who were offered CHESS accepted and used it with about the same frequency as women with breast cancer who were under the age of 60 [34]. Similarly, in a randomized trial of 246 younger (age <60 years) women with breast cancer, the one-third of subjects who were underserved inner-city African American women used CHESS as much as more affluent white women with breast cancer [35].

While total amount of use is about the same across population, different populations used CHESS very differently (Table 20.1). In particular, the underserved used computer-mediated communication services (such as electronic discussion groups) less frequently and information services (e.g., frequently-asked questions and library) and analysis services (e.g., decision analysis and health tracking) more. This is particularly important because a growing body of research discussed below, suggests that using CHIS for information and analysis is more important to quality of life than using CHIS for emotional support [36,37]. However, one of the important features of communication services is that they tend to be more "color blind" than face-to-face contacts. Underserved and affluent people interact with each other quite well in the anonymous environment of CHIS.

Impact of CHIS

A tentative picture is beginning to emerge about the impact of CHESS on diverse populations and the underserved people with lift threatening illnesses. Several research studies have been conducted on the impact with underserved African Americans. All results reported below are statistically significant at the 0.05 level or better, unless other wise stated.

TABLE 20.1. CHESS use by Caucasian, minority and elderly women with breast cancer [8]

	Elderly Caucasian	Younger Caucasian	Younger Minority
Total weekly use	6.8	5.9	6.2
% Communication	56	75	48
% Information	33	19	32
% Analysis	11	4	16

Impact on underserved African Americans. The NICHD/NCI funded randomized trial [38] of 246 younger women with breast cancer (30% underserved minorities) involved placing CHESS in the homes of experimental subjects for 6 months while controls received standard care plus a book on breast cancer. CHESS patients improved more than controls in confidence in physician, comfort in posing questions to clinicians, decision confidence and information competence. Four of six quality of life measures (emotional well being, functional well being, participation in healthcare and breast cancer concerns) showed significant interactions with characteristics associated with being underserved. Underserved minority women with CHESS moved to outcome levels similar to middle class whites.

Impact on the elderly. This HCFA-funded study [39] examined the ability to get a full population of Medicare eligible women with breast cancer to accept and use CHESS. Surgeons in a five-county, region (94% of them agreed to refer) referred 70% of the 73 patients they could have referred and 73% of those patients accepted CHESS. CHESS was used as much by this group as younger women (under 60 year) with breast cancer. As a population-based study no control group was available. However, emotional health, provider relations, active life and cognitive functioning improved more for the heaviest users of CHESS than for those who used it least. The changes in quality of life scores were similar to the findings for younger women with breast cancer. Using physicians and clinical staff as the only referral source gave nearly 50% penetration.

Impact on HIV+ patients. HIV infected people ($n = 204$) at all stages of disease (12% minorities) were randomly assigned to either no intervention (control) or CHESS in their homes [40]. Experimental subjects used CHESS extensively. No significant differences in use total use rates were found between minority patients and others. However, minority patients were more likely to use information and analysis services and less likely to use discussion group services. Five of eight quality of life measures (activity, reduced negative emotions, social support, cognition, and participation in health care) improved in those with CHESS compared to the controls. Average time spent with physicians dropped for CHESS users, as did average length of hospital stay.

Impact on AIDS patients. A randomized trial of 261 patients (35% minority) with advanced HIV disease (a CD4 count of <500), is notable because CHESS had little impact. Use rates were similar to the previous HIV+ study. Minority women used it most. But quality of life changes, while statistically significant, were modest. Health service use improved only between 8 and 12 months. Minority status had no effect on any results. One possible explanations for the relative lack of effect is that the discussion group was flourishing as usual when two subjects began an extended and heated argument (over religion). Many users dropped out of the discussion group and overall CHESS use dropped dramatically. This suggests discussion groups are fragile; requiring careful monitoring and facilitation.

Use that makes a difference. One qualitative study examined how men and women with HIV used CHESS. Because of the intensity of analysis only 14 subjects were used. Half of these subjects made substantial improvements in quality of life and half did not. Transcripts were analyzed to determine whether the discussion involved communicating information versus emotional support messages. Similarly, other services uses were divided into information versus support content. No tests of significant were run on the following results because of the small sample. However, people who use CHESS most were not those who benefited most. Instead, quality of life improvements were greatest in those who were most involved in information tools [41]. Similar results have been found by Brennan in a study of caregivers of Alzheimer's patients [42]. Hence, although computer services are frequently used to provide emotional support, this may not be their most important role.

These studies are beginning to demonstrate a pattern for people using CHESS to cope with serious disease. (1) Underserved minorities (African Americans in particular) and the elderly (two key groups often on the wrong side of the Digital Divide) are as likely to accept and will use CHIS as much as the younger, more affluent majority. (2) While they use CHESS services as frequently, they use them very differently. Less use in discussion groups and more information and analysis services. (3) Underserved groups benefit from CHIS more, partly because they have more to gain and partly because of the different style of use.

Other results simply raise questions. One is what happens if CHESS and psychotherapy are combined. A small pilot test (24 adult children of alcoholics) were randomly assigned to receive CHESS for 10 weeks or group psychotherapy for the same time period or receive both CHESS and psychotherapy. Average attendance at psychotherapy-only sessions was 39 versus 82% for those who also had CHESS. Total use of CHESS services increased by 20% when psychotherapy was combined with CHESS.

Summary

Based on current data, one would conclude that the underserved use CHIS differently from more affluent counterparts. This conclusion might change as one moves to other cultures. Studies are needed of how CHIS are used in different cultures and problems.

It appears that the different use patterns have worked the to the advantage of the elderly and underserved because they tend to use information and analysis services more and that use is most associated with improvements in outcome measures. But, what if communication services were easier to use for those of lower literacy (e.g. when voice recognition software is reliable without training) and if information were communicated verbally rather than in writing? Would underserved use the communication services more? Would that work to their detriment?

We know little about how the Internet is used by the patient. Unpublished data from one of our current grants suggests that training people to use the Internet and giving them URLs for high quality websites, leads to less use and impact than training them to navigate one comprehensive website (CHESS) with links to specific pages on other sites so they need not learn how to navigate a variety of sites. But do these results hold as well for prevention, disease management and disease coping programs? How do the underserved use the Internet? Can they discriminate high from low quality sites? What effect does access have on quality of life and behavior change? CHIS may have important interactive effects with existing treatments. Those effects need to be studied in depth.

Acknowledgments. CHESS research has been funded by public and private sources, including the W.K. Kellogg Foundation, the Agency for Healthcare Research and Quality, the National Cancer Institute, National Institute on Child Health and Human Development, National Institute on Aging, National Library of Medicine, Department of Defense, the American Cancer Society, the Robert Wood Johnson Foundation, the members of the CHESS Health Education Consortium, and former CHESS users.

References

1. Eng T, Gustafson D (Eds.). Wired for Health and Well-Being. The Emergence of Interactive Health Communication, US Department of Health and Human Services, Washington DC. 1999.
2. Slack W, Cybermedicine, San Francisco Josse-Baas, 1997.
3. Gustafson DH, Bosworth K, Hawkins RP, et al. Health education, and computers: the body awareness resource network (BARN). Health Education 1983;14(6): 58–60.
4. Bosworth K, Gustafson DH. CHESS: providing decision support for reducing health risk behavior. Interfaces 1991;21(3):93–104.
5. Kasper J, Mulley A, Wennberg J. Developing shared decision-making programs to improve the quality of health care. Quality Rev Bull 1992;18:183–90.
6. Jenkinson J, Wilson-Pauwels L, Jeweti M, Woolridge N. Development of a hypermedia program designed to assist patients with localized prostate cancer in making treatment decisions. JBC 1998;25(2):2–11.
7. Wagner E, Barrett P, Barry MJ, Barlow W, Fowler FJ. The effect of a shared decision making program on rates of surgery for begin prostatic hyperplasia: Plot results. Medical Care 1995;33(8):765–77.
8. Connelly M, Rusinal D, Racka L, Livingston W, Inui T. Randomized trial of intervention to support decision-making about postmenopausal hormone replacement therapy. J General Intern Med 1999;14(2):A2.
9. Glasgow RE, LaChance P, Toobern DJ, Brown J, Hampson SE, Riddle MC. Long term effects and cost of brief behavioural dietary intervention for patients with diabetes delivered from the medical office. Patient Education Counseling 1997;32:175–84.
10. Tibbles L, Lewis C, Reisine S, Rlppcy R, Donald M. Computer assisted instruction for pre-operative and post-operative patient education in joint replacement surgery. Comput Nursing 1992;10:208–12.
11. Peterson M. What are blood counts? A computer-assisted program for pediatric patients. Pediatr Nursing 1999;22(1):21–5.
12. Fieler VK, Borch A. Results of a patient education project using a touch-screen computer. Cancer Practice 1996;4:341–9.
13. Brennan P. Computer network home care demonstration: a randomized trial in persons living with AIDS. Comput Biol Med 1997;28:489–508.
14. Mercer ZB, Chiriboga D, Sweeney MA. Using computer technology with older adults: a pilot study on advanced directives. Gerontol Geriatrics Education 1997;18(1):61–76.
15. Taenzer P, Speca M, Arkinson M, et al. Computerized quality of life screening in an oncology clinic. Cancer Pract 1997;5(3):168–75.
16. DesJarlais D, Paone D, Milliken J, et al. Audio-computer interviewing to measure risk behaviors for HIV among injecting drug users: a quasi-randomized trial. Lancet 1999;353:1657–61.
17. Greist L, Gustafaon D, Stauss F, et al. A computer interview for suicide risk prediction. Am J Psychiatry 1973;130:1327–32.
18. Skinner H, Allen B. Does the computer make a difference? Computerized versus face-to-face versus self report assessment of alcohol, drug and tobacco use. Clin Psychol 1983;51:267–75.
19. Petrie A. Responses of para-suicides to a computerized interview. Comput Human Behav 1994;10:415–18.
20. Bosworth K, Gustafson D, Hawkins R. The BARN System, use and impact of adolescent health promotion by computer. Comput Human Behav 1994;10(4):467–82.
21. Hawkins R, Gustafson D, Chewning B, et al. Interactive computer programs as public information campaigns for hard-to-reach populations: the BARN project example. J Commun 1987.
22. Gustafson D, Bosworth K, Chewning B, Hawkins R. Computer based health promotion: combining technological advances with problem solving techniques to effect successful health behavior changes. Annu Rev Public Health 1987;8:387–415.
23. Pingree S, Hawkins R, Gustafson D, et al. Can the disadvantaged ride the information highway? Hopeful lessons from a computer assisted crisis support system. J Broadcasting Electronic Media 1996;40:331–83.

24. Gustafson D, Julesberg K, Stengle W, McTavish F, Hawkins R. Assessing costs and outcomes of providing computer support to underserved women with breast cancer: A work in progress Electronic. J Commun 2001;11(3).
25. Gustafson DH, Hawkins RP, Pingree S, et al. Effect of computer support on younger women with breast cancer. J General Intern Med 16:435–45.
26. Shaw B, McTavish F, Hawkins RP, et al. Experiences of women with breast cancer: exchanging social support over the CHESS computer network. J Health Commun 2000;5(2):135–49.
27. Gustafson DH, Hawkins RP, Boberg EW, et al. Impact of a patient centered computer-based health information/support system. Am J Preventive Med 1999;16(1):1–9.
28. Pingree S, Hawkins RP, Gustafson DH, et al. Will the disadvantaged ride the information highway? J Broadcast Electronic Media 1996;40:331–53.
29. Gustafson D, Wiso M, McTavish F, et al. Development and pilot evaluation of a computer based support system for women with breast cancer. Psychosocial Oncol 1993;11(4):69–93.
30. McTavish F, Gustafson D, Owens B, et al. CHESS an interactive computer system for underserved populations. J Ambulatory Health Care 1995.
31. McConnaughey J, Everette D, Reynolds T, Lader W (Eds.). Falling through the Net: Defining the Digital Divide (US Department of Commerce), National Telecommunications and Information Admin, Washington, DC, 1999.
32. Rhode G, McLean C (Eds.). Advanced Telecommunications in Rural America, National Telecommunications and Information Administration (Department of Commerce) and Rural Utilities Service (USDA), Washington, DC, 2000.
33. Boberg EW, Gustafson DH, Hawkins RP, et al. Development, Acceptance and Use Patterns of a Computer Based Education and Social Support System for people living with AIDS/HIV infection. Comput Human Behav 1995;11(2):289–311.
34. Gustafson DH, McTavish F, Hawkins RP, et al. Computer support for elderly women with breast cancer results of a population-based intervention. JAMA 1998;280(15):1305 (Letters).
35. Gustafson DH, Hawkins RP, Pingree S, et al. Effect of computer support on younger women with breast cancer. J General Intern Med 16:435–45.
36. Smaghk P, Hawkins RP, Pingree S, et al. The quality of interactive computer use among HIV infected individuals. J Health Commun 1998;3:53–68.
37. McTavish F, Pingree S, Hawkins R, Gustafson D. Can Discussion Group Account for the CHESS effect? Electronic J Commun (in press).
38. Gustafson DH, Hawkins RP, Pingree S, et al. Effect of computer support on younger women with breast cancer. J General Intern Med 16:435–45.
39. Gustafson D, McTavish F, Hawkins R, et al. Computer support for elderly women with breast cancer: results of a population-based intervention. JAMA 1998;280.
40. Gustafson DH, Hawkins RP, Boberg EW, et al. Impact of a patient centered computer-based health information/support system. Am J Preventive Med 1999;16(1):1–9.
41. Smaglik P, Hawkins RP, Pingree S, et al. The quality of interactive computer use among HIV infected individuals. J Health Commun 1998;3:53–68.
42. Brennan PF, Strombon I. Improving health care by understanding patient preferences: the role of computer technology. J Am Medical Informatics Association 1998;5(3):257–62.

Index